NEUROLOGICAL SPORTS MEDICINE:
A Guide for Physicians and Athletic Trainers

**Julian E. Bailes, MD, and
Arthur L. Day, MD, editors**

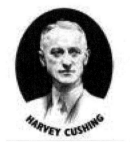

American
Association of
Neurological
Surgeons

Neurological Sports Medicine: A Guide for Physicians and Athletic Trainers
Julian E. Bailes, MD, and Arthur L. Day, MD, editors

Library of Congress Catalog
ISBN: 1-879284-75-8

Copyright © 2001 by the American Association of Neurological Surgeons

Printed in U.S.A.

American Association of Neurological Surgeons
5550 Meadowbrook Drive
Rolling Meadows, Illinois 60008
1-888-566-AANS (2267)

This publication is published under the auspices of the Publications Committee of the American Association of Neurological Surgeons (AANS). However, this should not be construed as indicating endorsement or approval of the views presented, by the AANS or by its committees, commissions, affiliates, or staff.

Warren R. Selman, MD, AANS Publications Committee Chair

Book Team
Publisher: K. Rynne
Project Manager/Editor: Gay L. Palazzo
Compositor: Barbara Jones
Proofreader: Joanne B. Needham
Cover photographs: courtesy of Batavia High School, Batavia, Illinois and
Batavia Park District, Batavia, Illinois
Printer: BookMart

AANS1.5M1100

Contents

List of Contributors

Julian E. Bailes, MD
Professor and Chair
Department of Neurosurgery
West Virginia University
    School of Medicine
Morgantown, West Virginia

Jeffrey T. Barth, PhD
John Edward Fowler Professor
Chief, Medical Psychology/
    Neuropsychology
Departments of Psychiatric Medicine
    and Neurosurgery
University of Virginia Medical School
Charlottesville, Virginia

Donna K. Broshek, PhD
Assistant Professor
Division of Neuropsychology
Department of Psychiatric Medicine
University of Virginia Medical School
Charlottesville, Virginia

Robert C. Cantu, MA, MS, FACS, FACSM
Chief Neurosurgery Service and
Director Service of Sports Medicine
Emerson Hospital
Medical Director National Center for
    Catastrophic Sports Injury Research
Chapel Hill, North Carolina

Michael W. Collins, PhD
Neuropsychologist
University of Pittsburgh Medical Center
    Sports Medicine Concussion Program
University of Pittsburgh
Pittsburgh, Pennsylvania

J. Christopher Daniels, MD
Naval Academy
Annapolis, Maryland

Arthur L. Day, MD
Department of Neurosurgery
University of Florida
Gainesville, Florida

Mark A. Giovanini, MD
Department of Neurosurgery
University of Florida
Gainesville, Florida

Kevin M. Guskiewicz, PhD, ATC
Assistant Professor
Director, Sports Medicine
    Research Laboratory
Department of Exercise and
    Sport Science
Department of Orthopaedics
University of North Carolina
    at Chapel Hill
Chapel Hill, North Carolina

T. Blaine Hoshizaki, PhD
Department of Human Kinetics
University of Windsor
LaSalle, Ontario, Canada

Vincent Hudson, MS, PT, ATC
Professor of Physical Therapy
University of Central Florida
Department of Health Professions and
    Physical Therapy
Orlando, Florida

Barry D. Jordan, MD, MPH
Director, Brain Injury Program
Burke Rehabilitation Hospital
White Plains, New York
Department of Neurology
Weill Medical College of
    Cornell University
New York, New York

David G. Kline, MD
Department of Neurosurgery
Louisiana State University
    Medical Center
New Orleans, Louisiana

Mark R. Lovell, PhD
Director, UPMC Sports Medicine
    Concussion Program
University of Pittsburgh
Pittsburgh, Pennsylvania

Michael McCrea, PhD
Neuropsychology Service
Waukesha Memorial Hospital
Waukesha, Wisconsin

Vincent J. Miele, BS, RPh Doctoral Candidate
West Virginia University
    School of Medicine
Morgantown, West Virginia

John Norwig, ATC
Head Athletic Trainer
Pittsburgh Steelers Football Club
Pittsburgh, Pennsylvania

Monique H. Olesniewicz, MS
American Academy of Neurology
St. Paul, Minnesota

John W. Powell, PhD, ATC
Michigan State University
East Lansing, Michigan

Robert J. Spinner, MD
Department of Neurologic Surgery
Mayo Clinic
Rochester, Minnesota

Charles H. Tator, CM, MD, PhD, FRCSC
Division of Neurosurgery
University of Toronto and
Toronto Western Hospital and
Think First Canada and
    SportsSmart Canada
Toronto, Ontario, Canada

Craig A. Van Der Veer, MD
Carolina NeuroSurgery and
Spine Associates
Charlotte, North Carolina

W. Lee Warren, MD
Department of Neurosurgery
Allegheny General Hospital
Pittsburgh, Pennsylvania

Preface

There have been numerous advances in the field of sports medicine in recent years, many of these affecting the central nervous system. Although the number of neurological athletic injuries seen today are increasing, there is greater understanding than ever before on the causation, diagnosis, and treatment. Neurosurgery is involved in the treatment of the most serious of athletic injuries. Termed "catastrophic injuries," these events often lead to quadriplegia, coma, or death. The time is upon us to continue to expand our knowledge and to assume a prominent and proper role, along with our athletic training colleagues, in the care of athletes with neurological injuries.

Our forefather in neurological surgery, Richard Schneider, M.D., was a pioneer in the discovery of the exact mechanisms involved in producing athletic injuries of the brain and spine. His research led to the appreciation of the causes of death in sports, particularly football, in which the head and neck striking an opponent in an incorrect manner could lead to fatal cerebral, brain stem, or spinal cord injury. Much has transpired in the interim, including changes in equipment, rules, and the size and quality of the players. However, we now realize that brain involvement, particularly concussion or mild traumatic brain injury, is all too common and has numerous implications. We are not only concerned with the acute effects of mild brain injury, but also with the long-term consequences such as suboptimal performance, premature retirement, persistent physical and/or emotional difficulties, ongoing postconcussion symptoms, and in some cases, dementia.

In addition to the large numbers of athletes involved in organized sports, many people throughout the world now have the time and opportunity to participate in recreational activities. In most recreational sports, injury to the head or spine is a potential risk and catastrophic injury is possible. For example, approximately 1300 persons annually in this country sustain fatal injuries while bicycling, with brain injury being the leading cause of death. Diving mishaps account for nearly 1000 instances of spinal cord injury every year. There are many minor and yet still popular recreational activities that contribute to the statistics of catastrophic head and spinal injuries. The extensive list emphasizes that there is a great role for prevention programs, systematic approaches, and neurological expertise to positively impact upon the rate of serious brain, vertebral column, or spinal cord injuries in sports.

There are many examples of the advances in neurological sports medicine within the last decade, including improved diagnosis, through appreciation of the syndromes of spinal injury in athletes, the classification of concussion, guidelines for proper onfield management, and return-to-play criteria. Neuropsychological assessment, balance testing, and various neuroimaging techniques give us an unprecedented ability to measure the degree of dysfunction to help those treating injured athletes in arriving at the correct diagnosis and treatment plan. There is also a greater appreciation of the metabolic abnormalities that occur secondary to mild traumatic brain injury, which allows a cellular level of understanding of the effects of these injuries. Neuroimaging and electrophysiological testing of the human spinal cord, as well as sophisticated reconstruction techniques, give the athlete with vertebral column or spinal cord injury hope for functional restoration and better outcomes.

In this book, we have attempted to assemble the country's experts for contributions to address the issues involved with modern-day neurological sports medicine and to give practicing neurosurgeons and athletic trainers a concise and reader-friendly format to access this information. We hope that it provides a reference for those practitioners caring for athletes and is a stimulus for further advances in these fields as we progress in time and complexity of athletic games and recreational activities.

The editors would like to thank the many people involved in the production of this book and especially Joyce Herschberger for her editorial assistance.

Julian E. Bailes, M.D.
Morgantown, West Virginia

Arthur L. Day, M.D.
Gainesville, Florida

Foreword

Neurological injuries are among the most complex and most feared of all sports injuries because of the likelihood of morbidity and mortality. In recent years we have gained much knowledge regarding mild brain injury, second impact syndrome, and the acute management of spine injuries. *Neurological Sports Medicine* is a comprehensive book that addresses a wide range of neurological disorders in a variety of settings, and is appropriate for practitioners of all levels. This book is appropriate as a text and a reference for physicians of all specialties, as well as for athletic trainers and other providers of sports health care.

Neurological Sports Medicine is a concise and detailed book with information on injuries to the brain and to the spine, and has unique sections detailing specific injuries in the sports of boxing, ice hockey, and recreational sports. The information on neuropsychological assessment of the professional athlete versus the amateur athlete is unique and very helpful. I also thought the chapter on helmet design for brain protection was unique to this book and very interesting. *Neurological Sports Medicine* bridges the gap between research and clinical practice in a way that few books can. Providing quality patient care, including the safe return of the athlete with a neurological injury, should be the goal of all providers of sports health care, and this book provides the foundation for the clinical decisions that each of us must make. This is an important contribution to the sports medicine and neurosurgery literature, and an asset to any clinician's library.

Douglas M. Kleiner, PhD, ATC, CSCS, EMT, FACSM
Chair, Inter-Association Task Force for
Appropriate Care of the Spine-Injured Athlete
Associate Professor
University of North Florida
Jacksonville, Florida

CHAPTER 1

The Management of Head Injuries in Athletes

JULIAN E. BAILES, MD

Much public scrutiny and media attention have been paid in recent years to the occurrence of head injuries in athletes. This has been highlighted by well-publicized coverage of professional athletes who have sustained a catastrophic brain or spinal cord injury. Recently, research has focused upon the improved characterization of minor head injury or concussion, which in fact, has a much greater impact considering the number of players involved. In addition, the long-term consequences of repetitive blows to the head are increasingly acknowledged to be deleterious to the future well-being of the athlete. Despite the rarity, the possibility of major brain injuries, and even fatality, remains a constant variable in nearly every sport and thus must be understood.

Considering the classification of recreational, nonorganized vs. organized, sanctioned sports helps us to analyze the frequency and degree of involvement of head injury. In recreational athletic activities, one of the highest rates of head injuries occurs in downhill skiing. Many of these are serious injuries, occurring as a result of collision with trees, boulders, and other skiers (often at high speed). Head injury is the leading cause of fatality at the majority of large alpine skiing resorts. Most of these traumatic lesions are extra-axial hematomas, often with associated parenchymal damage, cerebral edema, skull fractures, and resultant brain herniation syndromes.[24] Head injuries occur in most other sports only sporadically, with cycling, equestrian sports, and race car driving being important exceptions. In diving mishaps, intracranial injury is rare.[3]

The incidence and severity of head injury, as well as its impact on the player's role in the contest, vary greatly with the sport involved. Certain sports, by their design, are more likely to result in the occurrence of severe head injuries. These include the contact sports such as football, boxing, ice hockey, rugby, soccer, and the martial arts.

Head injuries in sports may be considered in two broad categories.[1] The first is severe head injuries that result in major skull fracture, intracranial bleeding, and diffuse axonal injuries. Along with the development of posttraumatic hydrocephalus or posttraumatic epilepsy, these are the major entities seen in this group. Although rare, they constitute a reproducible number of cases of severe neurological impairment and death on an annual basis in the United States. The second is minor head injuries, exemplified by cerebral concussion, that do not appear on first consideration to be of importance. However, it is now apparent that they may have a profound impact in sports medicine. This is a large public health issue because of the absolute number of players, particularly in football, who sustain cerebral concussions. In addition, we are now realizing that the cumulative effects of repeated minor head blows and concussions may have long-term sequelae and vast ultimate importance in chronic injury.

Historical Patterns

Through the years, the incidence of major injuries of the central nervous system has declined substantially.[57] Among the factors responsible for this trend is a recognition at the national level that an excessive amount of violence and serious injuries were occurring, initially recognized in football. The term "catastrophic injury" came to be recognized as representing trauma to the brain or spine/spinal cord, and thus was the focus of many of the impending reforms. Among the major improvements have been attention to the incidence and types of injuries, and study of those that led to the most serious of consequences. Despite this recognition, as late as 1968 the total annual incidence was 36 fatalities in high school and college football.[13]

Two areas have been addressed that contributed greatly to the substantial reductions in catastrophic injuries seen over the next two decades in organized football. First, there was implementation of performance standards for the manufacture and design of football helmets. In 1968, the National Operating Committee for Safety in Athletic Equipment (NOCSAE) was established as a nonprofit organization for safety research, performance guidelines, and testing. The manufacturers of football helmets, research engineers, and school administrators then set standards for cranial protection equipment. These standards were adopted by high school and college football programs beginning in 1973, leading to subsequent substantial reductions in the incidence of serious head injuries. Second is the rule changes that were found to be necessary to decrease the tendency of players to use the more substantially designed helmets as battering rams, so-called "spearing." This led to the prohibition of using the head as the initial point of contact in blocking or tackling.[14]

Injuries of the catastrophic category and fatalities gradually declined through the ensuing years. Cantu and Mueller,[13] through the National Center for Catastrophic Sports Injury at the University of North Carolina at Chapel Hill, have studied and trended these data during the recent decades. A recent report summarized the incidence of the most serious injuries in organized scholar sporting events. Football had the greatest number of direct fatalities and catastrophic injuries. During the reporting period of 1982 through 1996, there were 378 such injuries in high school and college sports, of which 374 (99%) were incurred during football. This led to a calculated annual incidence of less than one injury for every 100,000 participants. In general, there have been approximately four or five deaths annually in U.S. football in high school and college players for the last two decades.[13,60] This is contrasted to the nearly 800 deaths in boxing documented in this country since 1915.[44]

U.S. football has become the standard to which to compare incidence, equipment, performance, the effects of rule changes, and player behavior. The frequency of head injuries in football and other sports is undoubtedly related to the frequency and character of collisions that occur. Instances of head contact, which are numerous, intentional, and only partially mitigated by protective equipment, are inevitable. In contrast to other sports, in football the head often initiates contact, with blocking and tackling being the activities most often involved in producing head injury. The incidence of mild traumatic brain injury or concussion has recently been redefined. It occurs much more commonly than major head injury, but the consequences are perhaps equally as serious for many participants. This will be discussed in detail below.

Many of the advances that led to improvements in safety for athletes were made by Schneider[49] beginning in the 1960s. Schneider observed that vertex impact could transmit energy through the neural axis in a rostral-caudal direction, resulting in foramen magnum herniation or obliteration of the subarachnoid space, lateral sinuses, and bridging veins. He noted that the upper cervical spinal cord is relatively fixed by the dentate ligaments and that the brain is freely movable when pathologically displaced caudally by high-velocity forces. This movement can result in distortion of the upper cervical cord and lead to hemorrhage within it. This mechanism was believed to be the cause of death in several football players on which he reported. Schneider labeled "spearing" or "stick-blocking," the direct use of the cranium to tackle or block an opponent, as a main cause of these injuries (Figure 1). He also suggested that helmets may

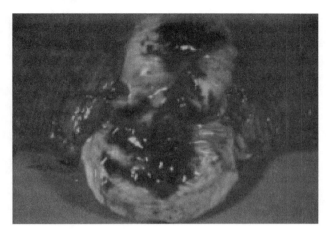

Figure 1: Autopsy specimen illustrating typical Duret hemorrhages that represented the terminal event in many football players due to cranial-caudal brain shifts. This phenomenon was recognized by Schneider and spurred his interest in redesigning football helmets.

actually have caused some cervical hyperextension injuries as the rear of the helmet struck the cervical spine, which he referred to as the "guillotine effect." This latter mechanism was subsequently refuted, as it has not been borne out in experience. Most severe central nervous system football injuries have been shown to have an axial compression mechanism. Schneider[49] frequently commented that the football field was where one could watch, record, and study neurological trauma, and represented a clinical trauma laboratory.

This research led to replacing leather football helmets with synthetic covering and inner suspension headgear. In the 1960s and 1970s, several manufacturers made further improvements with the development of thick foam padding suspended inside the helmets. Helmets came to be made of a hard polycarbonate shell with a "bird cage" facemask (iron bars covered with rubber) and suspension systems made of pneumatic, web, and hydraulic features. This was followed in 1972 by the four-point attachment chinstrap, which further improved stability and safety. Suggestions that football adopt helmets made of a highly absorptive material similar to rubber have been rejected because it would not be consistent with the desired collision effect or "hits" of the sport. More important, the biomechanics involved in redesigning the helmet shape and material are complex. In ice hockey, helmet use has been unequivocally shown to have reduced the incidence of severe brain injury.

The incidence of serious head injuries declined in football with the improvement in helmet design and the addition of the facemask. However, a simultaneous increase in serious cervical spine fractures and spinal cord injury occurred due to the instinct of the players to use their protective helmet as a battering ram.[25] Collisions occurred in which a player would strike a charging opponent with the crown of his protected head, placing his straightened cervical spine at risk for fracture or dislocation. This mechanism has been demonstrated with studies of impact on the helmeted heads of cadavers. It was determined that much greater strain is produced in the cervical spine when the neck is flexed and receives a vertex impact. Forces directed to the top of the head transferred more traumatic energy to the cervical vertebrae than did the impact to the areas of the head located farther forward.[49] Between 1971 and 1975, 54% of the quadriplegic injuries in football were caused by spearing techniques or making contact with the vertex of the helmet. In high school and college players, quadriplegia was sustained while making a tackle in 72% and 78%, respectively.[54] In 1976, the National Federation of State High School Associations (NFSHSA) and the National Collegiate Athletic Association (NCAA) made rule changes prohibiting making initial contact with an opponent with the top of the head using a spearing technique. Although not always enforced, it is believed that it has had a positive impact on reducing the previous upward trend of catastrophic cervical spine injuries in football.[4,7,13,14]

Owing to the violent nature of the game and the constant head impacts that occur, there is still a risk of serious head injury in football participation. In the reporting period from 1975 through 1984, 132 football players had intracranial hemorrhages. The apparent increase is somewhat related to the improved detection of clots with the advent and widespread use of computed tomography (CT) scanning during that period. The fatality rate from intracranial injuries in U.S. football averaged eight per year during this period, which on an exposure basis is small but nonetheless significant.[13] All medical attendants at football contests, especially at the high school and college level where significant high-velocity impacts occur, should be cognizant that severe head injury may still occur. Despite improvements in equipment and rule changes, every unconscious player must be considered a candidate for serious head injury, similar to the consideration of possible cervical fracture.[2]

Biomechanics of Head Injury in Athletes

Athletic injuries differ from other types of head trauma in several aspects. However, the primary difference is the intentional head impact that occurs and the fact that the player is subjected to repetitive cranial trauma. Despite the protection afforded by helmets, impact to the cranium and its contents still occurs along with pathophysiological alterations that follow acknowledged biomechanical principles.

The pathophysiology of brain injury has been divided into focal and generalized brain trauma. A focal brain injury often follows a direct blow or penetration of the brain and tearing of cerebral substance or vessels. This results in a localized area of bleeding (hematoma) or impact of the brain against bony irregularities of the inner surface of the skull, and eventually in macroscopic lesions that are hemorrhagic in nature. Focal injuries include cortical or subcortical brain contusions, hematomas in an extra-axial location, and intracerebral hematomas. These lesions result in the most serious form of neurological dysfunction. Patients may present with a wide spectrum of neurological deficits due to severe brain injury that results, in many cases, in neurological disability or death.

Diffuse brain injury is in contrast to focal brain injury and indicates that there has been a global insult to cerebral function and/or structure, usually resulting in widespread dysfunction. Diffuse injury exists along a continuum from mild concussion to more severe forms of concussion with alteration of consciousness. This type of injury also occurs with diffuse axonal injury, a clinical entity characterized by shearing of white matter fiber tracts as they course through the cerebral tissue from the cortex to the midbrain and brainstem to enter the spinal cord. At sites of relative tethering, such as the corpus callosum and brainstem, shearing of white matter tracts often occurs, especially with rotational energy forces. This leads to disruption of axons at these levels, sometimes marked by small areas of hemorrhage visualized on CT.

In its most severe form, diffuse brain injury consists of so-called "shear injuries," in which the patient is rendered deeply and often permanently comatose. Associated severe cognitive memory and motor deficits as well as greater than 50% mortality occur with severe shearing injury.[41]

Forces imparted to the cranium are generally considered to be of two types: acceleration-deceleration and rotational. Acceleration-deceleration injury, also considered as translational (linear) impact, most commonly occurs when the subject's body and head are traveling at a high rate of speed and strike a solid object. The resultant injury causes linear, tensile, and compressive strains that disrupt the cerebral cytoarchitecture. The brain, housed in a protective bony skull and bathed by a layer of cerebrospinal fluid (CSF), has freedom of movement before it abuts against the skull. Particularly in the anterior and middle cranial fossae, bone irregularities project at the undersurface of the frontal and temporal lobes and lead to the development of focal injuries. In addition, as the cerebral tissue shifts within the cranium, a vacuum phenomenon may occur, particularly in polar regions, leading to microscopic tearing of small vessels and capillaries that may result in the formulation of localized bleeding and hematoma.

Rotational (angular) movements are also a frequent etiology of cerebral injury. This occurs because of the fixation of the brain at the foramen magnum and craniospinal junction and the relative tethering of the midbrain and brainstem as they pass through the tentorial hiatus. Energy directed to the cranium may cause transmission of force in a rotatory direction. This often leads to diffuse brain injuries in which shearing of the white matter fiber tracts can occur. Rotational energy input is associated with diffuse white matter brain injuries, including those along the entire spectrum from concussion to the severe form of shearing injury.

Head injuries in sports thus occur as a result of both acceleration-deceleration (transitional, linear) and rotational (angular) factors. It is also possible for both of these pathogenetic mechanisms to coexist in a single patient's injury. However, usually one mechanism dominates. Contact sports, especially football, ice hockey, and boxing, have a high degree of acceleration-deceleration energy input. These injuries occur within the framework of the rules and often within a single contest. The same individual may be subjected to numerous insults during the course of one contest. Activities including blocking and tackling, checking, jabs, and cross-punches predominantly deliver acceleration-deceleration or linear energy vectors to the contestant. On the other hand, mechanisms exemplified by the boxing hook punch impart rotatory forces to the mandible and cranium. It is believed that the rotatory component of cranial impacts contributes most directly to injuries that include loss of consciousness and the etiology of many football cerebral concussions.

The maintenance of the conscious state implies that the person is awake and alert with the ability to interact with the environment. A normal level of consciousness is dependent on a complex interaction of cortical, subcortical, and brainstem nuclei. Alteration of the state of consciousness occurs when the integrity of this neurophysiological functional unit has been interrupted. The reticular activating system extending throughout the brainstem must interact with the hypothalamus and cerebral hemisphere in a normal feedback loop mechanism in order for consciousness to be maintained. Any alteration of this circuitry and feedback produces an alteration of the state of consciousness. This may be secondary to an anatomic disruption such as hematoma, contusion, swelling, or other focal injury. Diffuse brain injuries are believed to interrupt neurophysiological function on a more widespread or global basis involving mild, moderate, or severe cerebral dysfunction and injury.

Severe Head Injury

Epidural Hematoma

Epidural hematoma (EDH) is a collection of blood localized between the dura and skull. The dura becomes detached and blood accumulates beneath the skull and outside the dura. It dissects until the point of dural attachment to the overlying cranium. This results in the classic CT appearance of a biconvex or lenticular shape of the hematoma (Figure 2). An EDH is caused by head impact, usually of the acceleration-deceleration

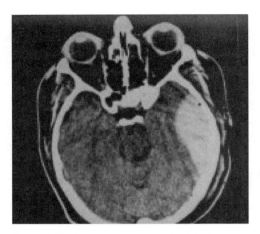

Figure 2: CT showing a left temporal epidural hematoma. In the athletic setting, and more commonly in nonhelmeted sports, this lesion is the most likely to be associated with a "lucid interval."

type, and may result in inward deformity, leading to dural detachment from the inner table of the skull. Often, EDHs are associated with skull fractures that lead to laceration of the middle meningeal artery or vein. In addition, bleeding may occur from the actual bone fragments or diploic space, leading to a collection of blood in the epidural location. A skull fracture is present in approximately 75% of patients who sustain an EDH.[32,42]

An EDH is usually an isolated injury to the skull, dura, and dural vessels that leads to the collection of blood and hematoma formation. In most acceleration-deceleration injuries, the skull has taken the brunt of the forces and absorbed the energy of the impact. There is often an associated loss of consciousness because the heavy force delivered to the cranium has disrupted the physiological substrate of consciousness.

Frequently, an EDH is not associated with a substantial primary brain injury, in contrast to other injuries, such as subdural hematoma, in which the brain often sustains a primary and massive injury. Another important distinguishing feature of this clinical entity is the concept of a lucid interval. This occurs when a substantial blow has been transmitted to the cranium and causes loss of consciousness. After awakening, the patient may appear asymptomatic and have a normal neurological examination. The problem arises when an injury to the skull and/or dural vessels leads to a slow accumulation of blood in the epidural space. The hematoma outside the brain may remain relatively asymptomatic until it reaches a critically large size and can cause compression of the underlying brain. The compression may be transmitted to the brainstem and rapidly progress to neurological dysfunction, brain herniation, and possibly death.

Any patient or athlete who has sustained a significant head impact should be observed in the awakened state and not allowed to retire for sleep until the longer-lasting effects of the head impact are known. Any patient with a significant loss of consciousness (minutes) or neurological abnormality should undergo a more thorough medical evaluation including CT scanning. The clinical manifestations of EDH depend on the type and amount of energy transferred, the time course of the hematoma formation, and the presence of simultaneous brain injuries. In addition to a lucid interval, patients with an EDH may present with no loss of consciousness, persistent unconsciousness, or any variation of these.

Subdural Hematoma

An acute subdural hematoma (SDH) presents within 48-72 hours after injury; a chronic SDH occurs in a later timeframe, with more variable clinical manifestations. An acute SDH is perhaps the most common major head injury seen and leads to severe neurological disability and death in many cases. It results from bleeding within the subdural space as a result of stretching and tearing of the veins located in the subdural space. These veins drain from the cerebral surface and connect to the dura or dural sinuses. In many people, especially older persons with brain atrophy, these veins are stretched and more easily subjected to a traumatic tear. Rupture of these venous channels results in blood escaping into the subdural space. With no subdural structure to apply tamponade to this flow of blood, this area accommodates the formation of an SDH. In addition, the bone irregularities of the middle cranial fossa, sphenoid bone, and frontal fossa form a rough surface over which inferior cortical surface contusions may form, resulting in hemorrhage in the subdural space.

An SDH may occur as an isolated collection of blood within the subdural space or as a more complicated hematoma associated with brain parenchymal injury.[27] Many patients with complicated acute hematomas sustain diffuse irreversible brain damage and do not improve after evacuation of the hematoma, the latter being something of an epiphenomenon in the injury process. Therefore, the outcome of the patient is influenced by the extent of parenchymal brain injury more than the hematoma collection per se.

The clinical presentation of any patient, including an athlete, with acute SDH may vary and include those awake and alert with no focal neurological deficits; typically, however, patients with any sizable acute SDH have a significant neurological deficit. This may consist of alteration of consciousness, often to a state producing coma, or focal neurological deficit. Skull fracture is much less commonly associated with SDH than EDH.[28,45] One case has been reported[50] and the author knows of another in which a football player with two mild concussions without loss of consciousness, separated by 7 and 10 days, resulted in acute SDH. Emergent CT diagnosis is mandatory for the expeditious and successful treatment of these patients.

Chronic SDH is defined as a hematoma present at 3 weeks or more after a traumatic injury. The pathogenesis of chronic SDH involves an injury that results in bleeding into the subdural space. The initial hemorrhage may be a small amount that fails to generate significant brain compression. However, bleeding or oozing of blood into the subdural space may continue. After 1 week, a chronic SDH involves infiltration of fibroblasts to organize into an outer membrane. Subsequently, an inner membrane may form, and this encapsulated hematoma may become a dynamic osmotic membrane that interacts with the production and absorption of CSF. Effusion of protein may occur, setting up an active process within the membrane.

The diagnosis of chronic SDH is often difficult because of the protean clinical manifestations (Figure 3). Patients may have clinical symptoms suggestive of increased intracranial pressure (ICP), mental disturbance such as personality change or even dementia, symptoms with focal transient neurological deficits similar to transient ischemic attacks, a meningeal syndrome with nuchal rigidity and photophobia, a clinical course with a slow progression of neurological signs reminiscent of cerebral neoplasm, or a progressive and severe headache syndrome only. Although not common in athletes, a chronic SDH must always be the differential diagnosis, especially in those presenting with a remote history of head impact. The diagnosis is confirmed by CT demonstrating the extra-axial low-density fluid collection in the subdural space.

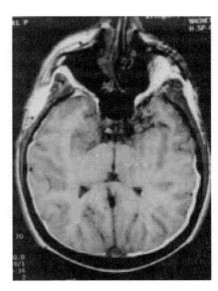

Figure 3: Axial T1-weighted MRI in a high school player who had persistent headache and diminished academic performance 6 weeks after sustaining a concussion. His cerebral CT was normal, but MRI detected extensive subdural hemorrhage across the hemisphere.

Intracerebral Hemorrhage

A cerebral contusion represents a heterogeneous area of brain injury that consists of hemorrhage, cerebral infarction, necrosis, and edema. Cerebral contusion is a frequent sequela of head injury and in some studies represents the most common traumatic lesion of the brain visualized on radiographic evaluation.[51] Contusions occur most often following acceleration-deceleration mechanisms as a result of the inward deformation of the skull at the impact site. This results in transient compression of the brain against the skull and the focal area of parenchymal injury. This energy is conducted to the underlying brain, resulting in cerebral contusion, the degree of which depends on the energy transmitted, the area of contact, the involved area of the cranium, and other factors.

Contusions may vary from small, localized areas of injury to large, extensive areas of involvement. There may also be evolution of a cerebral contusion injury, of which the size and hemorrhagic nature evolve over hours or days after the injury (Figure 4). Multiple small areas of contusions may coalesce into a large area resembling a lesion, more accurately classified as intraparenchymal hemorrhage. In addition, injuries remote from the site of impact may occur. The direct or coup lesion results from injury at the impact site, and the remote or contrecoup lesion occurs as the opposite pole of the brain re-

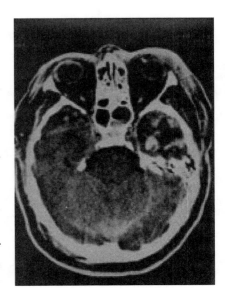

Figure 4: CT showing typical temporal lobe contusions resulting from a bicycle accident. This occurred as the inferior temporal lobe glides across the bony irregularities of the middle cranial fossa.

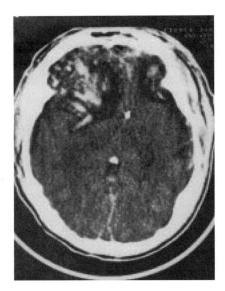

Figure 5: CT showing a bifrontal hemorrhagic contusion that occurred in a race car driver. It is important to consider that contusions may be found in those patients initially believed to have had a cerebral concussion.

bounds against the skull or because of a vacuum phenomena being set up within the parenchyma at that location. This leads to a hemorrhagic lesion in the area diametrically opposed to the impact site. The inferior surfaces of the frontal and temporal lobes are the areas most commonly seen with this type of injury. Contusions are often multiple and frequently associated with other extra- and intra-axial hemorrhagic lesions. Skull fracture is present in approximately 70% of patients with cerebral contusion.

The clinical course of these patients varies greatly, depending on the location, number, and extent of the hemorrhagic contusion lesions. The patient may present with essentially normal function or may experience any type of neurological deterioration, including coma. Frequently, behavioral or mental status changes are apparent because of the common involvement of the frontal or temporal lobes. The diagnosis of cerebral contusion is firmly established by CT, which is also useful for following patients as the lesions evolve throughout their clinical course (Figure 5).

An intracerebral hematoma is parenchymatous and is often similar in pathophysiology and radiographic appearance to a cerebral contusion. It represents a localized collection of blood within the brain. In this context, as a result of cranial trauma, the distinction between a hemorrhagic contusion and an intraparenchymal hematoma depends upon the latter being recognized as a confluent area of homogeneous bleeding within the brain. Intracerebral hematomas usually present with a focal neurological deficit but may progress to further neurological deterioration, including coma and death, resulting from brain herniation syndromes. Diagnosis is readily achieved by CT scanning, which demonstrates a hyperdense, localized collection of blood. Intracerebral hematoma has been, along with SDH, the most common cause of sports-related lethal brain injuries.

Another entity, delayed traumatic intracerebral hematoma, is a clot that forms hours to days after the initial trauma. Although most frequently seen in the older population, it must always be borne in mind when evaluating and attending to any patient who has sustained a significant head impact. The athlete is also at risk because these hematomas are seen more commonly when there has been rotational head trauma. Delayed traumatic hematomas are believed to be due to later bleeding into an already contused region of the brain, vascular injury, or the development of a coagulopathy.[17,20,29]

Skull Fracture

Cranial injury resulting in fracture of the skull is a common occurrence in sports, especially sports in which helmets are not regularly employed. Any recreational or sporting activity in which planned or inadvertent head impact occurs may result in skull fracture.

Skull fractures are considered in two categories: linear and depressed. Linear skull fractures are common entities involving the frontal, parietal, temporal, or occipital bones. They may occur in conjunction with an overlying scalp laceration, in which case they are considered to be a compound fracture. Linear skull fracture occurs as a result of a direct blow to the skull and is a fracture without malalignment of the bone edges. Most linear fractures are uncomplicated and, per se, not serious. They are more important as a harbinger of the patient sustaining an underlying cerebral injury and thus serve as a marker for potentially serious underlying neurological damage. When occurring over the major venous sinuses, or particularly in the temporal fossa overlying the groove for the middle meningeal artery and vein, it may be an indication that an underlying bleeding source exists. Most linear skull fractures do not require specific treatment other than the necessary observation for neurological dysfunction. They usually heal within several months to a year and often do not prevent the athlete from resuming participation, even in contact sports.

Depressed skull fractures ordinarily require a relatively small object of contact point that results in depression of the underlying bone. The bone fragments separate and are driven into the dura or penetrate the dura to touch or invade the brain surface. Many patients with depressed skull fractures do not have significant brain injury, although underlying hematoma, CSF leakage, or infection may occur. In addition, laceration leading to hemorrhage or thrombosis of a major dural venous sinus may be a concomitant injury. In contrast to linear skull fractures, depressed fractures often require treatment based on such features as the location, degree of depression, contamination, and cosmetic appearance. The diagnosis is made with skull radiographs and confirmed with CT. The latter is necessary to ascertain the degree of cerebral abnormality.

Epilepsy

It is thought that posttraumatic seizures are present in approximately 5% of all patients with cranial cerebral trauma and in approximately 15% of those with severe head injuries. Patients with an intracerebral lesion such as a contusion or hematoma, those with a depressed skull fracture impinging on the dural or cortical surface, and those experiencing seizures later than 1 week following trauma are believed to have a higher incidence of posttraumatic epilepsy.

Posttraumatic epilepsy is generally considered in several forms. *Impact seizures* occur immediately at the time of the trauma and are believed to result from the direct impact producing deranged electromechanical conductance. *Immediate seizures* occur within the first 24 hours after trauma. *Early seizures* occur within the first week after trauma and are believed to be acute reactions to trauma and not prognostic of the future development of epilepsy. *Later seizures* occur at a time remote from the initial injury and can be more accurately considered as posttraumatic epilepsy.

Prophylactic anticonvulsants have been administered to patients who are believed to be at high risk for posttraumatic epilepsy or to those who experience convulsions. Research has found that phenytoin reduced the incidence of seizures in the first week after trauma but not subsequently. This suggests that prophylactic anticonvulsants are not helpful after the first week after trauma.

The management of late posttraumatic seizures follows the guidelines for treatment of patients with epilepsy. Phenytoin has been the antiepileptic most commonly employed for treatment of posttraumatic epilepsy, but at times is not as effective for late-onset seizures. Phenobarbital has been commonly employed as a second agent; however, its sedative side effect is often a liability in recovering head-injured patients. Anticonvulsants are continued for a minimum of 1 year in most patients in whom seizures have occurred. The subsequent discontinuance of anticonvulsants would be on an individualized basis.

Posttraumatic Hydrocephalus

After the occurrence of head trauma, the cerebral ventricular system can become enlarged. This usually requires that a significant head injury has occurred. The incidence of posttraumatic ventriculomegaly has been reported to range from 30% to 86%.[28] It is always necessary to attempt to discern whether this anatomic ventricular enlargement represents ventriculomegaly alone or symptomatic hydrocephalus.[21]

After head trauma, especially in patients with severe head injury, it is not uncommon to have permanent cerebral injury. This results in the loss of cerebral tissue, which can be visualized on CT or magnetic resonance imaging (MRI) in the posttraumatic period as areas of porencephaly, areas of arterial or venous infarction, or atrophy. As this loss of cerebral tissue ensues, there can be passive dilatation of the ventricular system, in part to occupy the area of brain loss. As the ventricles expand to fill a void, this condition has been termed "hydrocephalus ex vacuo." In patients with significant head injuries, injuries such as subarachnoid hemorrhage, posterior fossa hematomas, supratentorial hematomas, and meningitis may cause disturbances in the normal CSF obstructive pathways. As the inexorable production of CSF continues at approximately 450 mL daily, the fluid accumulates and can result in ventricular dilatation. This active ventricular enlargement would be considered symptomatic and has been estimated to occur in approximately 18% of those with posttraumatic ventricular enlargement.[20]

In a comatose patient, the diagnosis of hydrocephalus is usually difficult to make on a clinical basis. At times, although unusual enough to be an isolated phenomenon in the posttraumatic period, hydrocephalus may produce an altered level of consciousness, even coma. Funduscopic examination may reveal blurring of the disc margins or papilledema. In these cases, the diagnosis is made most readily with radiological imaging. Enlargement of the lateral ventricles and frontal and temporal horns, periventricular edema, and effacement of the cerebral sulci are all seen on CT or MRI.

The diagnosis of hydrocephalus in an awake patient is characteristically made with the symptoms of aggressive mental status changes and dementia, sphincteric incontinence, and gait apraxia. It is also not uncommon to see posttraumatic hydrocephalus present as a leveling off of neurological improvement in the rehabilitation phase of head injury. The majority of patients with posttraumatic hydrocephalus improve after the placement of a CSF diversion device, most commonly a ventriculoperitoneal shunt. Because of the delicate and intricate function of a ventricular shunt, the active, constant production of CSF within the brain, and the shunt dependence and potential for rapid neurological demise in those who suffer an acute shunt malfunction, this author believes that the participation in contact sports by an athlete with an indwelling ventricular shunt should generally be prohibited.

Intracranial Hypertension

Elevated ICP is a common sequela in the pathophysiology of severe head injury. Due to the brain being housed in the cranium, which acts as a closed, rigid box, processes that lead to cerebral swelling can come to be associated with high ICP. In sports medicine, the second-impact syndrome has direct significance with these processes and is discussed below. The unyielding skull causes pressure to be turned within and directs displacement of CSF and blood as compensatory mechanisms. When this compensation is exhausted, brain tissue begins to shift, resulting in brain herniation syndromes as the brain is expelled through the tentorial hiatus and/or the foramen magnum. This leads to severe brain stem dysfunction and/or death.

The pressure of the CSF that surrounds and nourishes the brain is normally below 10 mm Hg. In certain disease states, including traumatic injury, the normal homeostatic mechanism is deranged, which can often lead to increased ICP, referred to as intracranial hypertension. The Monro-Kellie hypothesis helps explain the pathophysiological state that occurs in intracranial hypotension. When the compensatory mechanism of intracranial volume displacement has been exhausted, a linear and rapid increase in ICP occurs. Dramatic increases in pressure result in brain tissue displacement (herniation) and insufficient cerebral blood flow leading to ischemia.

Intracranial hypertension may exist in patients who have intracranial mass lesions. These become space-occupying masses that, together with a surrounding edematous brain reaction, lead to increases in ICP. It is possible to have severe generalized cerebral edema without intracranial mass lesions, and this also results in intracranial hypertension. The management of patients with intracranial hypertension involves strict adherence to set guidelines for minimizing the systemic insults (hypoxia, hypotension) and optimizing cerebral perfusion. This constant management is facilitated by the monitoring of ICP through one of various modalities such as ventricular catheters or subdural and epidural monitoring devices. Careful surveillance of ICP levels is necessary so that treatment may be instituted to reduce ICP and optimize the cerebral perfusion pressure (CPP). The CPP equals the mean systemic arterial blood pressure minus the jugular venous pressure, and the latter parameter is replaced by ICP whenever there is intracranial hypertension. Efforts are made to maintain the CPP at a level greater than 70 mm Hg. Numerous medical modalities, such as osmotic diuretics and hyperventilation, are employed to optimize the CPP by minimizing and controlling ICP, and hemodynamic support to augment systemic blood pressure.

The pathophysiological processes that occur with cerebral injury may be termed primary and secondary injuries. The primary injury is that which occurs at the moment of impact, leading to physical, anatomic injury and structural damage to the brain. This results in the formation of hematomas, such as parenchymal hematomas and contusions, or to diffuse trauma resulting in diffuse axonal injury and shear injury. Surgical treatment is often necessary to improve the patient's condition and subsequent clinical course by removing the primary injury if it is hematoma compression, depressed skull fragments, or a foreign body.

Secondary cerebral injury begins momentarily after the primary injury and consists of a series of biochemical steps that are set in motion by the primary injury. Secondary neurological injury involves a cascade of hypoxic and ischemic cellular events beginning with the loss of membrane integrity by the Na^+, K^+-ATPase-driven ionic pump. This subsequently leads to passive movements of ions following concentration gradients, the generation of electrical potential and activation of the voltage-dependent calcium channels, an influx of calcium, a breakdown of the cellular membrane, cellular swelling, and death. As clinicians, we can only intervene and minimize the degree of secondary brain injury. This involves treatments aimed at controlling hypoxia, hypotension, temperature, and other features of the patient's initial response to the injury. Pharmacological intervention may play a greater role in the future in minimizing the degree of secondary injury.

Minor Head Injury (Concussion)

Peculiar to sports medicine is the fact that head impact may occur intentionally or accidentally.[9,52,58,59] Although it was previously believed that the incidence of concussion in U.S. football was higher, recent research has shown that the most likely incidence is between 4% and 6%.[43] In the largest study to date, Powell and Barber-Foss[43] analyzed data from 23,566 reported injuries in 10 sports during a 3-year period. There were 1219 cases of mild traumatic brain injury, representing a 5.5% incidence. Football accounted for 63% of these concussions.[43]

The Definition of Concussion

The classical cerebral concussion is defined as a posttraumatic state that results in loss of consciousness.[22] This state is usually associated with various degrees of retrograde and posttraumatic amnesia. The patient regains full consciousness within 24 hours, and this condition may be accompanied by microscopic neuronal abnormalities.[41] However, in clinical terms, cerebral concussion has been defined as physiological without anatomic disruption of cerebral function. The concept of minor head injury is usually synonymous with concussion. Historically, 3% of patients with head injuries ultimately require neurosurgical intervention.[16]

Confusion has been considered to be the hallmark of concussion.[4,7,30] Although consciousness is preserved, there is dysfunction of cerebral processes whereby orientation, higher-thought processes, and memory are affected. This syndrome is completely reversible and, unless repetitive, is believed not to be associated with neurological sequelae. Various classification schemes have been devised to categorize and help understand and treat concussion. The gradation of severity of concussion has been especially pertinent for treating the athletic injury and for prognostication regarding return to play.

Cerebral concussion has been defined in various ways but generally means an alteration of cerebral function without associated pathological changes in brain structure. Experimental evidence has suggested, however, that reactive axonal swelling is seen on electron microscopy after even mild head injury. Concussion has also been defined as an "immediate and transient impairment of neural function such as alteration of consciousness, disturbance of vision, equilibrium and other similar symptoms." For athletic purposes, it has been defined as "a traumatically induced alteration of mental status." In the U.S., it has been estimated that approximately 150,000 concussions occur annually in football alone.

Grading Concussion

Concussion has most often been categorized into three types or grades for clinical purposes.[7,10,31] Other classification schemes have also been proposed. Using the Colorado grading system (see Chapter 2, Table 2), a mild concussion (Grade 1) is most common. It involves no loss of consciousness, and confusion is the hallmark sign. This type of concussion is often seen in football games and occurs to at least one player in nearly every game, if thoroughly searched for. It may be stated that the player was "dinged." The athlete, who is awake and alert, may function unnoticed during the course of the athletic contest. Management entails removing the player, who is sometimes identified by teammates because of his confusion or difficulty remembering plays, from the field of competition for 15 to 20 minutes. If significant disorientation, confusion, memory disturbance, dizziness, headache, or any neurological abnormality persists after this observation period, a return to play should not be allowed. If these features are absent, the athlete may be considered for return to play following a mild concussion.

A moderate or Grade 2 concussion is associated with the development of amnesia either initially or during the period of observation. There is no loss of consciousness. The athlete is removed from competition and not allowed to return. The athlete should be examined as soon as possible by the team physician and consideration given to consultation with a neurological or neurosurgical specialist, especially if disturbances in level of consciousness or other neurological signs develop. Brain radiological imaging studies (e.g., CT or MRI) are performed in all athletes who have neurological abnormalities, headaches, or other associated symptoms that either worsen or persist for more than 1 week.

A severe or Grade 3 concussion is associated with loss of consciousness. It may require emergent transport to the nearest facility with CT scanning, and consideration should be given for neurosurgical consultation. This is especially true for athletes in whom there is more than a brief loss of consciousness or a neurological deficit is suspected. The possibility of a concomitant cervical spine injury must always be considered in an unconscious patient and transport performed with cervical immobilization and maintenance of an adequate airway.[2] Often, unless the loss of consciousness has been very brief (i.e., less than 30 seconds), the athlete is admitted to the hospital overnight for observation and treated according to standard accepted procedure for closed-head injury. Caretakers should be aware of the phenomenon of the "lucid interval." This phenomenon has also occurred in baseball players and golfers struck on the head by a high-velocity ball.

Repeat Concussions

With a significant period of loss of consciousness, neurological and CT examination are usually required. If both are normal and there are no symptoms, and if the length of unconsciousness was less than 1 minute, it is believed that the athlete may return to competition within 2 weeks of being asymptomatic. With loss of consciousness for more than 1 minute, implying significant interruption of cerebral function, it is recommended that return be withheld for 1 month. A second severe concussion will terminate the athlete's season and consideration should be given to ending participation in any contact sport. These recommendations are based on the author's experience and that of others, and are reinforced by neurophysiological testing. With a single incident of minor athletic head injury, abnormalities on neurophysiological testing usually resolve by 1 month; however, with a second concussion, they may be present for up to 6 months.

The concern is not only concussion per se, but the cumulative effects of multiple cerebral impacts. Repeated concussions, especially within a short time span, may lead to headaches, visual disturbances, vertigo, and other symptoms typical of postconcussion syndrome. However, permanent injuries are also possible, such as neuropsychological abnormalities, cerebral atrophy, and even death. Cumulative effects of concussion may lead to cerebral edema and death, similar to the reactive hyperemia resulting from autoregulatory dysfunction seen in some pediatric head trauma cases. Children, adolescents, and young adults appear to be susceptible to this phenomenon of pathological vascular congestion.

Kelly et al[30] described a 17-year-old high school football player who sustained a loss of consciousness a week before being struck again on the left side of his helmet during a game. He subsequently collapsed on the field, never regained consciousness, and died 15 hours later. Detailed investigation showed cerebral edema on CT and uncontrolled intracranial hypertension. Necropsy findings were of cerebral edema. This demonstrated that serious, fatal injury can result from repeated concussions without loss of consciousness or any obvious preceding abnormality of the athlete. The previously concussed athlete is at perhaps a fourfold greater risk of sustaining another minor head injury. Gronwall and Wrightson[19] studied 20 young adults and found that information-processing capacity is reduced to a greater degree and for a longer period of time after a second concussion. Multiple concussions resulted in a longer interval before normal cerebral function returned. They concluded that the mechanism of concussion of all grades of severity involves neuronal damage.

Chronic Traumatic Brain Injury

Chronic traumatic brain injury has been associated with several sports and is most notably found among professional boxers.[36,47] Recent studies indicate that soccer players may also exhibit permanent cognitive deficits, usually detected on neurophysiological testing. Initial studies focused on the effects sustained in professional soccer players. It has been thought that repetitive "heading" of a soccer ball, which typically weighs 14 ounces and can travel at speeds of up to 50 miles per hour, may have a cumulative deleterious effect on the brain's higher cortical functions. Several studies have shown that chronic traumatic brain injury occurs in retired professional soccer players; whether the injury is due to repetitive head impacts with the soccer ball or collisions with an object such as a goal post or another player has been a source of ongoing debate.

Recent Clinical Research on Brain Injury in Athletes

Debate has recently shifted to the influence that chronic traumatic brain injury may have upon amateur athletes. This is particularly important in light of the large number of youths and adolescents who participate in soccer in this country. Even greater is the extreme popularity of this sport worldwide, as there are 200 million Fédération Internationale de Football Association soccer players.

Matser et al[37] studied 22 amateur soccer players with interviews and neuropsychological testing. Compared with control athletes, these soccer players exhibited performance impairment on assessments of memory and planning. Among these players, nine had sustained one soccer-related concussion and seven had incurred two to five concussions during their amateur careers. This study utilized the Complex Figure Test Immediate Recall for analyzing memory functioning and the Wisconsin Card Sorting Task for assessment of planning capability. Compared to controls who exhibited a 7% and 13% abnormality rate on memory and planning testing, respectively, the impairment rate for soccer players was 27% and 39%. Matser et al concluded that even amateur soccer participation is associated with mild cognitive impairment.

Macciocchi et al[35] prospectively studied neuropsychological functioning in 2300 collegiate football players at 10 NCAA universities, of whom 183 had suffered cerebral concussions. Players and control subjects were tested at 24 hours and 5 and 10 days following their injuries. It was found that neuropsychological dysfunction occurred after mild head injury, but was limited in scope and relatively brief in duration. Impairment was seen in auditory attention and concentration on detailed testing. These injured athletes also had a statistically and clinically significant increase in headaches, dizziness, and memory deficits when compared to control subjects. The majority of injured athletes had reversal of their deficits by Day 5 and all had resolution of neuropsychological testing abnormalities by Day 10.[35]

Gerberich et al[18] surveyed 103 secondary school football teams in Minnesota and reviewed data from 3063 players who participated in the study. There was a reported incidence of 74 concussions; however, an additional 507 players reported that they had sustained a loss of consciousness and/or loss of awareness. Many of these athletes did not associate transient amnesia, confusion, or other typical symptoms unless they were told that they had a "concussion." This resulted in a 19% incidence of one or more concussions during a single football season. In their study, a significant number (up to 24%) of all sports injuries were concussions. Loss of consciousness was experienced by 112 athletes during this one season, of whom 45 (40%) had previously been knocked out. If there was a prior episode, the incidence for a concussion with loss of consciousness was more than fourfold greater. Permanent neurological disability occurred in six athletes.[18]

In attending to these concussed athletes who were rendered unconscious, 41% reported that they had been examined by coaches, 33% by physicians, and 18% by athletic trainers. Players who experienced only a loss of awareness were not examined at all 58% of the time. Of the return-to-play decision, 60% reported that they made the decision to send themselves back into the contest, whereas an athletic trainer and physician made this decision only 5% and 3% of the time, respectively. There was a tendency for players to minimize symptom reporting to avoid peer pressure and ridicule as well as loss of playing time. Concussions with loss of consciousness occurred primarily while tackling, being tackled, or during blocking. Illegal techniques were reported as being associated with injuries in 23% of cases.[18]

Tegner and Lorentzon[52] prospectively studied 14 teams with 480 semiprofessional Swedish ice hockey players over a four-season time period. They reported that, of 805 total injuries, 52 (6%) were concussions. Of the 480 players, 43 (9%) had at least one concussion and three players (1%) each had two or three concussions. The risk of experiencing a concussion during league play was calculated to be 6.5/1000 player-game-hours, or roughly one concussion per team annually. The vast majority of concussions happened during game play and were caused by bodily contact, either body checking or boarding. Contact with the puck or stick caused only 10% of concussions. During the course of an ice hockey career, they estimated that 20% of players at the elite level of play would suffer a concussion.

Bohnen et al[7] studied nine patients who had sustained mild closed head injury and who had persistent postconcussion symptoms and compared them to a group with similar injuries who were asymptomatic at 6 months following their injury. Detailed neuropsychological testing demonstrated that patients who continued to have subjective symptoms after 6 months had deficits on tests of attention and information processing. This report gives credence to the subgroup of patients who complain of continued neurological symptoms despite a normal neurological examination.

Hugenholtz et al[26] studied 22 adults who had sustained mild concussions and compared them with matched controls, analyzing both the neurological and neuropsychological examination. They found that on choice reaction-time testing, which assesses attention and information processing, the concussed subjects were significantly slower than normal controls. This was especially true during the first month following injury, but also five (23%) patients had posttraumatic symptoms after the first month. Other studies have shown persistent posttraumatic symptoms in 20% to 80% of patients with mild head injuries after 3 months.[40,46,58]

The duration of loss of consciousness is of limited value in many instances primarily because of inaccuracy of the documentation, as patients, bystanders, and family members frequently overestimate the duration. If present, the length of posttraumatic amnesia is a more reliable indicator of severity.[26,40]

In 1973, Yarnell and Lynch[59] reported on four cases of marked short-term memory impairment in college football players who had not had alteration of consciousness. These players shared similar characteristics of a sense of bewilderment without marked cognitive difficulty and an inability to recall immediate events. While they were initially able to immediately recall what had happened, these memories would rapidly fail and thus indicated that the ongoing dynamic process of memory encoding was disrupted in these injuries. The term "ding," which had previously been an aphorism for a benign cerebral insult, was thus equated to being mildly concussed.

Second-impact Syndrome

Although well described, the second-impact syndrome is a fortunately rare syndrome in which massive cerebral edema and death occur in athletes who sustain relatively minor head injuries shortly after receiving similar head injuries. The athlete is usually still symptomatic from the first injury, such as a player who sustains a minor concussion and returns to play prior to complete clearing of the sensorium. This syndrome is believed to result from abnormal cerebrovascular sensitivity from the first injury. The second injury then leads to cerebral autoregulatory dysfunction, vascular congestion, and subsequent intracranial hypertension.[8] This can result in the precipitous death of the victim and has occurred in the setting of seemingly mild head injury without loss of consciousness.

The occurrence of a catastrophic and fatal brain injury after a relatively minor injury has been documented in contact sports. Most reported cases have been in football, but it also has been described in boxing and ice hockey.[12] In the usual sequence, a player receives a relatively minor blow to the head and suffers a mild concussion. Within approximately 1 week after the initial impact, the player sustains a second cranial energy input that results in rapid neurological demise and death, usually within several hours. Autopsy studies have demonstrated cerebral contusion and/or parenchymal hematomas. However, the overwhelming pathophysiological abnormality is diffuse cerebral edema with brain herniation.[39] Saunders and Harbaugh[48] reported the case of a 19-year-old college football player who was involved in a fist fight and received a blow to the head, resulting in a brief loss of consciousness. Four days later, while involved in a football game and despite receiving no unusual head impact, he collapsed on the field and died 4 days later with diffuse and uncontrollable cerebral edema. They postulated that loss of vasomotor tone allows increased intracranial vascular volume, provoking large increases in ICP and failure of intracranial compliance with a second minor head impact during the susceptible time. The exact pathophysiology of this entity is presently incompletely understood.

Approximately 50 cases of second-impact syndrome have been identified since 1980, although the true incidence is likely higher. This entity involves a head injury, which is a concussion or even worse injury (e.g., cerebral contusion), with the athlete experiencing continued postconcussion symptoms. The typical athlete will have had an incident in a game or practice that results in what appears to be a postconcussion syndrome. Prior to resolution of these symptoms, which may take up to several weeks, a second head impact is sustained when the athlete returns to competition. The subsequent collision, which precipitates rapid and fulminant cerebral edema and brain herniation, may not necessarily be a major blow. A minor impact, including one in which the head is not directly struck but undergoes rapid acceleration-deceleration, may occur via a blow to the chest or back. Usually within several minutes and often after leaving the field of play under his/her own power, the athlete collapses and the onset of the downward neurological course begins. Treatment for this condition requires rapid diagnosis and involves primarily medical treatment of intracranial hypertension, usually not surgical intervention.

Prevention through recognition of the initial injury is the key. Since there is ordinarily no space-occupying lesion, such as an intracranial hematoma, there is no life-saving surgery that can be performed. The patient is usually intubated and given medications to reduce cerebral swelling. With a mortality rate of 50% and a morbidity rate of nearly 100%, prevention is most important through early recognition of an athlete who may have the potential to develop the second-impact syndrome. The athlete with such a history should not participate in contact sports until concussion symptoms have resolved.

Postconcussion Syndrome

A postconcussion syndrome is not an uncommon problem after closed-head injury. It is most commonly seen in patients following motor vehicle accidents. It may also be seen in athletes, especially those with repeated or successive concussions during the course of one season. A multitude of common complaints occur with postconcussion syndrome, including persistent headache, irritability, inability to concentrate, dizziness, vertigo, memory impairment, and generalized fatigue. Many factors influence the duration and the extent and number of postconcussion syndrome complaints, including motivation, psychological factors, pending litigation, educational level, and degree of injury.

Postconcussion syndrome consists predominantly of deficits in cognition, the sense of physical well-being, and mood. This results in diminished memory and concentration, fatigue, dizziness, depression, anxiety, and irritability; headaches are also a common symptom. It appears that the incidence of postconcussion syndrome is highest for patients who have suffered mild head injuries. Mild head injury has been defined quantitatively by a Glasgow Coma Scale score of 13 to 15 (see Chapter 2, Table 10, for further information). However, the use of such a scale alone may be misleading in that it does not consider factors related to prior cortical function such as orientation and memory.

It is suggested that certain athletes involved in contact sports who have received repeated cerebral concussions may be at risk for developing a prolonged postconcussion syndrome. In most studies of postconcussion syndrome, patients have experienced a single episode of minor or at times even severe head injury. The potential for repeated cerebral concussion and minor head injury is almost unique to athletes who participate in contact sports. Whether they can develop a prolonged postconcussion syndrome or suffer cumulative effects is at present incompletely defined and under study.

It is believed that most of these symptoms run a self-limited and benign course, usually resolving by 6 to 8 weeks after the accident. Neuropsychological testing documents recovery in 1 to 6 months following the injury in most patients who are not athletes. Neurological examination as well as radiographic work-up are usually normal. Neuropsychological evaluation with a formal testing battery may be the best objective measure for documentation and serial follow-up in these patients and is invaluable for athletes who must perform at maximal physical levels.

Ancillary Testing

One of the greatest difficulties in managing athletes with concussions is arriving at the diagnosis when the person has had a normal neurological examination, has vague or minor neurological complaints, when significant time has elapsed between the injury event and the evaluation, or when all of these features are present. Concussion definitions and guidelines are most helpful in deciding upon the initial management of the athlete (i.e., removal from the contest) but often have limited utility in assisting the caregivers in determining when it is safe for the athlete to return to contact sport participation.

Because of the limited use of concussion guidelines, several ancillary testing maneuvers, some radiographic and others functional, are used to aid in arriving at a diagnosis of ongoing cerebral dysfunction that may predispose the athlete to another concussion, the second-impact syndrome, or cumulative brain injury with chronic effects on mental and physical performance. Athletes differ from the general population in that the latter ordinarily would sustain only a single concussion in a lifetime, most likely occurring as a result of a motor vehicle accident or a fall. However, they are not asked to return to an environment where they are subjected to repeated head impacts that can have cumulative effects. This becomes especially difficult when high physical and mental performance standards are expected of the athlete. Determining when it is safe to again participate in contact sports and knowing the propensity for exposure to more head impacts require that all appropriate and available ancillary testing be utilized to formulate an opinion.

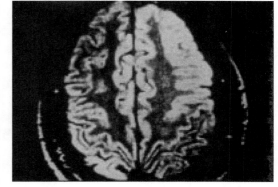

A detailed neurological examination must be performed to provide a baseline for future comparisons. In athletes who have sustained a loss of consciousness, especially for any significant length of time (i.e., greater than seconds), CT is often indicated. This excludes the possibility of a traumatic structural brain lesion such as a hematoma, which, if present, would necessitate neurosurgical evacuation. However, most athletes with persistent neurological symptoms after a concussion do not have abnormalities following either neurological examination or CT. Thus, more sensitive indicators of ongoing brain function must be utilized. Occasionally, MRI will disclose an abnormality not seen on CT, such as a deep white matter contusion or a small SDH (Figure 6). Consideration of MRI scanning if the symptoms persist or if anything unusual is detected and not clarified by CT is therefore recommended.

Figure 6: Axial T2-weighted MRI in a professional football player who had persistent postconcussion symptoms, a normal neurological examination, and no findings on CT. A high-intensity lesion was demonstrated on MRI in the right central semiovale that greatly assisted in the decision to end his playing career.

Other ancillary tests have shown significant value in assisting the documentation of ongoing brain involvement following a concussion. Neuropsychological testing has come to the forefront of supplementary methods of objectifying the cognitive deficits in athletes when the other aforementioned tests are not able to document an abnormality.

Neuropsychological Testing

In most instances, radiographic testing (CT or MRI) of athletes with concussion does not demonstrate evidence of intracranial hemorrhage, contusion, or other anatomic abnormalities. In addition, the neurological examination is often within normal limits. In the days and weeks following a cerebral concussion in the athlete, it has traditionally been difficult to obtain a measure of the degree of persistent cognitive and mental status dysfunction. However, with the implementation of a neuropsychological test battery, we have the ability to measure, quantify, and follow persistent and evolving cognitive and higher cortical function modalities in these patients. Even mild abnormalities on a formal neuropsychological evaluation indicate that there are persistent and ongoing brain effects of the prior concussion.[33]

Effective neuropsychological testing must be brief to administer, reproducible, and somewhat tailored for the examination. The importance of a baseline examination done in the preseason cannot be overemphasized. Orientation, attention, memory, information processing, and other modalities are the basis for neuropsychological testing of the athlete. Since 1990, a neuropsychological test battery has been utilized with the Pittsburgh Steelers football team members. This assessment has proved to be reliable, reproducible, and efficient. It has been helpful in following athletes with postconcussion symptoms and deciding when it would be safe to return to play. It has also been utilized successfully at the collegiate and high school football levels.[5,6,34]

Neuropsychological examination provides an objective measure to use for documentation of true brain dysfunction when all other tests, including physical and neurological examination, are normal. As the effects of the concussion resolve, reliable improvement in the neuropsychological test battery occurs. This objective demonstration of cognitive and mental status abnormality is valuable for the athletes, team physicians, trainers, coaches, officials, and parents in understanding and following the extent of the injury. Numerous neuropsychological testing instruments are available, and there is some disagreement about which are preferred. However, the ability to objectify the cognitive, visual, and memory disturbances have proved invaluable to the clinician caring for such athletes. Neuropsychological testing may be appropriate as early as 48 hours following the injury, provided that there is helpful objective evidence to guide management.

Since its inception, neuropsychological testing has enjoyed widespread utilization and is currently being administered to members of several National Football League teams and to every team in the National Hockey League during the 1997-1998 hockey season. Neuropsychological testing has been shown to be a very sensitive indicator of ongoing cognitive dysfunction in players who otherwise appear normal. Due to the heterogeneity of athletes and their respective socioeconomic backgrounds, baseline testing is optimal. Athletes who continue to be symptomatic following a concussion almost always show a change from baseline testing. When basic neurological and neuroradiological examinations are normal, the neuropsychological battery often indicates the concussive cognitive deficits. Results at the high school, collegiate, and professional levels have affirmed the important role of this modality. Usually, an uncomplicated concussion will revert to normal examination in 7 to 10 days.

Collins et al[14] reported their analysis of 393 college football players from four Division 1A football programs during a 2-year period. Their study was designed to discern not only whether neuropsychological testing was useful in diagnosing and defining recovery following concussion in athletes, but also to determine the effects of a learning disability on the presentation and analysis of concussion in their population. A learning disability represents a heterogeneous mixture of disorders in the acquisition and utilization of the skills of speaking, listening, reading, writing, and mathematical skills. Although usually discovered during childhood, learning disabilities are believed to be present in 12% of a general university population.

The findings of Collins et al[14] demonstrated that there appears to be an association between learning disability and multiple episodes of concussion, in an addictive manner. Importantly, individuals who sustained two or more concussions had long-term deficits in speed of information processing and executive functioning. In addition, there was correlation with self-reported symptoms of typical postconcussion states. However, a single concussion did not portend similar deficits. As in prior research, acute effects of concussion usually resolved by 5 days following injury. Their findings emphasized again the fact that the presence of any cognitive deficit, as detected by neuropsychological testing or neurological examination of postconcussion symptoms, indicates that full neurological recovery has not occurred and that return to play is contraindicated.

Other methodology has emerged and proved as useful as an adjunctive measure of brain dysfunction in the injured athlete. Single photon emission CT (SPECT) scanning has been shown to give additional information about the functional state of the cerebral cortex. A traceable agent, ordinarily a labeled amphetamine, is injected and its uptake measured in a brain map sequence. This gives an indication of neuronal function as evidenced by the uptake of the labeled agent, and asymmetry is indicative of focal brain metabolic depression. SPECT has been used successfully in the author's experience to document hypometabolism in one hemisphere in an athlete with postconcussion symptoms. Another method currently being reported is the use of postural stability measures to denote brain balance mechanism dysfunction.

Guskiewicz et al[23] reported a preliminary study of athletes following acute mild head injury, with no other documented abnormality, who had persistent and ongoing inability to maintain postural stability. They were tested for postural sway by dedicated measuring methods for stability. Their findings suggested that computerized dynamic posturography appears to be a reliable indicator of ongoing postural instability 1 to 3 days following concussion, even when other postconcussion symptoms are absent. More research may disclose that other brain areas, such as those involved with axial postural mechanisms or the motor skills, may also be indicators of continual cerebral dysfunction.[23]

Neurological Examination

When evaluating the athlete for possible head injury, the neurological assessment follows an abbreviated but definite examination. Any player who is downed or unconscious must be addressed with the basic principles of cardiopulmonary resuscitation in mind. As always, an unconscious player, who is thus unable to verbally report symptoms of spinal cord or spinal column injury, must be treated as having a possible cervical spine fracture or dislocation. Therefore, meticulous attention is given to spinal alignment during the onfield evaluation and in moving or transporting the athlete. Maintenance of the airway and ensuring adequate ventilation for air movement are of paramount importance. When a player is unconscious, there is no immediate treatment more important than maintaining good spinal alignment and guaranteeing adequate ventilation. In most athletes, the period of unconsciousness is very short, lasting from seconds to a few minutes. If there is a prolonged period of unconsciousness, arrangements should be made for rapid evaluation at a center that has appropriate trauma services and resources to deal with acute neurosurgical emergencies.[55]

Even with an unconscious or semiconscious athlete, important information may be gleaned from the neurological examination that will subsequently assist in determining the degree of injury and formulating an appropriate treatment plan. The neurological examination for suspected head injury in the athlete should begin with an assessment of the level of consciousness. For any patient who has an altered level of consciousness, a determination should be made of the degree of response to verbal, tactile, and painful stimulation. The Glasgow Coma Scale has improved our ability to quantitate the response of a patient who is comatose or has an altered level of consciousness and, in addition, ultimately allows prognostication. When the level of consciousness and degree of interaction of the patient with the environment have been determined, an examination of cranial nerve function should be carried out. The movement and conjugate deviation of the eyes should be assessed. The pupillary position and reaction to light and accommodation are very important signs in patients with head injury. The pupillary assessment can be carried out quickly and reproducibly. In conscious patients, the reported visual acuity, facial movement and sensation, degree of hearing, and tongue movement complete the cranial nerve examination. The patient's motor function in all limbs is assessed, with voluntary function noted in the conscious patient and involuntary and reflex activity noted in the unconscious patient. A brief sensory examination and reflex assessment complete the cursory neurological assessment of the athlete on the field. A more detailed and formal neurological examination is carried out when the patient has been transported to a definitive care facility.[56]

In patients being considered for cerebral concussion, the examination centers around mental status changes. The patient's orientation to person, place, and time is first acknowledged. A measure of memory for immediate, recent, and remote facts is then obtained. The ability to perform simple calculations and abstract reasoning and to solve simple practical problems can be assessed within 2 minutes. The author has found it particularly useful to quiz the player on particular game-day assignments, as these have added to recent memory and serve as a good benchmark for cerebral concussion. In addition, players have been found to be unable to remember key components of assignments and therefore would be unable to contribute adequately to the team effort. In a matter of minutes, even a brief mental status and neurological examination provides a reproducible and accurate assessment of the athlete's cerebral function, assists in appropriate triage for further medical diagnosis and care, and aids in making decisions regarding future return to competitive participation.[38]

Any patient with a serious head injury, including those with a Grade 3 concussion, requires hospitalization and appropriate diagnostic evaluation. The ultimate treatment plan is dictated by the pathophysiological processes that are discovered. Mass lesions of significant size, such as an EDH or SDH, usually require emergent evacuation. In patients with elevated ICP, monitoring is used to help guide in selecting and administering therapy.

Treatment and Return to Competition

The medical and neurosurgical treatment of the head-injured athlete does not differ significantly from those individuals with nonathletic-related head injuries.[53] Excellent emergency guidelines for the management of severe head injury have been published elsewhere. In general, onfield management follows the standard trauma and cardiopulmonary resuscitation guidelines. Impact or early seizures may occasionally be seen, are ordinarily self-limited, and are managed by standard procedures. Diffuse axonal injury, when severe, can be neurologically devastating and places the athlete who survives in need of long-term care and rehabilitation. EDH and significant SDH are typically managed surgically, as are intracerebral hematomas that cause mass effect. Although many patients with EDH recover well, acute SDH requiring surgery is associated with a very high mortality rate, up to 60% in some series. It is generally accepted that any athlete who requires operative intervention for head injury should not be allowed to return to contact sport competition in the future.[32] An athlete who has sustained a brain contusion or intracerebral hemorrhage is also ordinarily prevented from future competition.[11]

Return Following a Mild Concussion

In considering a mild concussion, where there is confusion but no loss of consciousness, the management entails removing the player (who is often identified by teammates because of his/her confusion or difficulty remembering plays) from the field of competition for 15 to 20 minutes. If disorientation, confusion, memory disturbance, dizziness, headache, or any neurological abnormality persists after this observation period, the athlete should not be allowed to return. This constellation of symptoms, if persistent, would be termed "a postconcussion syndrome," and most often clears by a maximum of 6 weeks. If these features are absent, the athlete may be allowed to return to play following a mild concussion, provided that the neurological examination is normal. The physician should keep in mind that concussion may be present and significant even without loss of consciousness. Ommaya and Gennarelli[41] showed in their animal model that three of six grades of concussion do not involve loss of consciousness. They postulated that, unless shearing forces reached the reticular activating system, cortical and subcortical structures could be affected to produce amnesia and confusion but not loss of consciousness.

If an athlete has been withheld from play because of a mild concussion, he/she should be examined as soon as possible by the team physician. With a single mild concussion, the athlete may return to competition within 1 week of being asymptomatic. If still symptomatic, the athlete should not be allowed to play until the symptoms abate and a head CT scan is performed. With a second mild concussion in the same season, the athlete should be withheld from contact sports for 2 weeks and consideration should be given to CT scanning, especially if the concussions occur in short succession. The athlete should be asymptomatic with a normal neurological examination and CT scan before being allowed to return to play. If a third concussion occurs in a single season, most experts recommend terminating the athlete's season. Appropriate neurodiagnostic tests are then indicated (Figure 7).

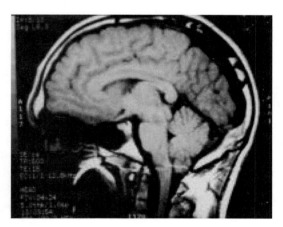

Figure 7: Sagittal MRI demonstrating low-lying cerebral tonsils in a high school football player who sustained several concussions in a single season. While not an absolute, it is suspected that in predisposed individuals, the normal "buffering" capacity of the CSF to provide buoyancy as the brain undergoes rapid acceleration-deceleration in contact sports may be compromised in the presence of a Chiari malformation. This finding may represent a relative contraindication to contact sports in symptomatic athletes.

The author recommends allowing return only after 1 full week without symptoms. In deciding whether the athlete is ready for competition, the author has found a "provocative exertional" practice session, in which the athlete participates fully in sports with the exception of avoiding head impacts, to be helpful. An athlete with a second moderate concussion in one season should be withheld for 1 month and have a normal CT scan prior to returning. A third moderate concussion would be grounds for terminating the season. Some suggest that at this point consideration should be given to not allowing return to contact sports.

Return Following a Moderate Concussion

Using the Colorado guidelines,[15] a moderate or Grade 2 concussion is associated with the development of amnesia either initially or during the period of observation. There is no loss of consciousness. The athlete is removed from competition and not allowed to return. He/she should be examined as soon as possible by the team physician and consideration given for consultation with a neurological specialist, especially if disturbances in the level of consciousness or other neurological signs develop. The guidelines recommend return to competition only after the patient has been asymptomatic for 1 full week.

An athlete with a second moderate concussion in one season should be withheld for 1 month after being asymptomatic and have had a normal CT scan before returning. A third moderate concussion would be grounds for terminating the season. Some experts suggest that at this point consideration should be given to not allowing the patient to return to contact sports.

Return Following a Severe Concussion

A severe or Grade 3 concussion is associated with loss of consciousness. It usually requires emergent transport to the nearest facility with CT scanning, and consideration should be given to a neurosurgical consultation, especially with any prolonged loss of consciousness or neurological deficit. The possibility of a concomitant cervical spine injury must always be considered in an unconscious patient, and transport should be performed with cervical immobilization and maintenance of an adequate airway. Unless the loss of consciousness has been very brief (i.e., less than 30 seconds), the athlete is most often admitted to the hospital overnight for observation. He/she is treated according to the standard accepted procedure for closed-head injury and observed for development of an expanding intracranial hematoma.

With any significant loss of consciousness, neurological and CT examinations are required. If both are normal and the athlete is asymptomatic, the athlete may return to competition within 2 weeks of being without symptoms, if the length of unconsciousness was less than 1 minute. With a loss of consciousness greater than 1 minute, which implies significant interruption of cerebral function, it is recommended that competition be avoided for 1 month. A second severe concussion will usually terminate the athlete's season, and consideration should be given to ending the patient's participation in any contact sport.

These recommendations are based on the author's experience and that of others, and are reinforced by neuropsychological testing. With a single incidence of minor athletic head injury, abnormalities on neuropsychological testing usually resolve by 1 to 2 weeks; however, with a second concussion, they may be present for a prolonged period.

The concept of "significant" loss of consciousness has come to be most important in understanding mild traumatic brain injury in the athlete. That is, a very brief loss of consciousness may be consistent with a limited residual on cognitive function, whereas other symptoms, notably posttraumatic amnesia, may portend more serious and ongoing cerebral dysfunction. This fact is taken into account more in the Cantu concussion scheme,[11] as it is more heavily weighted for amnesia than brief loss of consciousness.

References

1. Annegers JF, Grabow JD, Kurland LT, et al: The incidence, causes and secular trends of head trauma in Olmsted County, Minnesota, 1935–1974. **Neurology 30**:912-919, 1980
2. Bailes JE, Hadley MN, Quigley MR, et al: Management of athletic injuries of the cervical spine and spinal cord. **Neurosurgery 29**:491-497, 1991
3. Bailes JE, Herman JM, Quigley MR, et al: Diving injuries of the cervical spine. **Surg Neurol 34**:155-158, 1990
4. Bailes JE, Maroon JC: Neurosurgical trauma in the athlete, in Tindall GT, Cooper PR, Barrow DL (eds): **The Practice of Neurosurgery**. Baltimore, Md: Williams & Wilkins, 1996, pp 1649-1672

5. Barth J, Alves WM, Ryan TV, et al: Mild head injury in sports: neuropsychological sequelae and recovery of function, in Levin H, Eisenberg H, Benton A (eds): **Mild Head Injury**. New York, NY: Oxford University Press, 1989, pp 257-275
6. Barth JT, Macciocchi SN, Giordani B, et al: Neuropsychological sequelae of minor head injury. **Neurosurgery 13**:529-533, 1983
7. Bohnen N, Jolles J, Twijnstra A: Neuropsychological deficits in patients with persistent symptoms six months after mild head injury. **Neurosurgery 30**:692-696, 1992
8. Bruce DA, Alavi A, Bilaniuk L, et al: Diffuse cerebral swelling following head injuries in children: the syndrome of "malignant brain edema." **Neurosurgery 54**:170-178, 1981
9. Buckley WE: Concussions in college football. A multivariate analysis.

Am J Sports Med 16:51-56, 1988

10. Cantu RC: Cerebral concussion in sports: management and prevention. **Sports Med** 14:64-74, 1992
11. Cantu RC: Guidelines for return to contact sports after a cerebral concussion. **Phys Sportsmed** 14:75-83, 1986
12. Cantu RC: Second impact syndrome: a risk in any contact sport. **Phys Sportsmed** 23:27-34, 1995
13. Cantu RC, Mueller F: Fatalities and catastrophic injuries in high school and college sports, 1982-1997. **Phys Sportsmed** 27:35-48, 1999
14. Collins M, Grindel SH, Lovell MR, et al: Relationship between concussion and neuropsychological performance in college football players. **JAMA** 282:964-970, 1999
15. Colorado Medical Society: **Report of the Sports Medicine Committee: Guidelines for the Management of Concussion in Sports (revised).** Denver, Co: Colorado Medical Society, 1991
16. Dacey RG Jr, Alves WM, Rimel RW, et al: Neurosurgical complications after apparently minor head injury. Assessment of risk in a series of 610 patients. **J Neurosurg** 65:203-210, 1986
17. Fukamachi A, Kohno K, Nageseki Y, et al: The incidence of delayed traumatic intracerebral hematoma with extradural hemorrhages. **J Trauma** 25:145-149, 1985
18. Gerberich SG, Priest JD, Boen JR, et al: Concussion incidences and severity in secondary school varsity football players. **Am J Publ Health** 73:1370-1375, 1983
19. Gronwall D, Wrightson P: Cumulative effects of concussion. **Lancet** 2: 995-997, 1975
20. Gudeman SK, Kishare PR, Miller JD, et al: The genesis and significance of delayed traumatic intracerebral hematoma. **Neurosurgery** 5: 309-313, 1979
21. Gudeman SK, Kishare PRS, Becker DP, et al: Computed tomography in the evaluation of incidence and significance of post-traumatic hydrocephalus. **Radiology** 141:397-402, 1981
22. Gurdjian ES, Voris HC: Report of *Ad Hoc* Committee to Study Head Injury nomenclature. **Clin Neurosurg** 12:386-394, 1966
23. Guskiewicz KM, Riemann BL, Perrin DH, et al: Alternative approaches to the assessment of mild head injury in athletes. **Med Sci Sports Exerc** 29 (Suppl 7):213-221, 1997
24. Harris JB: Neurological injuries in winter sports. **Phys Sportsmed** 11:110-122, 1983
25. Hodgson VR, Thomas LM: Mechanisms of cervical spine injury during impact to the protected head, in: **24th STAPP Car Crash Conference.** Detroit, Mich: Society of Automotive Engineers, 1980, pp 15-42
26. Hugenholtz H, Stuss DT, Stethem LL, et al: How long does it take to recover from a mild concussion? **Neurosurgery** 22:853-858, 1988
27. Jamieson KG, Yelland JDN: Surgically treated traumatic subdural hematomas. **J Neurosurg** 37:137-149, 1972
28. Katz RT, Brander V, Sahgal V: Updates on the diagnosis and management of posttraumatic hydrocephalus. **Am J Phys Med Rehabil** 68: 91-96, 1989
29. Kaufman HH, Moake JL, Olson JD, et al: Delayed and recurrent intracranial hematomas related to disseminated intravascular clotting and fibrinolysis in head injury. **Neurosurgery** 7:445-449, 1980
30. Kelly JP, Nichols JS, Filley CM, et al: Concussion in sports. Guidelines for the prevention of catastrophic outcome. **JAMA** 266:2867-2869, 1991
31. Kelly JP, Rosenberg JH: Diagnosis and management of concussion in sports. **Neurology** 48:575-580, 1997
32. Kvarnes TL, Trumpy JH: Extradural haematoma. Report of 132 cases. **Acta Neurochir** 41:223-231, 1978
33. Levin HS, Mattis S, Ruff RM, et al: Neurobehavioral outcome following minor head injury: a three-center study. **J Neurosurg** 66:234-243, 1987

34. Lovell MR, Maroon JC, Bailes JE, et al: Neuropsychological assessment following minor head injury in professional athletes, in Bailes JE, Lovell MR, Maroon JC (eds): **Sports-Related Concussion.** St Louis, Mo: Quality Medical, 1999, pp 200-228
35. Macciocchi SN, Barth JT, Alves W, et al: Neuropsychological functioning and recovery after mild head injury in collegiate athletes. **Neurosurgery** 39:510-514, 1996
36. Martland HS: Punch drunk. **JAMA** 91:1103-1107, 1928
37. Matser EJT, Kessels AG, Lezak MD, et al: Neuropsychological impairment in amateur soccer players. **JAMA** 282:971-973, 1999
38. McCrea M, Kelly JP, Kluge J, et al: Standardized assessment of concussion in football players. **Neurology** 48:586-588, 1997
39. McQuillen JB, McQuillen EN, Morrow P: Trauma, sport, and malignant cerebral edema. **Am J Forensic Med Pathol** 9:12-15, 1988
40. Merskey H, Woodforde JM: Psychiatric sequelae of minor head injury. **Brain** 95:521-528, 1972
41. Ommaya AK, Gennarelli TA: Cerebral concussion and traumatic unconsciousness. Correlation of experimental and clinical observations on blunt head injuries. **Brain** 97:633-654, 1974
42. Phonprasert C, Suwanwela C, Hongsaprabhas C, et al: Extradural hematoma: analysis of 138 cases. **J Trauma** 20:679-683, 1989
43. Powell JW, Barber-Foss KD: Traumatic brain injury in high school athletes. **JAMA** 282:958-963, 1999
44. Putnam P: Going-going-gone. **Sports Illustrated**, June 6, 1983, pp 46-53
45. Richards T, Hoff J: Factors affecting survival from subdural hematoma. **Surgery** 75:253-258, 1974
46. Rimel RW, Giordani B, Barth JT, et al: Disability caused by minor head injury. **Neurosurgery** 9:221-228, 1981
47. Roberts AH: **Brain Damage in Boxers.** London: Pittman, 1969
48. Saunders RL, Harbaugh RE: The second impact in catastrophic contact-sports head trauma. **JAMA** 252:538-539, 1984
49. Schneider RC: Serious and fatal neurosurgical football injuries. **Clin Neurosurg** 12:226-236, 1966
50. Shell D, Carico GA, Patton RM: Can subdural hematoma result from repeated minor head injury? **Phys Sportsmed** 21:74-84, 1993
51. Sweet RC, Miller JD, Lipper M, et al: Significance of bilateral abnormalities on the CT scan in patients with severe head injury. **Neurosurgery** 3:16-21, 1978
52. Tegner Y, Lorentzon R: Concussion among Swedish elite ice hockey players. **Br J Sports Med** 30:251-255, 1996
53. Thorndike A: Serious recurrent injuries of athletes. Contraindications for further competitive participation. **N Engl J Med** 247:554-556, 1952
54. Torg JS, Quendenfeld TC, Burstein A, et al: National Football Head and Neck Injury Registry: report on cervical quadriplegia 1971 to 1975. **Am J Sports Med** 7:127-132, 1977
55. Torg JS, Vegso JJ, Sennett B, et al: The National Football Head and Neck Injury Registry: 14-year report on cervical quadriplegia, 1971 through 1984. **JAMA** 254:3439-3443, 1985
56. Warren WL Jr, Bailes JE: On the field evaluation of athletic head injuries. **Clin Sports Med** 17:13-26, 1998
57. Whitman S, Coonley-Hoganson R, Desai BT: Comparative head trauma experiences in two socioeconomically different Chicago-area communities: a population study. **Am J Epidemiol** 119:570-580, 1984
58. Wrightson P, Gronwall D: Time off work and symptoms after minor head injury. **Injury** 12:445-454, 1981
59. Yarnell PR, Lynch S: The "ding:" amnestic states in football trauma. **Neurology** 23:196-197, 1973
60. Zemper ED: Injury rates in a national sample of college football teams: a prospective study. **Phys Sportsmed** 17:100-113, 1989

CHAPTER 2

Classification and Clinical Management of Concussion

ROBERT C. CANTU, MA, MD, FACS, FACSM

Concussion is derived from the Latin *concussus*, which means "to shake violently." Initially, it was believed to produce only a temporary disturbance of brain function due to neuronal, chemical, or neuroelectrical changes without gross structural change. We now know that structural damage with loss of brain cells does occur with some concussions. In the last several years, the neurobiology of cerebral concussion has been advanced not only in animal studies but also in studies in man. It has become clear that, in the minutes to days following concussive brain injury, brain cells that are not irreversibly destroyed, remain alive but in a vulnerable state. These cells are particularly vulnerable to minor changes in cerebral blood flow (CBF) and/or increases in intracranial pressure and, especially, anoxia. Animal studies have shown that during this period of vulnerability, which may last for as long as a week with a minor head injury such as a concussion, a minor reduction in CBF that was believed to be well tolerated actually produces extensive neuronal cell loss.[10,11,15,17,26] This vulnerability appears to be due to an uncoupling of the demand for glucose, which is increased after injury with a relative reduction in CBF. While the precise mechanisms of this dysfunction are still in the process of being fully understood, it is now clear that although concussion in and of itself may not produce extensive neuronal damage, the surviving cells are in a state of vulnerability characterized in terms of a metabolic dysfunction that can be thought of as a breakdown between energy demand and production. Precisely how long this period of metabolic dysfunction lasts is not fully understood. Unfortunately, there are no current neuroanatomical or physiological measurements that can be used to precisely determine the extent of injury with concussion, the severity of metabolic dysfunction, or when it has cleared. It is this fact that makes return-to-play decisions following a concussion a clinical judgment.

There is no more challenging problem faced by team physicians, athletic trainers, and other medical personnel responsible for the medical care of athletes than the recognition and management of concussion. Indeed, such injuries have captured many headlines in recent years and have spurred studies within both the National Football League and the

TABLE 1

CANTU[1] GRADING SYSTEM FOR CONCUSSION

Grade I	No loss of consciousness; posttraumatic amnesia lasting less than 30 minutes in duration
Grade II	Loss of consciousness for less than 5 minutes in duration, or posttraumatic amnesia lasting longer than 30 minutes but less than 24 hours in duration
Grade III	Loss of consciousness for more than 5 minutes in duration, or posttraumatic amnesia lasting longer than 24 hours in duration

TABLE 2

COLORADO MEDICAL SOCIETY[5] GRADING SYSTEM FOR CONCUSSION

Grade 1	Confusion without amnesia; no loss of consciousness
Grade 2	Confusion with amnesia; no loss of consciousness
Grade 3	Loss of consciousness

TABLE 3

AMERICAN ACADEMY OF NEUROLOGY PRACTICE PARAMETER (KELLY AND ROSENBERG[14]) GRADING SYSTEM FOR CONCUSSION

Grade 1	Transient confusion; no loss of consciousness; concussion symptoms or mental status abnormalities on examination resolve in less than 15 minutes
Grade 2	Transient confusion; no loss of consciousness; concussion symptoms or mental status abnormalities on examination last more than 15 minutes
Grade 3	Any loss of consciousness, either brief (seconds) or prolonged (minutes)

National Hockey League. When discussing concussion, it must be realized that there is no universal agreement on the definition and grading of concussion.[1,5,14,21-23,28] In Tables 1 to 8 are eight different attempts at grading concussion. As can be seen, each system tends to focus on loss or no loss of consciousness and amnesia as hallmarks. Furthermore, perhaps not enough attention has been given to the other signs and symptoms of concussion. As is well known with concussion, any combination of the following signs and symptoms may be encountered: a feeling of being stunned or seeing bright lights, a brief loss of consciousness, lightheadedness, vertigo, loss of balance, headaches, cognitive and memory dysfunction, tinnitus, blurred vision, difficulty concentrating, lethargy, fatigue, personality changes, the inability to perform daily activities, sleep disturbance, and motor or sensory symptoms.

The lack of a universal definition or grading scheme for concussion renders the evaluation of epidemiological data extremely difficult. As a neurosurgeon and a team physician, the author has evaluated many football players who have suffered a concussion. In most instances, the injuries were mild and were associated with retrograde amnesia, which is helpful in making the diagnosis, especially in mild cases. The author has developed a practical scheme for grading the severity of a concussion based on the duration of unconsciousness and/or posttraumatic amnesia, which has worked well both on the field and on the sidelines (Table 1). The most mild concussion (Grade I) occurs without loss of consciousness, and the only neurological deficit is a brief period of confusion or posttraumatic amnesia which, by definition, when present, lasts less than 30 minutes. With a moderate concussion (Grade II), there is usually a brief period of unconsciousness, by definition not exceeding 5 minutes. Less commonly, there is no loss of consciousness but only a protracted period of posttraumatic amnesia lasting over 30 minutes but less than 24 hours. Severe concussion (Grade III) occurs with a more protracted period of unconsciousness lasting over 5 minutes. Rarely, it may occur with a shorter period of unconsciousness, but with a very protracted period of posttraumatic amnesia lasting over 24 hours.

In 1991, Kelly et al[13] proposed another guideline regarding the severity of concussion in which the most mild concussion (Grade 1) had no loss of consciousness and no posttraumatic amnesia, but rather just a brief period of disorientation or confusion. A moderate concussion (Grade 2) was one in which there was no loss of consciousness but posttraumatic amnesia was present. This essentially split the Grade I of the Cantu system into two grades depending on whether amnesia was present. In their guideline, athletes rendered unconscious were placed in the Grade 3, or severe concussion, category. This guideline essentially has been adopted by the American Academy of Neurology and subsequently published by that organization. While it can be debated that posttraumatic amnesia of over 24 hours may reflect a more severe brain insult than 30 seconds of unconsciousness, both guidelines will prevent the second-impact syndrome, as no athlete still symptomatic from a prior head injury is allowed to return to competition.

Today, it is recognized that the ability to process information after a concussion may be reduced,[8] and the functional impairment may be greater with repeated concussion, suggesting that the damaging effects of concussion may be cumulative.[8,27] Furthermore, in proportion to the degree to which the head is accelerated and such forces are imparted to the brain, concussion may produce a shearing injury to nerve fibers and neurons.

The late effects of repeated head trauma of concussive or even subconcussive force lead to anatomical patterns of chronic brain injury with correlating signs and symptoms. Martland[18] introduced the term "punch drunk" (dementia pugilistica) in 1928. Although first described in boxers, this traumatic encephalopathy may occur in any person subjected to repeated blows to the head from any cause.

The characteristic symptoms and signs of the punch-drunk state (Table 9) include the gradual appearance of a fatuous or euphoric dementia with emotional lability, with the victim displaying little insight into the deterioration. Speech and thought become progressively slower. Memory deteriorates considerably. There may be mood swings, intense irritability, and sometimes truculence leading to uninhibited violent behavior. Simple fatuous cheerfulness is, however, the most common prevailing mood, although there may be depression with paranoia. From the clinical standpoint, the neurologist may encounter almost any combination of pyramidal, extrapyramidal, and cerebellar signs. Tremor and dysarthria are two of the most common findings. Corsellis et al[6] described necropsy findings in the brains of men who had been boxers. They described a characteristic pattern of cerebral change that appeared not only to be the result of boxing but also to underlie many features of the punch-drunk syndrome. They documented changes in the middle of the brain, which may shear into two layers or even be shredded by the distortions that follow blows to the head. Corsellis et al found that destruction of the limbic system, a portion of the brain that governs emotion and has a role in memory and learning, was present. There was a characteristic loss of cells from the cerebellum, a part of the brain that governs balance and coordination. Finally, there was an unusual microscopic change throughout the brain resembling changes that occur with Alzheimer's disease, which causes progressive loss of intelligence, but is sufficiently different (neurofibrillary tangles only and no senile plaques) to be regarded as a distinct entity, unique to subjects suffering from blows to the head.

Management Guidelines

Immediate Treatment on the Field

The major purpose of the on-the-field evaluation is to rule out a life-threatening injury, especially a head injury, a cervical spine fracture, or a spinal cord injury. A decision is then made regarding the most appropriate and safest method of transport of the injured athlete off the field and whether this transport is to the sideline or directly to a facility with definitive neurosurgical capabilities.

After reaching the athlete with a cerebral concussion, the initial evaluation should include the ABCs of first aid (airway, breathing, and circulation). Is the airway obstructed? Is the athlete breathing? Does the athlete have a pulse? This evaluation must take place before a neurological examination is undertaken. Only after the treating physician has determined that the airway is adequate and that circulation is being maintained should attention be directed to the neurological assessment. If the athlete complains of neck pain or is unconscious, it must be assumed that there is a cervical spine fracture and that the cervical spine must be immobilized and the athlete transported as if there is a cervical spine fracture. Similarly, if the athlete is found to be without a pulse and is unconscious, the head and neck must be immobilized while cardiopulmonary resuscitation is initiated.

Once the ABCs have been determined to be unimpaired and the athlete noted to be conscious, a brief neurological exam should then be carried out on the field, particularly including a brief mental examination with orientation to time, person, place, and situation. It is preferable that a Glasgow Coma Scale assessment (Table 10) be quickly carried out and that eye contact with the individual and the briskness of the patient's responses to commands be documented. If the athlete is alert, the brief neurological exam is normal, and there are no neck symptoms, the athlete may be allowed to sit, then stand, and then walk off the field. If there are cervical symptoms, despite a neurological exam being normal, the neck should be immobi-

TABLE 4

JORDAN ET AL[12] GRADING SYSTEM FOR CONCUSSION

Grade 1	Confusion without amnesia; no loss of consciousness
Grade 2	Confusion with amnesia lasting less than 24 hours; no loss of consciousness
Grade 3	Loss of consciousness with an altered level of consciousness not exceeding 2-3 minutes; posttraumatic amnesia lasting more than 24 hours
Grade 4	Loss of consciousness with an altered level of consciousness exceeding 2-3 minutes

TABLE 5

OMMAYA[22] GRADING SYSTEM FOR CONCUSSION

Grade 1	Confusion without amnesia (stunned)
Grade 2	Amnesia without coma
Grade 3	Coma lasting less than 6 hours (includes classic cerebral concussion, minor and moderate head injuries)
Grade 4	Coma lasting 6 to 24 hours (severe head injuries)
Grade 5	Coma lasting more than 24 hours (severe head injuries)
Grade 6	Coma, death within 24 hours (fatal head injuries)

TABLE 6

NELSON ET AL[21] GRADING SYSTEM FOR CONCUSSION

Grade 0	Head struck or moved rapidly; not stunned or dazed initially; subsequently complains of headache and difficulty in concentrating
Grade 1	Stunned or dazed initially; no loss of consciousness or amnesia; sensorium clears in less than 1 minute
Grade 2	Headache; cloudy sensorium longer than 1 minute in duration; no loss of consciousness; may have tinnitus or amnesia; may be irritable, hyperexcitable, confused, or dizzy
Grade 3	Loss of consciousness for less than 1 minute in duration; no coma (arousable with noxious stimuli); demonstrates Grade 2 symptoms during recovery
Grade 4	Loss of consciousness for more than 1 minute; not comatose; demonstrates Grade 2 symptoms during recovery.

TABLE 7

ROBERTS[23] GRADING SYSTEM FOR CONCUSSION

Bell Ringer	No loss of consciousness; no posttraumatic amnesia; symptoms less than 10 minutes
Grade 1	No loss of consciousness; posttraumatic amnesia less than 30 minutes; symptoms greater than 10 minutes
Grade 2	Loss of consciousness less than 5 minutes; posttraumatic amnesia greater than 30 minutes
Grade 3	Loss of consciousness greater than 5 minutes; posttraumatic amnesia greater than 24 hours

TABLE 8

TORG[28] GRADING SYSTEM FOR CONCUSSION

Grade 1	"Bell rung"; short-term confusion; unsteady gait; dazed appearance; no amnesia
Grade 2	Posttraumatic amnesia only; vertigo; no loss of consciousness
Grade 3	Posttraumatic retrograde amnesia; no loss of consciousness; vertigo
Grade 4	Immediate transient loss of consciousness
Grade 5	Paralytic coma; cardiorespiratory arrest
Grade 6	Death

lized and the athlete transported to a facility where x-rays can be obtained and neuroradiological capability is present.

Once the athlete has been transported or walks off the athletic field unassisted, a more detailed neurological exam should be carried out on the sideline, with recording of a detailed mental exam including repeating the months of the year backward, repeating serial digits backward, and/or other mini-neuropsychological mental status studies, such as the Galveston Orientation and Amnesia Test (Table 11)[16] and the Standardized Assessment of Concussion (see Chapter 8, Figure 1).[20] The sideline neurological exam should also include a detailed evaluation of cranial nerve function and motor strength, coordination, and sensation. Balance should be tested with the Romberg test and tandem gait. Symptoms of concussion, including lightheadedness, vertigo, headaches, tinnitus, blurred vision, difficulty concentrating, or a feeling of lethargy, fatigue, or vagueness, should be determined.

Once the patient becomes asymptomatic with a normal neurological evaluation at rest, exertional tests of having the individual do either sprints, repetitive sit-ups, or push-ups should be carried out to see if exertional tests provoke postconcussion or other neurological symptoms.

Just as there are no lack of grading systems for concussion, there are a number of return-to-play guideline recommendations after an initial concussion, as outlined in Tables 12, 13, and 14.[1,5,12,13] Although within the different guidelines there are minor differences in the duration of holding an athlete from athletic competition, all of the guidelines agree that no athlete who still has postconcussion symptoms should be allowed to return to competition.

Tables 15 and 16 provide guidelines for return to competition after a cerebral concussion of Grades 1, 2, or 3 and whether this was the first, second, or third concussion sustained by the patient in a given season.[1,5,13] The author believes that it is important to recognize, as indicated and shown in other tables, that such multiple concussion guidelines for return to play exist.[1,5,12,13] While there is no precise agreement as to the timing of return to play after various degrees and numbers of concussions received in a given season, and all are truly only guidelines, all agree on the one most salient point, that is, no athlete still symptomatic from a previous injury at rest or exertion should be allowed to risk incurring a second head injury, either by practice or by participation. Therefore, while grading and return dates may vary slightly, all of the guidelines prevent the dreaded "second-impact syndrome."

In December 1997, the American Orthopedics Society for Sports Medicine hosted "A Concussion in Sports Workshop" with representatives from the American Academy of Neurology, the American Academy of Pediatrics, the American Academy of Orthopedic

TABLE 9

DEMENTIA PUGILISTICA: AREAS OF BRAIN DAMAGE AND RESULTANT DEFICIT

Area	Deficit
Altered affect and memory	Abnormalities of the septum pellucidum and the adjacent periventricular gray matter
Slurred speech, loss of balance and coordination	Cerebellar scarring and nerve cell loss
Tremor	Degeneration of the substantia nigra
Loss of intellect	The regional occurrence of neurofibrillary tangles

Surgeons, the American Association of Neurological Surgeons, the American College of Emergency Physicians, the American Medical Society for Sports Medicine, the Congress of Neurological Surgeons, the American College of Sports Medicine, the American Osteopathic Academy of Sports Medicine, the National Athletic Trainers Association, the National Collegiate Athletic Association, the National Football League, the National Hockey League, and other interested sports medicine specialists. While that group was not able to settle the issue of a universal classification scheme for concussion, it did define concussion as "a brain injury produced by direct or indirect head trauma and manifesting one or more of the following signs or symptoms." The signs and symptoms that fell into the acute group included posttraumatic amnesia, alteration of cognitive function or "memory/concentration," headache, nausea, vomiting, photophobia, balance disturbance, and "dizziness/vertigo." Delayed signs and symptoms included any of the acute signs and symptoms that persisted plus sleep disturbance, fatigue, depression, and the feeling of being slowed down in a fog.

Concussion was broken down into essentially two groups: athletes who could return to play the same day and athletes who could return to play after being asymptomatic for 7 days at rest and exertion. To qualify as "safe to return to the contest the same day," the following criteria had to be present: 1) signs and symptoms had cleared within 15 minutes at rest and exertion; 2) the neurological evaluation was normal; and 3) no loss of consciousness was documented.

The criteria required to be categorized in the "safe to return to competition only after being asymptomatic for 7 days both at rest and exertion" group included: 1) signs and symptoms had not cleared by 15 minutes at rest and exertion; 2) there was documented loss of consciousness; and 3) at the time of return to play, the individual been asymptomatic for 7 days at rest and exertion and also the neurological evaluation was normal.

TABLE 10
GLASGOW COMA SCALE

Verbal Response	
None	1
Incomprehensible sounds	2
Inappropriate words	3
Confused	4
Oriented	5
Eye Opening	
None	1
To Pain	2
To Speech	3
Spontaneously	4
Motor Response	
None	1
Abnormal extension	2
Abnormal flexion	3
Withdraws	4
Localizes pain	5
Obeys verbal commands	6
Normal	15

TABLE 11
GALVESTON ORIENTATION AND AMNESIA TEST[16]

Instructions: Error points (in parentheses) are scored for incorrect answers and are entered in the two columns in the right column. Enter the total error points accrued for the different items in the lower right corner. The GOAT (Galveston Orientation and Amnesia Test) score equals 100 minus the error points. A score of 85 or less should be considered to be a priority for special consideration and follow-up. Recovery of orientation can be plotted daily using the GOAT scores.

Error Points

1. What is your name? (5) Where were you born? (4) Where do you live? (4) _____
2. Where are you now? Participation area? (5) City? (5) _____
3. What is the *first* event you can remember *after* injury? (5) _____ _____
   Can you describe (type of play, teammates, etc.) the first event following injury? (5)
   _____ _____
4. What is the *last* event you can remember *before* the injury? (5) _____ _____
   Can you describe (type of play, teammates, etc.) the last event prior to the injury? (5)
   _____ _____
5. What time is it? (1 point for each half hour up to 5 points) _____
6. What day of the week is it? (1 point for each day up to 5 points) _____
7. What day of the month is it? (1 point for each day up to 5 points) _____
8. What month is it? (5 points for each month up to 15 points) _____
9. What year is it? (10 points for each year up to 30 points) _____

If the patient is hospitalized, add the following question.
10. On what date were you admitted to this hospital? (5) _____
    How did you get here? (5) _____ _____

TABLE 12

CANTU[1] GUIDELINES FOR RETURN TO PLAY AFTER A FIRST CONCUSSION*

Grade 1	May return to play if asymptomatic for 1 week
Grade 2	May return to play if asymptomatic for 1 week
Grade 3	Should not be allowed to play for at least 1 month; may then return to play if asymptomatic for 1 week

*A patient is considered asymptomatic if there are no physical symptoms at rest and exertion.

TABLE 13

COLORADO MEDICAL SOCIETY[5,13] GUIDELINES FOR RETURN TO PLAY AFTER A FIRST CONCUSSION

Grade 1	May return to play if asymptomatic at rest and exertion after at least 20 minutes observation
Grade 2	May return to play if asymptomatic for 1 week
Grade 3	Should not be allowed to play for at least 1 month; may then return to play if asymptomatic for 2 weeks

TABLE 14

JORDAN ET AL[12] GUIDELINES FOR RETURN TO PLAY AFTER A FIRST CONCUSSION

Grade 1	May return to play if asymptomatic at rest and exertion
Grade 2	May return to play if asymptomatic for 1 week
Grade 3	Should not be allowed to play for at least 1 month; may then return to play if asymptomatic for 1 week
Grade 4	Should not be allowed to play for at least 1 month; may then return to play if asymptomatic for 2 weeks

Second-impact Syndrome and Cumulative Brain Injury

The reason that no athlete still symptomatic from a prior head injury should be allowed to return to practice or participation in a contact collision sport is that the brain in this situation is vulnerable not only to cumulative injury, as pointed out by Hovda, but also to the rare but frightful second-impact syndrome.

Recognizing the Syndrome

What Saunders and Harbaugh[24] called the "second-impact syndrome of catastrophic head injury" in 1984 was first described by Schneider in 1973.[25] The syndrome occurs when an athlete who has sustained a head injury—often a concussion or a worse injury, such as a cerebral contusion—sustains a second head injury before the symptoms associated with the first have cleared. Typically, the athlete suffers postconcussion symptoms after the first head injury. These may include visual, motor, or sensory changes as well as difficulty with thought and memory processes. Before theses symptoms resolve—which may take days or weeks—the athlete returns to competition and receives a second blow to the head.

The second blow may be remarkably minor, perhaps only involving a blow to the chest that jerks the athlete's head and indirectly imparts accelerative forces to the brain. Affected athletes may appear stunned but usually do not lose consciousness and often complete the play. They usually remain on their feet for 15 seconds or more but seem dazed, like someone suffering from a Grade I concussion without loss of consciousness. Often, the affected athlete remains on the playing field or walks off under his/her own power.

It is what happens in the next 15 seconds to several minutes that sets this syndrome apart from a concussion or even a subdural hematoma. Usually within seconds to minutes of the second impact, the athlete—conscious yet stunned—quite precipitously collapses to the ground, semicomatose with rapidly dilating pupils, loss of eye movement, and evidence of respiratory failure.

The pathophysiology of second-impact syndrome is believed to involve a loss of autoregulation of the brain's blood supply. This loss of autoregulation leads to vascular engorgement within the cranium, which in turn markedly increases intracranial pressure and leads to herniation either of the medial surface (uncus) of the temporal lobe or lobes below the tentorium or of the cerebellar tonsils through the foramen magnum. Animal research has shown that vascular engorgement of the brain after a mild head injury is difficult, if not impossible, to control. The time from second impact to brainstem failure is rapid, usually taking 2 to 5 minutes. Once brain herniation and brainstem compromise occur, ocular involvement and respiratory failure precipitously ensue.

Demise occurs far more rapidly than usually seen with an epidural hematoma. Magnetic resonance imaging (MRI) and computed tomography (CT) are the neuroimaging studies most likely to demonstrate the second-impact syndrome. While MRI is more sensitive to traumatic brain injuries, especially true edema, CT is usually adequate to show bleeding or midline shifts of the brain requiring neurosurgical intervention. This is important because CT scanning is cheaper, more widely available, and more quickly performed than MRI.

Incidence

The precise incidence of second-impact syndrome per 100,000 participants is not known because the precise population at risk is unknown; nonetheless, it occurs more frequently than previous reports have suggested.[2,4] Between 1980 and 1993, the National Center for Catastrophic Sports Injury Research in Chapel Hill, North Carolina, identified

TABLE 15

CANTU[1] GUIDELINES FOR RETURN TO PLAY AFTER A SECOND OR THIRD CONCUSSION

First Concussion Grade	Second Concussion*	Third Concussion*
Grade 1	Return to play in 2 weeks if asymptomatic at the time for 1 week	Terminate season; may return to play next season if asymptomatic
Grade 2	Minimum of 1 month; may return to play then if asymptomatic for 1 week; consider terminating season	Terminate season; may return to play next season if asymptomatic
Grade 3	Terminate season; may return to play next season if asymptomatic	

*A patient is considered asymptomatic if there are no physical symptoms at rest and exertion.

TABLE 16

COLORADO MEDICAL SOCIETY[5,13] GUIDELINES FOR RETURN TO PLAY AFTER A SECOND OR THIRD CONCUSSION

First Concussion Grade	Second Concussion	Third Concussion
Grade 1	Terminate contest or practice; may return to play if without symptoms for at least 1week	Terminate season; may return to play in 3 months if without symptoms
Grade 2	Consider terminating season; may return to play in 1month if without symptoms	Terminate season; may return to play next season if without symptoms
Grade 3	Terminate season; may return to play next season if without symptoms	Terminate season; strongly discourage return to contact or collision sports

35 probable cases among American football players alone. Necropsy or surgery and MRI findings confirmed 17 of these cases. An additional 10 cases, although not conclusively documented with necropsy findings, most probably are cases of second-impact syndrome. Careful scrutiny excluded this diagnosis in 22 of 57 cases originally suspected.[3]

Second-impact syndrome is not confined to American football players. Head injury reports of athletes in other sports almost certainly represent the syndrome but do not label it as such. Fekete,[7] for example, described a 16-year-old high school hockey player who fell during a game, striking the back of his head on the ice. The boy lost consciousness and afterward complained of unsteadiness and headaches. While playing in the next game 4 days later, he was checked forcibly and again fell, striking his left temple on the ice. His pupils rapidly became fixed and dilated, and he died within 2 hours while in transit to a neurosurgical facility. Necropsy revealed contusions of several days' duration, an edematous brain with a thin layer of subdural and subarachnoid hemorrhage, and bilateral herniation of the cerebellar tonsils into the foramen magnum. Although Fekete did not use the label "second-impact syndrome," the clinical course and necropsy findings in this case are consistent with the syndrome.

Other examples include an 18-year-old male downhill skier described by McQuillen et al,[19] who remains in a persistent vegetative state, and a 17-year-old football player described by Kelly et al,[13] who died. Such cases indicate that the brain is vulnerable to accelerative forces in a variety of contact and collision sports. Therefore, physicians who cover athletic events, especially those in which head trauma is likely, must understand the second-impact syndrome and be prepared to initiate emergency treatment.

Prevention is Primary

For a catastrophic condition that has a mortality rate approaching 50% and a morbidity rate nearing 100%, prevention takes on the utmost importance. An athlete who is symptomatic from a head injury must not participate in contact or collision sports until all cerebral symptoms have subsided and preferably not for at least 1 week after the injury. Whether it takes days, weeks, or months to reach the asymptomatic state, the athlete must never be allowed to practice or compete while still suffering postconcussion symptoms.

Players and parents as well as the physician and medical team must understand this. Files of the National Center for Catastrophic Sports Injury Research include cases of young athletes who did not report their cerebral symptoms. Fearing that they would not be allowed to compete and not knowing they were jeopardizing their lives, they played with postconcussion symptoms and tragically developed second-impact syndrome.

Postconcussion Symptoms

A second late effect of concussion is the postconcussion syndrome. This syndrome—consisting of headache (especially with exertion), dizziness, fatigue, irritability, and especially impaired memory and concentration—has been reported in football players, but its true incidence is not known. In the author's experience, it is uncommon. The persistence of these symptoms reflects altered neurotransmitter function and usually correlates with the duration of posttraumatic amnesia.[9]

When these symptoms persist, the athlete should be evaluated with a CT scan and neuropsychiatric testing. Return to competition should be deferred until all symptoms have abated and the diagnostic studies are normal.

A Final Comment on Concussion

Following a concussion, a thorough review of the circumstances resulting in the concussion should occur. In the author's long experience as a team physician, athletes subjected to repeated concussions were often using their head unwisely, illegally, or both. If available, videotapes of the incident should be reviewed by the team physician, trainer, coach, and player to see if this was a factor. Equipment should also be checked to be certain that it fits precisely, that the athlete is wearing it properly, and that it is being maintained, especially the air pressure in air helmets. Finally, neck strength and development should be assessed.

The author is very well aware that lawyers read medical publications and it should be bluntly clear that guidelines listed for return to competition in contact sports after a concussion are just that, guidelines. The final decision is a clinical judgment in every case, and deviations based on the clinical judgment of the treating physician may be entirely appropriate. However, there is agreement that it is not appropriate for an athlete still symptomatic from a previous concussion to be allowed to return while symptomatic, and any athlete still symptomatic will require further medical evaluation to determine that he/she has become asymptomatic before being allowed to return to practice or competition.

References

1. Cantu RC: Guidelines for return to contact sports after a cerebral concussion. **Phys Sportsmed** 14(10):76-79, 1986
2. Cantu RC: Minor head injuries in sports, in Dyment PG (ed): **Adolescent Medicine: State of the Art Reviews.** Philadelphia, Pa: Hanley and Belfus, 1991, Vol 2, pp 141-148
3. Cantu RC: Second impact syndrome: immediate management. **Phys Sportsmed** 20:55-66, 1992
4. Cantu RC, Voy R: Second impact syndrome: a risk in any contact sport. **Phys Sportsmed** 23:27-34, 1995
5. Colorado Medical Society: **Report of the Sports Medicine Committee. Guidelines for the Management of Concussion in Sports.** Denver, Co: Colorado Medical Society, 1990 (revised May 1991), Class III
6. Corsellis JAN, Bruton CJ, Freeman-Browne D: The aftermath of boxing. **Psychol Med** 3:270-303, 1973
7. Fekete JF: Severe brain injury and death following minor hockey accidents. The effectiveness of the "safety helmets" of amateur hockey players. **Can Med Assoc J** 99:1234-1239, 1968
8. Gronwell D, Wrightson P: Delayed recovery of intellectual function after minor head injury. **Lancet 2:** 605-609, 1974
9. Guthkelch AN: Posttraumatic amnesia, post-concussional symptoms and accident neurosis. **Eur Neurol** 19:91-102, 1980
10. Jenkins LW, Marmarou A, Lewelt W, et al: Increased vulnerability of the traumatized brain to early ischemia, in Baethmann A, Go GK, Unterberg A (eds): **Mechanisms of Secondary Brain Damage.** New York, NY: Plenum Press, 1986, pp 273-282
11. Jenkins LW, Moszynski K, Lyeth BG, et al: Increased vulnerability of the mildly traumatized rat brain to cerebral ischemia: the use of controlled secondary ischemia as a research tool to identify common or different mechanisms contributing to mechanical and ischemic brain injury. **Brain Res** 477:211-224, 1989
12. Jordan BJ, Tsairis PT, Warren RF (eds): **Sports Neurology.** Rockville, Md: Aspen Publications, 1989
13. Kelly JP, Nichols JS, Filley CM, et al: Concussion in sports. Guidelines for the prevention of catastrophic outcome. **JAMA** 266:2867-2869, 1991
14. Kelly JP, Rosenberg JH: Diagnosis and management of concussion in sports. **Neurology** 48:575-580, 1997
15. Lee SM, Lifshitz J, Hovda DA, et al: Focal cortical-impact injury produces immediate and persistent deficits in metabolic autoregulation. **J Cereb Blood Flow Metab (Suppl)** 15:S722, 1995 (Abstract)
16. Levin HS, Williams DH, Eisenberg HW, et al: Serial MRI and neurobehavioural findings after mild to moderate closed head injury. **J Neurol Neurosurg Psychiatry** 55:255-262, 1992
17. Lifshitz J, Pinanong P, Le HM, et al: Regional uncoupling of cerebral blood flow and metabolism in degenerating cortical areas following a lateral cortical contusion. **Neurotrauma** 12:129, 1995 (Abstract)
18. Martland HS: Punch drunk. **JAMA** 91:1103-1107, 1928
19. McQuillen JB, McQuillen EN, Morrow P: Trauma, sport, and malignant cerebral edema. **Am J Forensic Med Pathol** 9:12-15, 1988
20. McCrea M, Kelly JP, Kluge J, et al: Standardized assessment of concussion in football players. **Neurology** 48:586-588, 1997
21. Nelson WE, Jane JA, Gieck JH: Minor head injury in sports: a new system of classification and management. **Phys Sportsmed** 12:103-107, 1984
22. Ommaya AK: Biomechanics of head injury: experimental aspects, in Nahum AM, Melvin J (eds): The **Biomechanics of Trauma.** Norwalk, Conn: Appleton and Lange, 1985, pp 245-269
23. Roberts WO: Who plays? Who sits? Managing concussions on the sidelines. **Phys Sportsmed** 20:66-76, 1992
24. Saunders RL, Harbaugh RE: The second impact in catastrophic contact-sports head trauma. **JAMA** 252:538-539, 1984
25. Schneider RC: **Head and Neck Injuries in Football: Mechanisms, Treatment, and Prevention.** Baltimore, Md: Williams & Wilkins, 1973
26. Sutton RL, Hovda DA, Adelson PD, et al: Metabolic changes following cortical contusion: relationships to edema and morphological changes. **Acta Neurochir Suppl** 60:446-448, 1994
27. Symonds C: Concussion and its sequelae. **Lancet** 1:1-5, 1962
28. Torg JS (ed): **Athletic Injuries to the Head, Neck and Face.** St Louis, Mo: Mosby-Year Book, 1991

CHAPTER 3

Cervical Spine Injuries in Athletes

JULIAN E. BAILES, MD, and W. LEE WARREN, MD

Spinal injury is perhaps the most feared complication of athletic activities. Every participant in a sporting or recreational activity is at potential risk for sustaining an injury to the spine. The vertebral column may be solely involved, either with or without the spinal cord itself suffering neurological damage. Therefore, an entire spectrum of soft tissue, bony structural elements, or spinal cord injury (SCI) can be seen. There is no other sports-related injury that is potentially more catastrophic than a cervical spinal cord lesion. In contrast to other injuries encountered in sports medicine, spinal injuries often result in significant disability and time lost from competition, and can become the source of chronic pain with functional limitation. Unique and important facets of an optimal response to the athlete with suspected or proven neck injury are detailed in this chapter.

Incidence and Classification

Spinal injuries in athletes may be considered in two broad groups. The first includes those injuries occurring during participation in nonsupervised recreational sports such as diving, surfing, and skiing. In these sports, there are limited degrees of training, rules, participation, and supervision, which make it difficult to achieve improvement in injury patterns. There is also a limited ability to enforce safety guidelines and manufacturing standards in these recreational activities. The second group of injuries includes those occurring in supervised, organized sports with a higher level of bodily contact, velocity or torque forces, competition, and team participation. These injuries happen primarily in athletes participating in football, wrestling, ice hockey, gymnastics, and rugby.

Of the approximately 10,000 cases of SCI in the United States each year, it is estimated that 10% occur during athletic events. The majority of spinal trauma, which constitutes 2%-3% of all sports-related injuries, occurs during activities such as diving, surfing, skiing, and "sand lot" games.[7] Much more visible, however, are injuries that occur during football, wrestling, soccer, rugby, ice hockey, and gymnastics.[5-7] Spinal injuries among professional football players are the most highly profiled. For the thousands of physicians and athletic trainers who are responsible for the medical care of these athletes, no situation is fraught with more danger or elicits more anxiety than that of the injured player who manifests symptoms of a cervical fracture and/or spinal cord dysfunction.

Caretakers of patients with athletic injuries of the spine and spinal cord attempt to characterize the athlete's injury, render appropriate treatment, and make recommendations about future activity restrictions. Although the frequency of serious neck injuries among athletes is low, instances of relatively mild vertebral column injury or temporary neurological disability do arise and require difficult decisions to be made by the physician. The group of athletes most likely to sustain cervical trauma is football players. Data concerning the frequency and incidence of injury in this group are also the most reliable, yet statistical estimates of the incidence rate vary significantly, ranging from one quadriplegic injury per 7000 participants in organized football to one injury per 58,000 participants.[27] These data include football players from pre-high school to the professional level but do not include injuries with no quadriplegia or injuries sustained only transiently.

Cantu and Mueller[8] reported that since 1977, there has been an annual incidence of fewer than 10 cases of permanent injury to the cervical spinal cord among football players. The ongoing risk is emphasized, however, by four high school football players in Louisiana who sustained cervical SCIs during the 1989 football season alone.[9] These accidents occurred in a state where, based on the national average, only one such injury would be expected during a 14.5-year period.

At the high school, college, and professional levels over the last 20 years, there has been a decrease in the incidence of permanent catastrophic injuries to the cervical spine in terms of fracture, dislocations, and irreversible SCIs. Over this same time period, however, there has been an increased awareness of sports-related injuries with newly recognized syndromes associated with quadriplegia, quadriparesis, and central cord abnormalities that involve two or more extremities.[11]

Activities in Which Cervical Injuries are Commonly Seen

Athletic injuries to the cervical vertebral column and spinal cord have similar biomechanics but vary somewhat with the sport involved.[5] Diving and water sports such as surfing may result in cervical fractures and/or SCI if, for instance, the forehead of the participant strikes the bottom of the swimming pool, lake, or ocean. This usually results in a hyperflexion mechanism injury.[6] Skiers and surfers are also susceptible to a variety of impact positions because they are propelled by falls or tidal action, which initiates different mechanisms of injury to the vertebral column. Among football players, neck injuries occur most commonly by axial loading, frequently combined with hyperflexion forces. Hyperextension, lateral flexion, compressive, and rotational mechanisms, however, may all be involved.[7] Gymnasts sustain neck injuries as a result of missed maneuvers or landing askew during dismounts, which produces a mechanism of injury consistent with an uncontrolled fall. Wrestling participants sustain injuries that usually consist of hyperflexion but may simulate the biomechanics of a fall. They are also subjected to tremendous axial, rotational, and horizontal shearing forces that place great stress on the facet joints, intervertebral discs, and ligaments.

Cervical injury in football, gymnastics, ice hockey, martial arts, rugby, skiing, water sports, and wrestling are discussed below.

Football

Football players are the most likely athletes to sustain cervical trauma and are the group for whom the most reliable records of the frequency and incidence of injury are available, although reporting in the past has varied. There are approximately 1.4 million athletes participating annually in junior and senior high school football, 75,000 in college football, and 1000 in professional play. This contrasts to roughly 60,000 rugby players in the U.S. With the innumerable high-velocity collisions that occur every year during practice and games, football is the most dangerous sport for SCI in terms of exposure. Although more than 1 million preadolescents and early adolescents participate in organized football programs such as Pop Warner leagues, disabling spinal injuries are almost nonexistent among them. This is due to their small size and the relative lack of high-velocity collisions.

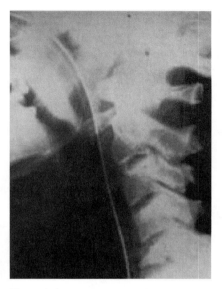

Figure 1: Lateral radiograph of a high school football player with a quadriplegia-producing C5 compression fracture.

The vast majority (83%) of cervical SCIs are sustained by high school players (Figure 1). This may be largely explained by discrepancies in player size, age, maturity, and speed among those on the high school field of competition. Most football players are injured during the course of tackling, and thus defensive players are usually involved. Defensive backs, members of the kickoff and receiving teams, and linebackers constitute the majority of those injured. The annual incidence of fewer than 10 cases reported by Cantu and Mueller[8] represents a 50% reduction from the rate reported by Torg and coworkers[52] in the early 1970s.

Apart from position, players with long, slender necks in high school appear to be most vulnerable. Almost all cervical spine injuries occur with high-velocity impact, usually with the player striking the opponent by using the vertex of the helmet or with the head down.[5,51] This results in an axial-loading mechanism, often with a minor or major component of flexion (Figure 2). In football, impacts with the head may involve a hyperflexion, hyperextension, lateral flexion, rotational, or an axial compression mechanism, or a combination of these. The cervical musculature responsible for maintaining such extension is much stronger than that used in maintaining flexion. When a player lowers his head in blocking or tackling, the cervical spine is placed in a position that is less able to absorb the opponent's energy, and the player is therefore vulnerable to cervical injury. Recent laboratory and clinical evidence has shown that in almost every sport where collisions occur, axial loading is the primary method of sustaining cervical fracture or fracture-dislocation.

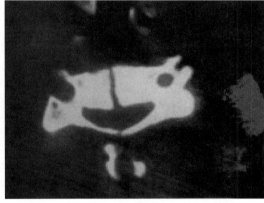

Figure 2: CT scan showing C6 vertebral body fracture in a high school football player that resulted in quadriplegia.

A group of athletes who are at high risk for the development of cervical quadriplegic injury are those subjected to "spear-tackler's spine." Torg et al[50] emphasized that when the spine is straightened and associated with a narrow canal, impact at the top or crown of the helmet causes buckling of the neck, as the head is momentarily stopped and the trunk continues to accelerate forward. These athletes are habitual users of spear-tackling techniques and had evidence of characteristic radiographic abnormalities (vide infra).

Gymnastics

The use of the trampoline, including the minitrampoline, has become controversial and the source of debate even within the medical profession. The trampoline is the leading cause of serious spinal injuries in gymnastics. Since the earliest report of trampoline cervical spine injuries approximately 40 years ago, there have been numerous instances of documented cervical spine fractures and fracture-dislocations, with and without SCI, both in the U.S. and abroad. Several reports implicated causative factors as being related to the athlete's inexperience, fatigue, loss of concentration, carelessness, poor technique, or improper assistance.

One of the most enlightening articles was reported from Denmark, in which Hammer and associates[15] described eight patients with severe SCI from trampoline mishaps. Seven of the accidents occurred on minitrampolines; in six of these, spotters were present and thick (30-cm) dismounting mats utilized. These authors noted that, although injuries can occur with any jump or dismount, they usually occurred in maneuvers with a rotation component. The neurological injuries associated with the trampoline were independent of the environment in which it was used and occurred despite the use of safety and preventive measures (including mats and spotters); also, they occurred independent of the jumper's experience. It was determined that transient periods of "blackout" may have preceded the accidents.[15] This may have contributed to the accidents and explains why, to a great extent, these injuries may not be preventable.

Torg and Das,[46] in their recent review of the world literature, identified 114 quadriplegic injuries resulting from the trampoline and minitrampoline. The vast majority of lesions occurred at the C4-5 and C5-6 levels. Because of the nature of the activity and the reporting of these injuries, it was not possible for them to calculate a rate-of-exposure likelihood of trampoline-related injury. Torg and Das commented on the observation that there appears to be a strong increase in trampoline-related sports mishaps. These injuries tended to occur while a highly skilled and experienced trampolinist attempted to perform a forward or backward somersault. The widespread notion that major cervical spine injuries can be prevented by better trampoline training, more experience, better equipment, and safety harnesses is seriously challenged by the evidence presented in the review of Torg and Das and both the U.S. and European experience.

The American Academy of Pediatrics (AAP) in 1977 issued a policy statement recommending that trampolines be "banned from use as part of the physical education programs in grammar schools, high schools and colleges, and also be abolished as a competitive sport."[2] However, presumably because of studies suggesting that each individual participant must rely on his/her abilities and those of a spotter, and purporting that there was a decline in recent years in this type of injury, the AAP revised its position 4 years later to support trampoline use under certain conditions.[3] This was termed a trial period, but no data were presented to explain this change of policy.

The authors concur with the belief expressed by Torg and Das[46] that the incidence of quadriplegic injury from trampolining is low; however, its very nature predisposes the user to injury that is catastrophic and associated with great human and economic loss. The unpredictability of such injury, and its association with experienced and highly trained performers, make trampolining a very risky athletic endeavor. As Torg[44] concludes, "the trampoline and minitrampoline are dangerous devices when used in the best of circumstances, and their use has no place in recreational, educational, or competitive gymnastics."

Ice Hockey

In recent years, ice hockey has been noted to be a significant cause of athletic spinal injury. Tator has discussed brain and spinal cord injuries in hockey in Chapter 15 of this book. Largely due to the research of Tator and coworkers[41,42] in Canada, the true incidence and causative factors of the injuries have been elucidated. Curiously, there were no reported cases of spinal injury from ice hockey prior to the 1970s. However, since the establishment of an organized reporting system, spinal injury has been documented to occur at a substantial rate in the sport. Tator[41] described the characteristics of spinal injury incurred during ice hockey participation, which were 85 in number by 1987. These injuries were seen almost exclusively in male players approximately 20 years of age. The majority of these happened during competitive, organized games and involved the C5 spinal level. The usual injury was a push, a check from being pushed, or falling onto the ice. This resulted with the player striking the head with a vertex axial-loading mechanism. The impact against the player's head usually occurred when striking the ice or the boards around the rink. As in other sports, such as football and rugby, the usual position of the head was one of flexion.[41]

Several factors have been elucidated as contributing to this apparent increase in serious spinal injuries in ice hockey players. Among these are the increasing size and speed of the players, the use of helmets, a more aggressive style of play, the lack in enforcement of rules, and poor shock absorption of the boards. Prevention programs and efforts at improving equipment and safety guidelines are in place; it is hoped that they have a positive effect on this sport.

Martial Arts

Different but mechanistically related to wrestling, judo players are at risk of sustaining spinal injuries. The vast majority are minor and nonosseous in nature. However, judo players may sometimes be subjected to tremendous forces and vertex impact associated primarily with takedowns. Koiwai[23] reported in an international survey that four of 10 judo-related deaths were consequent to cervical fracture-dislocation. These injuries occurred during "sweeping ankle," "drawing down turn," and "winding inner thigh" throws. It appears that the injured player most likely sustains impact with the head and/or neck, not dissipating the kinetic energy of the fall with a body roll or arm rollout. Regulations now require that any player with significant neck symptoms or any neurological symptoms be withheld from competition. In addition, the International Judo Federation Directing Committee enacted rule changes that severely penalize contestants who dive into the mat headfirst or throw a competitor headfirst during the execution of certain maneuvers. These rules also penalize the player for intentionally falling backward while the opponent is clinging to his/her back. Other martial arts such as hapkido, kenpo karate, and aikido at times place the player at risk because of frequent throws or violent takedowns.

Rugby

Although not as popular in the U.S. as in other countries, Rugby carries a certain risk of spinal injury. Of all organized sports in South Africa, Rugby has the greatest incidence of SCI. Scher[33,34] reported 50 cases of cervical injury that occurred during Rugby matches. He concluded that most of these injuries are sustained during certain phases of the game. While formed in the scrum, Rugby players are susceptible to hyperflexion injuries, at times with a rotational component, the latter accounting for instances of unilateral facet dislocation. The "collapsing scrum" and "crashing of the scrum" are particularly dangerous aspects of the game, again where a player's head may be pushed into the ground, often with the tremendous weight of many bodies driving the player. While in the scrum, the three front-row players join with interlocking arms and push against the front row as the ball is brought into them. Simultaneously, five additional members of each team also push from behind the front-row line. More than half of the 30 catastrophic cervical injuries in the U.S. in this sport since 1976 have occurred in this manner. Tackling is another common mechanism of producing cervical injuries, comprising 55% of Rugby injuries in one review. Three types of tackling have been cited as being particularly causative. A high tackle may occur whereby the tackler wraps his arms around the opponent's neck and drags the opponent to the ground, causing hyperextension, often with a rotational mechanism of injury. The double, or "sandwich," tackle is a rarer cause of cervical injury in which tacklers, usually high and low, down the ball carrier. The tacklers also collide with one another, a common mechanism that can be seen in U.S. football. As with football, Rugby players may be injured while tackling an opponent, especially with their heads down, producing a hyperflexion injury with or without an axial component.

Recommendations have been made to help reduce the incidence of catastrophic spinal injuries in Rugby. These involve the elimination of certain dangerous techniques such as the high or late tackle. As in every sport, proper coaching, education, player technique, and neck conditioning are paramount to success in injury prevention. Unfortunately, as in other contact sports such as football, there is an inherent risk of serious spinal injury because of the violent impacts and collisions that occur. However, in the 4-year period between 1984 and 1988, New Zealand reported no SCIs occurring in Rugby as a result of modifying the rules of the scrum.[12]

Skiing

Injuries occur more often during alpine snow skiing than water skiing. The latter sport has a slower speed, relatively friendly surface (water), and there are usually fewer objects with which to collide. Alpine snow skiers are probably at greater risk today than in the past because of improvements in ski equipment design, plastic materials, and manufacturing processes.[21] Although skiing is also dependent upon trail grooming and climatic conditions, these improvements have led to the attainment of greater skiing speeds. In a 14-year study from a major U.S. ski resort, Harris[16] found an average annual incidence of two SCIs. Overall, there were 13 instances of quadriplegia, 10 of diplegia, and three each of paraplegia and hemiplegia. These skiers were usually younger males of expert ability and were traveling at high rates of speed. Harris noted that as the skill of an alpine skier increases, the incidence may be reduced but the severity of neurological injury is increased. Except in competition, it is recommended that there be strong enforcement of safety guidelines for speed. Helmets provide some means of protection against head injuries but not SCIs. Safety programs should emphasize cognizance of the fact that collisions with trees or boulders and high speeds are responsible for most catastrophic injuries in snow skiing.[16]

Water Sports

Diving injuries tend to occur in teenage males who are involved in unsupervised recreational activities during the summer months.[32] Diving accidents have been reported to comprise between 2% and 22% of all spinal injuries, with the incidence increasing when the reporting center lies in close proximity to an area of high water-sport activity frequented by younger age groups or in times of seasonal droughts.[31] Up to 75% of recreation-related SCIs are due to diving mishaps.[13,14] Although diving injuries usually contribute to the majority of all sports-related spinal injuries, the true incidence is believed to be even higher, because injuries are likely to have occurred in drowning victims. In addition, alcohol consumption is often a contributing factor in diving injuries.

In reviewing the medical literature, it is seen that flexion, often with axial compression, is the usual mechanism of diving injuries; other mechanisms include lateral flexion or hyperextension. Divers may occasionally enter the water in an unconventional manner, producing a mechanism which is essentially that of a fall.[20] The most common method of injury in diving is when the diver strikes his/her head on the bottom of a pool, lake, or ocean after having miscalculated the depth of the water (Figure 3). Diving injuries have also been reported after one swimmer strikes another swimmer or a submerged object. For example, persons have sustained broken necks after diving into murky water, striking their heads on a submerged object such as a boulder or a nonvisible picnic table that had been thrown in during the winter months. Surfing-related cervical injuries are usually due to a variety of impact positions, as surfers are propelled by falls or tidal action, striking their heads and necks. This initiates different mechanisms of injury to the vertebral column.[40]

Diving injuries occur almost exclusively in the cervical spine and usually result in quadriplegic injury. The C5 level has the highest frequency of injury (70% in our recent series[6]); this is attributed to the range of motion that occurs in association with the relatively smaller size of the vertebral canal at the midcervical level. Most multilevel injuries also have involvement at the C5 level. In four patients, the C1 vertebra was also fractured due to an axial load, resulting in a Jefferson fracture in each case. In only two patients were odontoid fractures identified, emphasizing the relative rarity of diving injuries of the upper cervical spine.[6]

Diving injuries constitute a unique entity for several reasons. First, they are essentially completely isolated cervical spine injuries. They are ideal for preventive programs, and in fact, were the impetus for the "Think First" injury-prevention program sponsored by organized neurosurgery. Prevention can occur along several lines, including warnings about diving in shallow water and above-ground pools or in places where there may be submerged objects; the use of proper diving technique and not diving while under the influence of alcohol should also be stressed. It is calculated that when a person is diving from deck level or higher, it takes almost double the diver's height in water depth to cause complete deceleration.[1] It is believed that just as the public is cautioned against the dangers of drinking and driving, it should be warned against drinking and diving.[6]

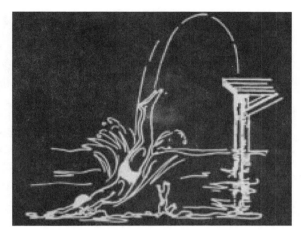

Figure 3: Diving accidents are the leading cause of recreational spinal injuries, occurring as the head strikes the bottom of a swimming pool or a natural body of water. In teenage males, many of these injuries have been caused by diving off a diving board far enough out so that the head strikes the upslope of the pool.

Wrestling

Neck injuries in wrestling are common, but few are catastrophic in nature. Although the participants are usually in superior physical condition and have strong cervical soft-tissue support, they are subjected to high degrees of cervical stress. Wrestling can place great pressure on the intervertebral discs, ligaments, joints, and vertebrae as a result of rotational and horizontal shearing vectors during certain maneuvers, holds, and positions. In addition, techniques that drive the opponent's head into the mat, "spearing," are particularly dangerous. Prevention of such injuries is facilitated by rules in amateur wrestling that make it illegal to throw a wrestler to the mat "out of control" or to spear the opponent with his head and shoulders striking the mat.[5,55]

The vast majority of spinal injuries in wrestling occur in the soft tissues of the neck. Acute cervical strains result in tearing of one of the musculotendinous segments of the paraspinal musculature. Most commonly involved are the rhomboids, trapezius, sternocleidomastoid, scalenes, and erector spinae. These injuries occur primarily with takedowns, as the extensor musculature is overloaded by stress forces with hyperflexion, hyperextension, rotational, and lateral flexion mechanisms. The acute sprain syndrome may be seen either with or without simultaneous muscle strain syndromes. In these injuries, the ligamentous and capsular structures of the spine are involved, with pain being confined to the neck and interscapular area. Brachial plexus involvement resulting in the so-called "stinger" or "burner" injury may occur in wrestling; the categorization and mechanisms of such injury are described below. Wrestlers may suffer from a traumatic herniated intervertebral disc syndrome, with a descending order of frequency being cervical, lumbar, and thoracic. In summary, although spinal injuries are common in wrestling and more common in the neck than the low back, catastrophic SCI is rare.

Injury Patterns

The musculotendinous structures of the cervical and lumbar spine are commonly injured in athletic activities. A strain is the result of mechanical overloading with forces that exceed the extensor musculature capacity. There is a characteristic response of the muscle to injury. Initially, there is localized pain, tenderness, and diminution or inhibition of voluntary muscle contraction. Weakness may be the only initial sign. Within several hours, there is usually swelling of musculature and limitation of motion. Stretching of the musculature by flexing the neck to the opposite side may cause pain.

Injury to the ligaments or capsular structures of the spine is termed a "sprain" and may occur without muscular strain. In cervical injuries, the pain is located in the neck, interscapular area, and occasionally the upper arm. A lumbar ligamentous sprain is usually located in the lumbar paraspinal and midline positions. In all true sprain syndromes, the pain is nonradicular and there is no sensory disturbance.

The ligamentous supporting structures of the spine may be damaged by repeated insult, leading to chronic tears, calcification, and the development of fibrous tissue. A cumulative effect of ligamentous hemorrhage causes fibrous tissue reaction that may lead to restricted motion and chronic pain. In both strain and sprain syndromes, vertebral column and neurological injury must be excluded. With sprain injuries, one must be certain to exclude ligamentous damage resulting in spinal instability.

The mechanism of spinal injuries in football was initially believed to be primarily hyperflexion. Research has shown that axial loading is a leading factor in placing the cervical spine at risk. Often, an athlete will improperly flex his/her neck, eliminating the cervical lordosis and making the spine a straight-segmented column. When a player strikes an opponent or some other rigid surface, energy is transmitted directly to the osseous spine. With improper neck positioning, this energy transfer cannot be absorbed by the cervical musculature and supporting structures, which are the ordinary buffers for such energy. Forces of sufficient magnitude may cause failure of the intervertebral discs, ligaments, and vertebrae, resulting in neurological injury in the majority (58% in the authors' series[5]) of athletes. The C5 level is the most common region involved in athletic vertebral and neurological injuries. Fracture-dislocation injury is seen in 33% and anterior compression fracture in 22%. As observed in football as well as wrestling, ice hockey, and diving, the C5 level is the most commonly involved because of the greater degree of motion there.

Syndromes of Spinal Cord Injury

Trauma to the spinal column may cause a variety of clinical syndromes depending on the type and severity of the impact and bony displacement as well as secondary insults such as hemorrhage, ischemia, and edema.

Complete Injury

Complete SCI results in a transverse myelopathy with total loss of spinal function below the level of the lesion. This is caused either by anatomic disruption of the spinal cord at the site of injury or by hemorrhagic or ischemic injury. Complete injury patterns are rarely reversible; however, with long-term follow-up, improvement of one spinal level may be seen as a result of resolution of initial segmental traumatic spinal cord swelling.

Incomplete Injury

There are several patterns of incomplete SCI, usually produced on a vascular basis.

Central Cord Syndrome

The central cord syndrome, originally described by Schneider et al,[37] results in an incomplete loss of motor function, with a disproportionate weakness of the upper extremities as compared with the lower extremities. This is believed to be the result of hemorrhagic and ischemic injury to the corticospinal tracts because of their somatotopic arrangement. Nerve fibers that participate in cervical nerves innervate the upper extremities and are arranged more medially than those subserving function to the lower extremities. The original central cord syndrome also includes a nonspecific sensory loss and bladder and sexual dysfunction. This injury pattern is often seen in older persons with spondylitic bony changes and in hyperextension injuries in which, in the absence of fracture, a hyperextension mechanism causes an infolding of the ligamentum flavum with transient compression of the spinal cord and its blood supply. However, recently, it has been stressed that the central cord syndrome probably best indicates only the site of SCI, for there is a wide range of clinical expression and overlap with other incomplete spinal injury syndromes, especially the Brown-Séquard syndrome. Merriam et al[28] found that, in contrast to the original description, the central cord syndrome occurring in a younger group of patients (mean age 34.6 years, with half of the patients being less than 30 years old) has fewer long-tract findings, motor deficits limited primarily to the upper limbs, and a good recovery. Therefore, the central cord syndrome is probably best thought of as an injury pattern based on an insult, either hemorrhagic or ischemic, to the central portion of the cord and associated with a variety of clinical manifestations.[35,38] The characteristic finding remains, however, selective weakness in the upper extremities. Overall, there is a good prognosis for some degree of recovery, if not for total recovery.

Anterior Spinal Cord Syndrome

The anterior spinal cord syndrome describes injury that occurs to the anterior two thirds of the spinal cord in the region supplied by the anterior spinal artery. The neurological deficit usually consists of a complete loss of all motor function below the level of injury in addition to loss of sensation conveyed by the spinothalamic tracts (i.e., pain and temperature). In contrast to the disproportionate motor deficit seen in the central cord syndrome, there is usually an equal amount of deficit in the upper and lower extremities. The anterior cord syndrome usually includes impairment of sphincteric and sexual function as well. Although the precise mechanism of the pathological process is not known, the final common insult is ischemia in the distribution of the anterior spinal artery, which is seen with a variety of spinal column injuries. Thus, there is not the strong association with hyperextension injury without fracture as in the central cord syndrome. Although there is relative preservation of the posterior funiculus of the spinal cord and dorsal column function, this sparing has little importance in determining functional outcome because there is usually permanent motor function loss.

Brown-Séquard Syndrome

The Brown-Séquard syndrome is classically described as a hemisection of the spinal cord with loss of ipsilateral motor function and contralateral spinothalamic (pain and temperature) modalities. This latter finding occurs because of the decussation of spinothalamic fibers one or two spinal levels above their entry site into the cord, whereas the corticospinal tracts have already crossed higher in the medullary pyramids and maintain their ipsilateral course to spinal levels for innervation of anterior horn cells.

Although theoretically sound on an anatomic basis and occasionally seen as a result of penetrating injuries, the Brown-Séquard syndrome usually occurs not in a pure form, but as a combination with other types of incomplete injury. Most commonly seen is a mixture of central cord and Brown-Séquard syndromes in which the patient has some degree of unilateral motor function loss and contralateral sensory deficit, but relatively greater weakness in the upper extremities. The posterior spinal cord syndrome is an often mentioned but seldom seen clinical entity in which there is loss of dorsal column function with preservation of the corticospinal and spinothalamic tracts; this is believed to be due to selective ischemia in the distribution of the posterior spinal artery.

Burning Hands Syndrome

In addition to these syndromes of SCI, some injuries are incomplete but not classifiable into any distinct pattern. Usually, these injuries consist of loss of all or nearly all useful motor function below the level of injury, with a sensory loss that does not fit any specific pattern. However, this sensory preservation does portend a better recovery than does complete functional loss.

The "burning hands" syndrome, characterized by burning dysesthesias and paresthesias in both hands, is commonly seen in athletes who participate in contact sports, especially football and wrestling, with repeated cervical trauma. It was proposed that the burning hands syndrome was a variant of the central cord syndrome in which there was selective injury to the central fibers of the spinothalamic tract that subserve pain and temperature sensation to the upper limbs.[26] Because this injury does not result in permanent loss of either function or in pain states, it probably occurs as a result of edema or vascular insufficiency. Credence to this theory has been given by the case reports of burning hands in which somatosensory evoked potentials and magnetic resonance imaging (MRI) following cervical injury demonstrated a reversible insult to sensory pathway conduction in the spinal cord, implicating a contusion as the pathogenetic mechanism.[54] The burning hands syndrome has been known to occur both with fractures and dislocations of the cervical spine and in patients without demonstrable radiographic abnormality.

Carotid Injury

In addition to persons with syndromes caused by blunt trauma directed to the spinal column and underlying neural structures, a small group of patients are at risk for neurological injury on the basis of vascular involvement. The carotid and vertebral arteries are at risk from direct compression or as a result of traumatic fracture-subluxation. However, a patient with a vascular injury may radiographically show only chronic degenerative changes or have a normal spine.[25] The carotid arteries are rarely injured in athletic competition, but it must be kept in mind whenever signs or symptoms suggest cerebral hemispheric dysfunction (hemiparesis, hemiplegia, hemianesthesia, dysphasia, or homonymous visual fields defects). A delay in the appearance of the neurological defect, even up to several days, is most characteristic. Transient ischemic attacks in the territories of the anterior or middle cerebral arteries may occur secondary to distal embolization of the thrombotic material, forming at a site of intimal tear in the vessel.[17]

Vertebral Injury

More likely than carotid injury is an injury to the vertebral artery, seen with a fracture or fracture-dislocation at or above the C6 vertebra. This may result from direct compression by bony elements, by stretching of the artery by vertical movements, or by an expanding traumatic hematoma within the foramen transversarium.[36] Any insult that compresses the structural component of the vessel wall, the tunica intima, or the bony foramen transversarium may lead to potentiation of thrombosis or vasospasm, with resultant ascending thrombotic occlusion and hindbrain ischemia. Such an injury to the vertebral artery could likely be symptomatic immediately after the traumatic insult, with the developing neurological deficit ranging from gradual and mild to sudden and severe.

The clinical manifestation may be any of a variety of cerebellar or brainstem syndromes. The signs of vertebrobasilar insufficiency or infarction include dysarthria, emesis, ataxia, vertigo, diplopia, and long-tract deficits. Although rare, complete brainstem infarction may occur. There is a lower incidence of altered level of consciousness and lateralizing signs as compared with ischemia in the anterior cerebral circulation. Computed tomography (CT) scanning is less likely to show an abnormality in hindbrain ischemic injury than in anterior circulation ischemia; however, in either case, if a vascular injury is suspected, emergent angiography must be performed to make the diagnosis.

Cervicomedullary Injury

Schneider et al[38] reported seven cases of cervicomedullary injury in football players and stressed the causative role of spearing techniques, where the head is used to make initial contact in tackling or blocking an oncoming opponent. Five of the seven had no evidence of spinal fracture or dislocation, whereas two had hyperextension injury with atlantoaxial dislocation. Of two possible mechanisms that are proposed, the first involves vertebrobasilar insufficiency from occlusion or hypoperfusion of either the major arteries (vertebral or basilar) or the smaller vessels and microcirculation, especially in zones of poor collateral flow. With vertebrobasilar insufficiency, temporary neurological deficits or complete lesions can be seen. The diminution or lack of circulation to the cervical and upper thoracic spinal cord can produce intramedullary cavitation and hemorrhage.

A second cause of these serious injuries is an impact to the cranial vertex, transmitting the forces in a caudal direction and producing several pathological features. As the freely movable brain travels first cephalad, then rebounds in a caudal direction, the cerebral hemispheres may be displaced so that there is uncal herniation through the tentorial notch. This may cause either acute arterial inflow or venous outflow obstruction leading to acute stroke, cerebral edema, and death. In addition, shift of the brainstem and cerebellum through the foramen magnum may cause direct compression of the medullary centers for respiration and cardiovascular control. Vascular insufficiency can also be generated by vertebral or basilar artery compression. Finally, with high-velocity vertex impact, the interaction of the freely movable brain with the upper cervical cord (which is tethered by the dentate ligaments) causes a pressure discrepancy that produces petechial hemorrhages of the upper cervical region. These examples emphasize that cervical injuries in contact sports do not require that a fracture or dislocation take place if the blood supply to the brain or cord is significantly compromised. It is important to remain cognizant of other causes in addition to intracranial mass lesions (e.g., vascular injury) if there is a deterioration in mental status following craniocervical injury.[38]

Classification for Management of Spinal Injuries

The author (J.E.B.) has designed and prospectively applied a classification system for the management of athletic spinal injuries.[5] This classification consists of three types of athletic cervical spine injuries. Each type is observed often by physicians and may cause difficulty in diagnosis and management (Figure 4).

Type I Injuries

Type I injuries are those that cause permanent spinal cord damage, varying from immediate and complete paralysis below the level of injury to various patterns of incomplete SCI syndromes. As discussed above, in patients who have anterior spinal cord syn-

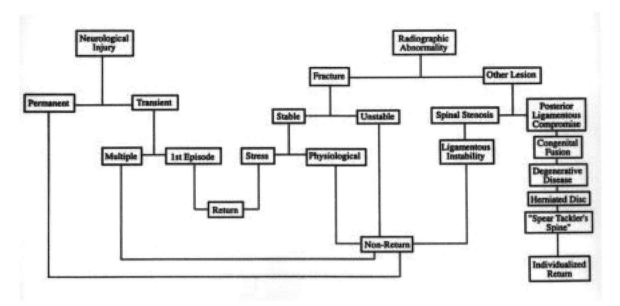

Figure 4: Classification system for the types of spinal athletic injuries.

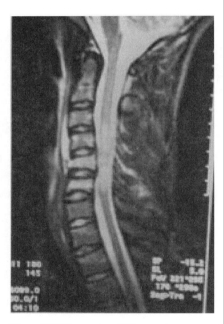

Figure 5: MRI showing C5-6 spinal cord contusion in a patient with a combination central cord/Brown-Séquard syndrome.

drome, there is preservation of only posterior column function. Patients with central cord injury syndrome experience selective weakness of the upper extremities with relative preservation of lower-extremity function. Often, there is an overlap of SCI syndromes, rather than the classic anatomical presentation. A central cord/Brown-Séquard combination, which consists of motor-sensory deficit on different sides of the body with a relatively greater weakness in the upper extremities, is frequently diagnosed on neurological examination.

At times, the symptoms may be minor but are associated with radiological evidence of SCI. Typically, the latter is documented by MRI or myelography suggestive of intrinsic spinal cord contusion, which is seen most clearly on intermediate MRI as a high-intensity lesion within the spinal cord (Figure 5). Usually, there is little argument that documentation of SCI, either clinically or radiologically, contraindicates the athlete's return to contact sports.[5,7]

Type II Injuries

Type II injuries exist transiently after athletic trauma and are related to the spinal cord, but occur in individuals in whom the neurological examination and radiological surveys, including MRI, yield normal results. Transient SCIs tend to occur in the cervical spine (90%), may have a pure motor, sensory, or combined sensorimotor deficit, and resolve within minutes to hours.[5,56] Because there is no evidence of vertebral fracture, spinal column instability, or intrinsic cord injury or contusion, it may be difficult for the physician to judge whether or not to recommend a return to sports activities.

Symptoms of spinal cord involvement in a patient must be actively sought by the physician.[48,50] A diagnostic problem often involves a distinction between the "burner," or "stinger," injury and SCI. The former is a common injury that, in some studies, is seen in as many as 50% of collegiate football players during the course of a season.[10] A burning, dysesthetic pain is usually present and begins in the region of the shoulder and radiates unilaterally into the arm and hand; at times, it is associated with numbness and/or weakness, usually in the C5 and C6 distribution (Figure 6). Several mechanisms for the burner or stinger injury have been proposed; the most common etiology is believed to be traction on the upper trunk of the brachial plexus occurring when a force is applied that depresses the ipsilateral shoulder when the neck is laterally flexed to the contralateral side.[10,30] These injuries usually resolve within several minutes, but may persist for days or weeks. Burner injuries usually leave no residual neurological damage unless they become a chronic injury. All radiological studies yield normal results, and there are no findings suggestive of spinal cord involvement, such as bilaterality, lower-extremity symptoms, long-tract findings, sphincter disturbance, or sexual dysfunction. Electromyography may be useful several weeks after the injury in confirming brachial plexus involvement by showing denervation potential.[10] It is also believed that some players with repetitive trauma to the nerve root within the neural foramen may develop a chronic burner syndrome.[24]

The burner or stinger injury is different from the burning hands syndrome, which is thought to be a mild variant of the central cord syndrome. The burning hands syndrome causes a burning dysesthesia and associated weakness in arms and hands. It is believed that the anteroposterior compressive forces result in injury to the corticospinal and spinothalamic tracts, both of which are somatotopically arranged; the latter accounts for the dysesthetic pain. Reversible abnormalities documented by MRI and electrophysiology have been described in conjunction with this syndrome.[54] In the authors' experience, most of these patients have a normal radiographic work-up and complete resolution of symptoms within 24 hours. Athletes who experience burning hands syndrome are allowed to return to competition once they are asymptomatic.[26,54]

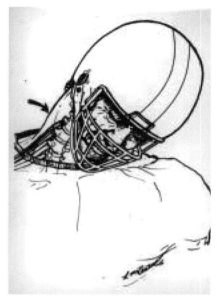

Figure 6: Diagram showing the usual mechanism of producing a "burner" or "stinger" injury by traction on the upper roots of the brachial plexus.

Temporary spinal cord dysfunction, including transient quadriplegia, is not completely understood on a pathophysiological basis.[45] It has been referred to as "neurapraxia," a term that ordinarily implies peripheral nerve dysfunction secondary to a physiological block in conduction, with no anatomical axonal interruption. Peripheral nerve neurapraxia is usually caused by mild degrees of compression or contusion (Figure 7). Gross inspection reveals a healthy peripheral nerve, whereas microscopically the nerve may have segmental demyelination and preservation of continuity of the axis cylinder.[22] The term "spinal cord concussion" was first used by Obersteiner in 1879 to describe SCIs that resulted in complete neurological recovery within 24-48 hours. Since then, few experimental models of reversible SCI have been developed. It has been postulated that spinal cord concussion could be secondary to a prolongation of the absolute refractory period of long-tract axons, which exaggerates the normal time during which axonal segments are unresponsive to any subsequent impulse.[56]

Available data indicate that athletes who experience spinal cord concussion usually have no significant spinal abnormalities that predispose the spinal cord to a direct compressive effect, nor does this transient dysfunction secondary to athletic injury necessarily predispose them to subsequent permanent SCI. The combined results of studies by Zwimpfer and Bernstein[56] and Torg et al[48] showed that 49 patients with transient spinal cord dysfunction experienced recurrent symptoms but did not have permanent neurological sequelae. Conversely, in interviews with 117 athletes who sustained permanent SCIs from football injuries, none recalled a prodromal experience of transient motor paresis.[48] Transiently injured athletes, therefore, have a good prognosis but must be carefully scrutinized before being allowed to resume competition. Often, they are allowed to return to full participation in contact sports if there is no neurological deficit or radiologically demonstrable injury or congenital cervical spine anomaly. If the athlete becomes a "repeat offender," however, with multiple episodes of spinal cord dysfunction, the risk for catastrophic injury is high, and thought should be given to curtailing future participation in contact sports.

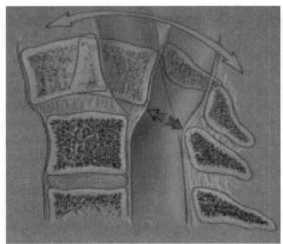

Figure 7: Artist's drawing showing the concept suggested by Penning, who theorized that transient SCI could result from high-velocity forces causing a "pincer" effect between adjacent vertebrae.

Type III Injuries

Injuries that are solely radiographic are termed Type III injuries. In athletes with an unstable fracture or fracture-dislocation, surgical stabilization or external orthosis is required. Further participation in contact sports by these patients ordinarily should not be allowed. A skeletal injury that appears to be stable on dynamic radiographs and during normal physiological ranges of motion may not be stable under stress. A more difficult management issue is posed by bony injuries involving other portions of the vertebrae that have healed and appear stable during physiological range of motion testing (flexion-extension radiographs), but exist in an area of the spine that normally contributes significantly to spinal column stability.[49]

The ability of the vertebral column and associated musculature to withstand and absorb the large amount of linear and angular forces involved in contact sports is not well quantitated. In addition, there are few experimental or clinical data that can be used to assess the degree of stability of a healed fracture or ligament injury of the cervical spine when it is placed under extreme degrees of stress. It is known that the cervical posterior ligamentous structures contribute more to stability in flexion, whereas the anterior ligaments are most important in extension.[53] It has been generally accepted that cervical instability exists when there is a more than 3.5-mm horizontal or 11° angular displacement between adjacent vertebrae.[29,53] There are no definitive data concerning the contribution of individual vertebral components to the stability of the cervical spine, especially when one includes such variables as the possibility of either partial or complete ligament injuries, the healing process, the insertion of a bone graft, and the exceptional stress forces to which the athlete may be subjected.[53]

Other spinal fractures, however, are considered inherently stable. Fractures that occur with no neurological injury need not necessarily prevent the athlete from further participation in contact sports. These fractures include isolated lamina or spinous process fractures. Depending on the given situation, a healed minor vertebral body fracture that is stable according to flexion-extension films also may be considered stable, and further participation by the patient in contact sports may be allowed.

Injuries showing radiological evidence of abnormality other than fracture are included among the Type III injuries. An example of a Type III injury is one that results in evidence of spinal motion on dynamic radiographs, which suggests a ligamentous injury requiring an orthosis or surgical stabilization. In that instance, the authors usually would not recommend further participation in contact sports because the likelihood of injury would be significantly higher than in a healthy patient.[29] Other Type III injuries include radiological abnormalities that ordinarily would not be considered unstable but that assume a greater importance in individuals who participate in contact sports. Compromise by the posterior ligaments, most commonly diagnosed with myelography or MRI, is considered to functionally narrow the size of the cervical canal, especially under high degrees of motion or stress forces. Combined with a congenitally narrow or relatively narrow cervical canal, this finding would place the athlete at a higher risk for further injury.

Historically, a diagnosis of congenital stenosis of the cervical spine has been made when the anteroposterior (AP) diameter of the spinal canal is less than 14 mm, a finding believed by some to predispose athletes to injury.[47,48] Torg,[43] however, related the ratio of the AP diameter of the spinal canal to the AP size of the vertebral body and concluded that a canal-to-body ratio of 0.80 or less, which indicates congenital cervical spine stenosis, is not a contraindication to participation in contact activities by otherwise asymptomatic athletes (Figure 8). Torg further concluded that football players with narrowed cervical canals are not necessarily predisposed to subsequent injury if they return to contact sports after an episode of transient sensory symptoms of cord origin.

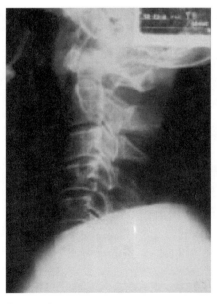

Figure 8: Lateral cervical radiograph in a patient with symptomatic cervical spinal stenosis.

The recent report by Torg et al[45] of 110 cases of athletic transient cervical cord injury associated with canal stenosis sites the latter as a causative factor. Permanent SCI was not seen with return to contact sports, although 56% of these players had recurrent episodes that were best predicted by sagittal canal diameter. However, there was no correlation with subsequent SCI, and Torg et al recommended that an athlete with an uncomplicated transient cord injury and canal stenosis ordinarily be allowed to return to contact sports. The canal:body ratio is sometimes still used as a sensitive screening device for stenosis; however, there are two major pitfalls in relying on such a ratio. First, athletes have been shown to have significantly larger vertebral bodies than those of control individuals, which gives an abnormal ratio in at least one cervical level.[18] Second, a bone measurement does not elucidate the relative size and accommodation of the cervical spinal cord. A "functional" MRI is relied on to clarify the spinal canal-to-cord relationship (Figure 9). In summary, the available medical literature indicates that the presence of cervical spinal canal stenosis, per se, does not indicate a high probability that catastrophic SCI will occur. On the contrary, it appears that there is no increased risk that the spinal cord is unusually susceptible, just as most athletes who have had a cord injury have not had prior warning episodes.[45] In the absence of complicating factors, instability, existing neurological deficit, and repetitive episodes, most athletes with canal stenosis who have had transient or "neurapraxic" spinal cord symptomatology may be individually considered for return-to-contact participation.

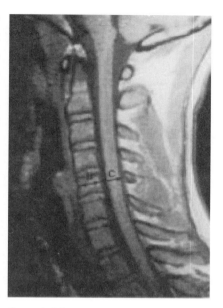

Figure 9: A "functional" sagittal MRI used to discern the relationship between the vertebral canal (C) and spinal cord (B).

Also common among Type III injuries are herniated intervertebral cervical discs, which are frequently difficult to manage (Figure 10). The symptoms of a herniated intervertebral cervical disc are usually radiculopathy, cervical pain, and occasional myelopathic signs, regardless of whether the injury occurs spontaneously or traumatically. There is little controversy about treatment because most symptomatic herniated cervical discs are surgically removed, via either an anterior approach if they are central or a posterior or anterior approach if they are lateral. There are no absolute guidelines that indicate whether a bony fusion should be performed. It has been suggested, however, that healed anterior interbody fusion results in preservation of strength in the cervical spine when tested in flexion and extension.[19] A posterior surgical approach maintains the integrity of the anterior and posterior longitudinal ligaments. In such a case, it may be possible for the patient to return to contact sports after 6-12 months of recuperation and demonstration of stability on flexion-extension radiographs. If the patient has congenital spinal fusion, some increase in movement at the motion segments above and below the fused level would be expected. Unless congenital spinal fusion is associated with more widespread abnormalities consistent with Klippel-Feil syndrome, a narrowed spinal canal, multilevel fusion, motion on flexion-extension radiographs, or recurrent neurological symptoms, this entity alone should not preclude engagement by the patient in contact sports.

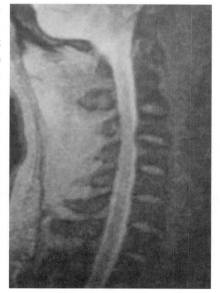

Figure 10: MRI demonstrating a bulging cervical disc in a National Football League defensive back player who had repetitive neck pain with contact activities. After several months rest, he became asymptomatic and was able to return to competition without recurrence.

Spear-tackler's Spine

Torg et al[50] described a group of athletes who are at high risk for cervical quadriplegic injury with the clinical term "spear-tackler's spine." Spear-tackler's spine is believed to be a contraindication for participation in contact sports activities. Torg et al found that football players with the following are predisposed to injury from cervical spine axial energy forces: 1) developmental cervical canal stenosis; 2) persistent straightening or reversal of the normal cervical spine lordotic curve; 3) evidence of pre-existing, post-traumatic radiographic abnormalities of the cervical spine; and 4) documentation of having previously used spear-tackling techniques. When a spine with a congenitally narrowed canal is straightened, impact at the top or crown of the helmet causes buckling of the neck because movement of the head is momentarily stopped while the trunk continues to accelerate forward.

Radiographic documentation of prior traumatic cervical spine injuries, such as healed cervical compression fractures, ligamentous instability, and intervertebral cervical disc bulge or herniation, indicates that athletes with these injuries are habitual users of spear-tackling techniques. In their study, Torg et al[50] reported a series of 15 athletes whose playing techniques were examined because the athletes had cervical spine or brachial plexus symptoms; four of these athletes sustained permanent neurological injuries. It was concluded that axial-loading impact to the persistently straightened cervical spine, which occurs when athletes deliberately engage in frequent head impact, resulted in permanent SCI in these athletes. Occasionally, if no significant bone or ligamentous instability is present, cervical lordosis is restored through physiotherapy. If the player can be coached against using head vertex impact, a return to competition may be allowed. Otherwise, the authors of this study concur with the recommendation that individuals with symptoms of spear-tackler's spine be withheld from participation in contact sports.

Onfield Evaluation and Management

Perhaps the most important fact in dealing with a potentially injured athlete is that an unstable spine injury can be easily converted into an injury with permanent neurological deficit if the athlete is mishandled. Since severe athletic-related injuries are relatively rare, the experience of the on-site medical staff is usually limited. Thus, everyone who shares responsibility for managing a spine-injured athlete should be adequately trained and frequently refreshed in the care of any situation that may arise. Prior preparation should ensure that all of the proper equipment, such as a spine board, cervical collars or immobilization devices, and stretcher, are available. There should be a clear hierarchy among the medical staff, indicating one member as the "captain" who directs the efforts of the team. In addition, arrangements should be made in advance to have ambulance services on site or close at hand. Preparation allays discomfort among providers and fosters efficiency and good decision-making on behalf of the injured participant.[22]

It should also be mentioned that those who manage injured athletes place themselves in legal responsibility for their actions, and precedent exists for legal action against team physicians and trainers who fail to properly handle players.[39]

Primary neurological injury is that sustained at the time of impact. The primary injury is treated once the player reaches a medical facility. Secondary neurological injury is sustained after the occurrence of the primary injury and results from a biochemical cascade of events, such as hemorrhage, release of vasoactive amines, and edema formation. As previously discussed, the prevailing goal among the medical team members should be the prevention of secondary neurological injury as a result of improper handling of the fallen athlete. Cervical spine injury should be suspected and the athlete managed as if a neurological injury were present whenever the mechanism of injury involves forced movement of the head and neck, even in the absence of a neurological deficit. The head and neck of the player should be immediately immobilized in a neutral position. As in any resuscitation, assessment of airway, breathing, and circulation should proceed, as well as evaluation of the athlete's level of consciousness. Unless unconscious or airway or breathing considerations exist, the player should be left in the position in which he/she is laying until there is safe transferring onto a spine board. If the player is wearing a helmet, it should be left in place until adequate immobilization of the head and neck can be instituted. The helmet can then be gently removed in line with the neck without flexion or extension, but only in conjunction with simultaneous shoulder pad removal. The occiput should be firmly supported during and after helmet removal.[56] It is ordinarily not necessary to remove the helmet for airway access.

If unconscious, the athlete is usually best managed by log-rolling him/her into a supine position, removing the mouthpiece (if present), and evaluating the breathing pattern. If no breathing is present, any type of facemask worn by the player must be removed to facilitate rescue breathing. The techniques of rescue breathing follow general guidelines as taught in cardiopulmonary resuscitation courses. It should be noted, however, that significant structural or neurological injury can occur with an injured cervical spine as a result of improper rescue breathing and subsequent intubation. Thus, any unconscious athlete should be treated as though a significant cervical spine injury exists until proven otherwise.[56]

As soon as the adequate airway, breathing, and circulation of the player are ensured, a thorough neurological examination should be undertaken. The level of consciousness, pupillary response, response to pain, abnormal movements or posturing, and flaccidity or rigidity should be noted as obvious indicators of head or spinal injury. Often, however, the team physician or trainer must actively seek clues to the spine or spinal cord injury, as the findings may be much more subtle. Neck pain, numbness, dysesthetic pain, or weakness all imply cervical spine or spinal cord injury. Especially foreboding is involvement of both upper extremities or neurological deficits in both the arms and the legs.

The athlete with any signs or symptoms of bony or neural element cervical injury must be completely immobilized until radiographic studies and further assessment can be completed. A cervical collar should be placed to immobilize the cervical spine. Once the equipment and personnel are available to transport the player off the field, the log-roll technique may be used to safely place the athlete onto a spine board. This is ordinarily accomplished with four individuals working together. The leader of the medical team should apply gentle in-line immobilization of the cervical spine. This person counts and directs the movement of the athlete. A second person is responsible for the torso, pelvis, and hips, and a third is responsible for the pelvis and legs. A fourth individual moves the spine board into place. Teamwork, prior rehearsal, and coordination are essential. Circumstances surrounding the downed athlete with cervical injury are often fraught with fear, excitement, and confusion, making the medical teamwork's synergy of utmost importance.

The leader of the team maintains immobilization of the head and neck while the others grasp the opposite side of the injured player. On the count of the leader, the two assistants gently and slowly roll the patient toward themselves, maintaining the spine in a straight line. The degree of roll should be as minimal as possible to allow the fourth team member to slide the spine board under the player. Caution must be exercised at all times to avoid excessive movement and maintain the neutral position of the spine. Once the player is on the board, straps and pads are used to secure the position to avoid movement. It should be mentioned that the player should be removed from the board as soon as possible to avoid pressure-sore development (Figure 11).

After immobilization and placement on the spine board, the athlete is transported to a hospital where radiographic and clinical assessment can define the injury, and appropriate therapy instituted.

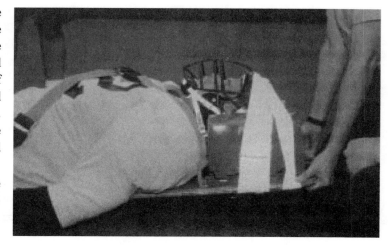

Figure 11: Proper positioning and immobilization is critical when transporting any downed athlete with suspected SCI. Helmet removal is not recommended on the field.

Treatment and Return to Competition

The treatment of the various forms of cervical spine injury has been previously summarized by Bailes and others[4] and follows established guidelines.[5,43] As mentioned, the emphasis must be on preventing secondary or further neurological injury through suboptimal management. Proper management begins with immobilization of the spine and withdrawal of the player from competition until the exact nature of the injury is delineated. When a vertebral column or a neurological injury is identified, the athlete must be transferred promptly to a facility for definitive management.[29]

The initial caregivers of the spine-injured athlete must be aware of the potential for respiratory failure and hemodynamic instability, as well as associated lesions, such as head injuries, which may affect the timing and order of needed treatments. Because of these concerns, patients with acute neurological deficit from SCIs usually are initially managed in an intensive care environment. The neurological deficits from SCI may be improved by methylprednisolone administration, which is believed to be beneficial if given in the first 8 hours from the time of injury.[18]

After initial resuscitation and radiographic evaluation of the player has been accomplished, informed decisions concerning management of the specific injuries can be made. Some bony injuries, such as spinous process fractures or unilateral laminar fractures, may require no treatment or only immobilization in a cervical collar. Others, such as the bilateral pars interarticularis fracture of C2 ("hangman's fracture"), are often treated with a cervical collar or, in some cases, halo vest immobilization. Unstable injuries should initially be reduced and temporarily stabilized with cervical traction using Gardner-Wells tongs or a halo ring device. Contrast-enhanced CT or MRI of the cervical spine should often be obtained before fracture reduction to rule out the presence of retropulsed intervertebral disc material. Unrecognized retropulsed disc material has been implicated in the sudden neurological deterioration of patients undergoing reduction of a cervical fracture. Surgical treatment may subsequently be required for severe comminuted vertebral body fractures, unstable posterior element fractures, type 2 odontoid fractures, incomplete SCIs with canal or cord compromise, and in those patients with progression of their neurological deficit to higher levels of spinal cord function.

Any athlete with a permanent neurological injury should be prohibited from further competition. However, those without cord injury who have stable fractures as evidenced by flexion-extension radiographs should be allowed to return to their normal daily activities. Athletes with burning hands syndrome or brachial plexus injuries may be considered healed and safe for return to play when their neurological examination returns to normal and they are symptom free.[30] Those whose fractures require halo vest or surgical stabilization are usually considered to have insufficient spinal strength to safely return to contact sports, although there may be exceptions (Figure 12). Even after the fracture has healed, the altered biomechanics in surrounding spinal segments and loss of normal motion produce a high risk of future sports-related injury.

Managing athletes with traumatic spine or spinal cord injury presents unique challenges for the spinal surgeon. The classification scheme previously described is useful in decision-making regarding optimal treatment and ultimate playing status of these athletes. Type I athletic injuries are those with permanent neurological injury; the player is precluded from further participation in contact sports. Type II injuries consist of transient neurological disturbances with normal radiographic studies. If the complete workup reveals no injury, the player may return to competition once he/she is symptom-free. Type III injuries include all players with radiographic abnormalities. Those athletes with bony or ligamentous spinal instability or spinal cord contusion are advised not to return to contact sports. Athletes with other radiographic abnormalities, such as spear-tackler's

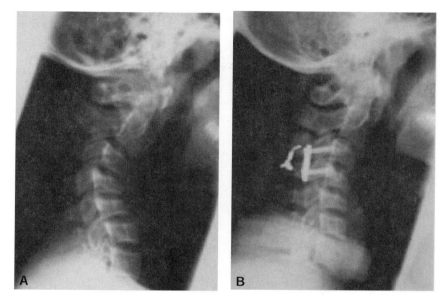

Figure 12: Ligamentous injury at C3-4 **(A)** in a hockey goalie who was allowed to return to competition following posterior cervical fusion **(B)**. (Photographs courtesy of Dr. Craig Coccia)

spine, posterior ligamentous injury, congenital fusion or stenosis, herniated discs, or degenerative spondylitic disease, require consideration on an individual basis.

Conclusion

SCI is devastating for the victim and the victim's family. The nature of contact sports ensures that there will be the occasional spine or spinal cord injury. When this occurs, it is the role of the team physician and athletic trainers to rapidly assess the situation, immobilize the spine, and prepare the athlete for transport to a facility where a definitive diagnosis can be made and treatment begun. Most importantly, the medical staff must do nothing that places the athlete in danger of further injury. Nowhere is the adage *primum non nocere* more applicable than in dealing with neurological injury, and athletic endeavors are no exception.

Prevention of sports-related spinal injuries is far more satisfying than any management scheme. Much has been accomplished in recent years to improve equipment, coaching, education of players, and rule changes. However, for those athletes who still suffer from spinal column or spinal cord injury, the team medical staff must be prepared for immediate and proper response.

References

1. Albrand OW, Watter J: Underwater deceleration curves in relation to injuries from diving. **Surg Neurol 4**:461-464, 1975
2. American Academy of Pediatrics: **Committee on Accident and Poison Prevention: Policy Statement. Trampolines.** Evanston, Ill: American Academy of Pediatrics, Sept 1977
3. American Academy of Pediatrics: Trampolines II. **Pediatrics 67**:438, 1981
4. Bailes JE, Cerullo LJ, Engelhard HH: Injuries, in Meyer PR Jr (ed): **Surgery of Spine Trauma.** New York, NY: Churchill Livingstone, 1989, pp 137-156
5. Bailes JE, Hadley MN, Quigley MR, et al: Management of athletic injuries of the cervical spine and spinal cord. **Neurosurgery 29**:491-497, 1991
6. Bailes JE, Herman JM, Quigley MR, et al: Diving injuries of the cervical spine. **Surg Neurol 4**:155-158, 1990
7. Bailes JE, Maroon JC: Management of cervical spine injuries in athletes. **Sports Med Clin North Am 8**:43-58, 1989
8. Cantu RC, Mueller FO: Catastrophic spine injuries in football. **J Spinal Disord 3**:227-231, 1990
9. Centers for Disease Control Communication: Football-related spinal cord injuries among high school players—Louisiana, 1989. **MMWR 39**:586-587, 1990 (reprinted in **JAMA 264**:1520, 1990)
10. Clancy WG, Brand RL, Bergfield JA: Upper trunk brachial plexus injuries in contact sports. **Am J Sports Med 5**:209-216, 1977
11. Clarke KS: Epidemiology of athletic neck injury. **Clin Sports Med 17**:83-97, 1998
12. Duda M: Reducing catastrophic injuries in rugby. **Phys Sports Med 16**:29-35, 1988
13. Frankel HL, Montero FA, Penny PT: Spinal cord injuries due to diving. **Paraplegia 18**:118-122, 1980
14. Good RP, Nickel VL: Cervical spine injuries resulting from water sports. **Spine 5**:502-506, 1980
15. Hammer A, SchwartzBack DL, Darre E: Svaere neurologiske skader some folge af trampolinspring. **Ugeskr Laegr 143**:2970-2974, 1981
16. Harris JB: Neurological injuries in winter sports. **Phys Sports Med 11**:110-122, 1983
17. Hart GR, Easton JD: Dissection of cervical and cerebral arteries. **Neurol Clin North Am 1**:155, 1983
18. Herzog RJ, Wiens JJ, Dillingham MF, et al: Normal cervical spine morphometry and cervical spinal stenosis in asymptomatic professional football players. **Spine 16**:S178-S186, 1991
19. Johnson RM, Wolf JW Jr: Stability, in Bailey RW (ed): **The Cervical Spine.** Philadelphia, Pa: JB Lippincott, 1983, pp 35-53
20. Kewalramini LS, Kraus JF: Acute spinal cord lesions from diving: epidemiological and clinical features. **West J Med 126**:353-361, 1977
21. Kip P, Hunter RE: Review. Cervical spinal fractures in alpine skiers. **Orthopedics 18**:737-741, 1995
22. Kline DG, Hudson AR: Acute injuries of peripheral nerves, in Youmans JR (ed): **Neurological Surgery.** Philadelphia, Pa: WB Saunders, 1990, pp 2423-2510
23. Koiwai EK: Fatalities associated with judo. **Phys Sports Med 9**:61-66, 1981
24. Levitz CL, Reilly PJ, Torg JS: The pathomechanics of chronic, recurrent cervical nerve root neurapraxia. The chronic burner syndrome. **Am J Sports Med 25**:73-76, 1997
25. Lyness SS, Simcone FA: Vascular complications of upper cervical spine injuries. **Orthop Clin North Am 9**:1029, 1978
26. Maroon JC: "Burning hands" in football spinal cord injuries. **JAMA 238**:2049-2051, 1977
27. Maroon JC, Steele PB, Berlin R: Football head and neck injuries. An update. **Clin Neurosurg 27**:414-429, 1980
28. Merriam WF, Taylor TKF, Ruff SJ, et al: A reappraisal of acute traumatic central cord syndrome. **J Bone Joint Surg (Br) 68**:708-713, 1986
29. Meyer PR Jr, Heim S: Surgical stabilization of the cervical spine, in Meyer PR Jr (ed): **Surgery of Spine Trauma.** New York, NY: Churchill Livingstone, 1989, pp 397-523
30. Poindexter DP, Johnson EW: Football shoulder and neck injury: a study of the "stinger." **Arch Phys Med Rehabil 65**:601-602, 1984
31. Raymond CA: Summer's drought reinforces diving's dangers. **JAMA 260**:1199-1200, 1988
32. Scher AT: Diving injuries to the cervical spinal cord. **S Afr Med J 59**:603-605, 1981
33. Scher AT: Rugby injuries of the spine and spinal cord. **Clin Sports Med 6**:87-99, 1987
34. Scher AT: Spinal cord concussion in Rugby players. **Am J Sports Med 19**:485-488, 1991
35. Schneider RC, Cherry GR, Pantek H: Syndrome of acute central cervical SCI with special reference to mechanisms involved in hyperextension injuries of cervical spine. **J Neurosurg 11**:546, 1954
36. Schneider RC, Crosby EC: Vascular insufficiency of brain stem and spinal cord in spinal trauma. **Neurology 9**:643, 1969
37. Schneider RC, Crosby EC, Russo RH, et al: Traumatic spinal cord syndromes and their management. **Clin Neurosurg 20**:424-435, 1973
38. Schneider RG, Gosch HH, Norrell H, et al: Vascular insufficiency and differential distortion of brain and cord caused by cervicomedullary football injuries. **J Neurosurg 33**:363, 1970
39. Sonntag VKH, Hadley MN: Nonoperative management of cervical spine injuries. **Clin Neurosurg 34**:630-649, 1988
40. Steinbruck K, Paeslack V: Analysis of 139 spinal cord injuries due to accidents in water sports. **Paraplegia 18**:86-93, 1980
41. Tator CH: Neck injuries in ice hockey. **Clin Sports Med 6:1**, 101-114, 1987
42. Tator CH, Edmonds VE: National survey of spinal injuries in hockey players. **Can Med Assoc J 130**:875-880, 1984
43. Torg JS: **Athletic Injuries to the Head, Neck and Face.** St Louis, Mo: Mosby-Year Book, 1991
44. Torg JS: Trampoline-induced quadriplegia. **Clin Sports Med 6**:73-85, 1987
45. Torg JS, Corcoran TA, Thibault LE, et al: Cervical cord neurapraxia: classification, pathomechanics, morbidity, and management guidelines. **J Neurosurg 87**:843-850, 1997
46. Torg JS, Das M: Trampoline-related quadriplegia: review of the literature and reflections on the American Academy of Pediatrics' Position Statement. **Pediatrics 74**:804-812, 1984
47. Torg JS, Naragja RJ Jr, Pavlov H, et al: The relationship of developmental narrowing of the cervical spinal canal to reversible and irreversible injury of the cervical spinal cord in football players: an epidemiological study. **J Bone Joint Surg (Am) 78**:1308-1314, 1996
48. Torg JS, Pavlov H, Genuario SE, et al: Neurapraxia of the cervical spinal cord with transient quadriplegia. **J Bone Joint Surg (Am) 68**:1354-1370, 1986
49. Torg JS, Ramsey-Emrhein JA: Suggested management guidelines for participation in collision activities with congenital, developmental, or postinjury lesions involving the cervical spine. **Med Sci Sports Exerc 29 (Suppl)**:S256-S272, 1997
50. Torg JS, Sennett B, Pavlov H, et al: Spear tackler's spine. **Am J Sports Med 21**:640-649, 1993
51. Torg JS, Truex R Jr, Marshall J, et al: Spinal injury at the level of the third and fourth cervical vertebrae from football. **J Bone Joint Surg (Am) 59**:1015-1019, 1977
52. Torg JS, Truex R Jr, Quedenfeld TC, et al: The National Football Head and Neck Injury Registry. **JAMA 241**:1477-1479, 1979
53. White AA, Johnson RM, Panjabi MM, et al: Biomechanical analysis of chemical stability in the cervical spine. **Clin Orthop Relat Res 109**:85-96, 1975
54. Wilberger JE, Abla A, Maroon JC: Burning hands syndrome revisited. **Neurosurgery 19**:1038-1040, 1986
55. Wu WQ, Lewis RC: Injuries of the cervical spine in high school wrestling. **Surg Neurol 23**:143-147, 1985
56. Zwimpfer TJ, Bernstein M: Spinal cord concussion. **J Neurosurg 72**:894-900, 1990

CHAPTER 4

Lumbar Spine Injuries in Athletes

ARTHUR L. DAY, MD, and MARK A. GIOVANINI, MD

Approximately 15% of all sports-related injuries involve the spine, most of which affect the lumbar region. The majority of injuries are caused by bruising, overstretching, or tearing of paraspinal soft tissues (e.g., muscles or ligaments), and the avoidance of aggravating activities may allow continued athletic participation while the pain resolves. Other injuries, however, pose a major obstacle to continued competition and require specific intervention to expedite full recovery. This chapter examines the unique clinical features of athletics-related lumbar spine problems and presents the types of evaluation and treatment that separate athletes from the general population.

Common Lumbar Injuries

Lumbar spine injuries differ from those in the cervical or thoracic region in that the brainstem, spinal cord, and cerebral vasculature are not at risk. The risks and extent of neurological injury are substantially milder and, when present, are usually limited to a single nerve root. One or more elements of the spine may be affected, including soft tissues (e.g., muscles or ligaments), intervertebral discs, bones, and neural elements. Lumbar spine injuries are separated into four categories: soft-tissue injuries, fractures, disc injuries, and pars interarticularis defects. Each type of injury has unique mechanisms of development, signs and symptoms, radiographic features, treatment, and return-to-play decisions.

Soft-tissue Injuries

Most acute low back pain problems are caused by soft-tissue injuries that resolve with time and rest without subsequent restrictions.[16] Symptoms that persist beyond the acute stage may represent a more serious process, needing additional investigation. Soft-tissue injuries include contusions, strains, and sprains.

Incidence, Clinical Features, and Differential Diagnosis

Contusions (or bruises) are usually the result of direct trauma, such as a knee or helmet striking the lumbar area during football, during which blood extravasates into subcutaneous structures or muscles. Physical findings include focal low back pain and tenderness, sometimes confirmed by later discoloration over the painful area. Back spasm may be an early accompaniment and may last for several days. Extensive bruising may indicate deeper injuries to a transverse process, the kidneys, and/or ureter. No neurological abnormalities accompany this type of injury, as the nerve roots are well protected by the thick lumbar paraspinous musculature.

A "sprain" refers to a ligamentous injury, while a "strain" indicates damage to a muscle, tendon, or musculotendinous junction.[16] Differentiation between the two conditions may be quite difficult (and probably unnecessary), as the clinical findings for both are quite similar. Sprains and strains are often caused by improper body mechanics, conditioning, or stretching, and their onset is most commonly associated with weightlifting or improper warm-up or stretching. Symptoms typically develop suddenly following an overload of the musculotendinous units during sprints or heavy weightlifting exercises. A chronic form can also occur following repeated overload during endurance training or highly repetitive activities. Clinical findings include back and paraspinous pain without radiculopathy that is accentuated by bending, twisting, or weight bearing. The pain may be located on one or both sides of the midline and may extend into one or both hips secondary to spasm of the lumbodorsal fascia extending into the tensor fascia lata. Neurological findings are absent and, if present, should prompt a search for an intraspinal cause.

Evaluation

Radiographic studies are generally normal, other than straightening of the lumbar spine from spasm or the other chronic osseous abnormalities often seen following longstanding athletic endeavors (accelerated degenerative changes in the endplates, facet joints, pars interarticularis, or disc spaces).

Treatment and Return To Play

Contusions may initially be treated with ice and cold packs to reduce pain and swelling. Heat, massage, and restricted activity are advised later until the discomfort is largely resolved, usually within a few days, at which time the athlete may return to play without restrictions.[4,18] When there are sprains or strains, however, the healing phase may vary depending on the severity of the injury and can sometimes be prolonged for up to 6 to 8 weeks. The initial treatment includes relative immobilization and ice to the affected area, with avoidance of extreme ranges of motion. In severe cases, bracing may provide some comfort. After the initial discomfort has improved, a rehabilitation process consisting of stretching, flexibility, and strengthening of the lumbar axial and abdominal muscles is begun, with return to competition once the discomfort and restricted motion have resolved. The exercises should be maintained so as to reduce the chances of repetitive injury.

Fractures

Major fractures threatening the stability or neural elements of the lumbar spine are quite uncommon in athletics-related activity. With the exception of sports such as auto racing or skiing, most lumbar fractures in athletes are "minor," as the lumbar vertebrae are quite large and well supported by ligamentous and muscular structures. Several types of fractures can be identified, including those to the transverse or spinous processes, facets, vertebral bodies, and endplates.

Incidence, Clinical Features, and Differential Diagnosis

Transverse process fractures are usually the result of a direct blow to the back and are generally accompanied by a severe muscular contusion. Spinous process fractures are exceedingly rare in the lumbar spine, as the forces necessary to generate these types of injuries are not experienced in most types of athletic activity. Lumbar facet injuries primarily occur in athletes performing repeated forceful hyperextension motions, such as football linemen, gymnasts, wrestlers, and golfers.[16]

Mild compression fractures of the vertebral body are common, particularly in individuals who have been undergoing heavy weightlifting training for many years. The anterior portion of the vertebral body lacks horizontal trabeculations, and exercises such as squats or military presses can generate significant flexion-compression forces that lead to repetitive endplate fractures, collapse of the disc space, and ultimately to compression fractures of the vertebral bodies.[43] When the endplate fails, the nucleus pulposus may herniate into the fracture, producing a Schmorl's node.

Younger, skeletally immature athletes are quite susceptible to endplate fractures or transient syndromes where bony growth of the spine surpasses that of the adjacent ligaments and tendons (during the second or pubertal growth spurt). Such imbalances may cause excessive tightness, postural alterations, or even spinal deformity. Scheuermann's disease, an entity usually identified in the thoracic spine of adolescents, may represent a congenital disorder of endochondral ossification or may be due to repetitive axial flexion forces.[2,26,45,47] Typical Scheuermann's disease occurs most commonly from T7 to T10 and results in progressive thoracic kyphosis due to anterior wedging (>5°) of three or more consecutive vertebral bodies. Atypical Scheuermann's disease affects the thoracolumbar junction, most commonly L1, and is more strongly associated with athletes, implicating training and repetitive endplate trauma as potential causative factors. Clinically, the athlete presents with a kyphotic posture that may or may not be associated with back pain. If back pain is prominent, it usually begins during the growth spurt, becomes maximal at the end of bone maturity, and resolves when growth is completed. Neurological deficits are rare but may become manifest with severe degrees of kyphosis.

Most fractures produce acute back pain very similar to that associated with contusions or sprains. Paraspinous muscle spasm is common, usually bilateral, may extend into the buttocks, and may be re-stimulated by movement or palpation of the affected region. The clinical findings of facet fractures are more unilateral and include ipsilateral paralumbar tenderness and hip and buttock pain referred to the groin, hip, and posterior thigh, and the pain is exacerbated by hyperextension. The neurological examination is usually normal, although a transverse process or facet fracture may uncommonly contuse an adjacent exiting nerve root.

Evaluation

Diagnostic evaluation should include plain films and, possibly, computed tomography (CT) scanning, with the addition of a urinalysis and intravenous pyelography if a transverse process fracture is identified (Figure 1). Bone or SPECT (single photon emission CT) scanning may help delineate acute from chronic osseous injuries.[1,3] In Scheuermann's disease, radiographic findings include irregular upper and lower endplates, loss of disc space height, greater than 5° of wedging in one or more vertebrae, and kyphosis of greater than 40°.

Treatment and Return To Play

With conservative care, most patients with lumbar spine fractures have an excellent prognosis, with little or no residual discomfort.[4,18] Treatment is similar to that of severe sprains and strains. Movement and axial loading are restricted until the acute pain resolves, followed by progressively increasing activities and range of motion until the athlete can return to former levels of activity without significant pain. Radiographic follow-up is usually not necessary, as instability is

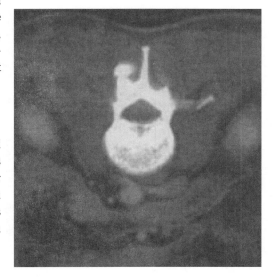

Figure 1: Upper lumbar CT demonstrating a transverse process fracture in a 19-year-old football player (wide receiver) struck by a defender's helmet in the flank while extended to catch a pass. After turning a somersault and landing hard on the ground, the athlete complained of upper lumbar pain and tenderness. Plain x-rays suggested fracture, confirmed by CT. Later urinalysis demonstrated microscopic hematuria. The athlete returned to play in 2 weeks without sequelae.

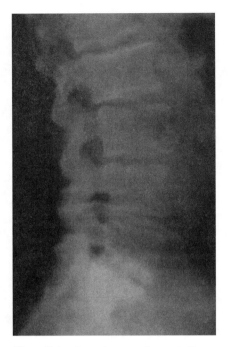

Figure 2: Lumbar spine x-ray demonstrating accelerated lumbar spondylosis in a 30-year-old former Olympic-caliber gymnast. The patient had a prior history of intermittent lower back pain that resolved with rest and a recent onset of increasingly frequent episodes, now associated with neurogenic claudication symptoms, in both lower extremities. Note multiple level disc collapse and compression of the vertebral bodies.

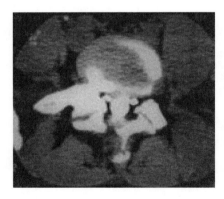

Figure 3: CT scan demonstrating degenerative facet changes in a 19-year-old collegiate sprinter with recurrent lower back and paraspinous pain, associated with vague numbness in both legs, precipitated by running. Marked degenerative changes in facets at L4-5 can be seen.

not likely to be progressive. A course of anti-inflammatory medications may reduce the general discomfort and inflammation during rehabilitation and promote an earlier return to play. Surgical intervention is not indicated unless other conditions accompany the fracture. For symptomatic Scheuermann's disease, treatment ranges from withdrawal from the activity to bracing. Surgical correction of the kyphosis is rarely required and is generally considered only in extreme cases for cosmetic reasons.

Disc/Endplate Injuries

Most younger athletes do not experience clinically significant disc degeneration during their competitive years. The adolescent disc is substantially more viscous, malleable, and forgiving than the mature (and aging) specimen. In sports that are particularly stressful on the spine, such as gymnastics, wrestling, weightlifting, and football, however, radiographic evidence of disc injury is far more common and appears earlier than expected in similar age-matched general populations.[3,17,27,45,46] Intensive weight training and repetitive axial loading appears to significantly accelerate the degenerative process and can lead to failure of even nondegenerated discs. Excluding the consequences of endplate fractures described in the previous section, lumbar disc disease in athletes clinically manifests in three forms, including disc rupture, spondylosis, and lumbar stenosis.

Incidence, Clinical Features, and Differential Diagnosis

Lumbar disc disease is very uncommon in young athletes and accounts for fewer than 10% of athletics-related chronic lumbar spine injuries that arise in persons younger than 18 years.[15,20,24,52] When athletics is begun at young ages, however, heavy stress is placed on the developing discs, which may accelerate the degenerative process and lead to premature lumbar disc desiccation and collapse, osteoarthritis, and lumbar stenosis at ages considerably earlier than that seen in the general population.[50]

By age 30, disc herniation and degeneration become more clinically relevant.[36,46,53] This age transition interval occurs in part because the disc becomes avascular by the mid-teens. Thereafter, the disc begins to lose its water content, and its viscoelastic and structural properties begin to degenerate, making it more susceptible to rupture.

Disc Herniation. The onset of symptoms often begins during weight training or some sudden pivot, turn, or strain. In other situations, there is no preceding event, indicating that the final disc rupture followed the accumulation of multiple smaller injuries over an extended interval of time.

Older athletes tend to present with the classical findings of disc herniation, including back and unilateral leg/hip pain with neurological radicular findings on examination depending on the level of disc disruption. Younger athletes usually present with subtle clinical findings and complain of back pain, mild stiffness or scoliosis, and unilateral hamstring tightness and spasm with little or no radicular components.[7,8,11,14,46,51] The straight-leg raising test is often not strikingly positive. Motor deficits are difficult to elicit, given the great strength of these well-conditioned athletes. The reasons for the indistinct clinical findings in younger athletes are unclear, but may reflect the younger age, increased flexibility, or increased pain threshold of the affected individuals. Pathologically, the younger athlete invariably has a protruded disc bulge contained within the annulus rather than a free-fragment herniation, which could lessen the amount of nerve root impingement.[7,36]

Spondylosis. Spondylosis occurs as an end result of multilevel or repetitive disc or endplate injuries. Usually, individuals who develop this problem have been chronic heavyweight lifters or involved in activities with repetitive hyperextension or axial loading. Spondylosis often mimics an arthritic process, with many episodes of back discomfort but none particularly dramatic. The individual often "plays through" the pain, as it is not severe or associated with neurological signs. Symptoms usually begin with an episode of lower back pain, associated with unilateral or midline paraspinous pain and spasm that refers to one or both hips or thighs.

Evaluation

Plain films of the lumbar spine should be done as part of the workup of any athlete with back and leg pain, and should include anteroposterior, lateral, and oblique views. The demonstration of one or more bony abnormalities is common, but their presence is no assurance that the offending lesion has been identified with certainty.[25] With spondylosis, plain x-rays demonstrate multiple asymmetrically collapsed discs, Schmorl's nodes, and osteophytes extending from the disc margins (Figure 2). Spondylolysis must be considered, especially in young athletes, and bone or SPECT scans may be required in complex cases. Plain CT is very helpful in further differentiating chronic bony conditions, and bone windows can distinguish facet fractures not apparent on plain films which could clinically mimic a ruptured disc (Figure 3).

Magnetic resonance imaging (MRI) and myelography and post-myelography CT are useful in defining disc herniation (Figure 4). Electromyography/nerve conduction velocity studies can occasionally be helpful in confirming a suspected radiculopathy, but are superfluous in most instances. In spondylosis, MRI often shows accelerated degenerative changes and loss of water content at multiple disc spaces (Figure 5). The discs appear to bulge, but do not compromise the spinal canal and neural foramen (lumbar stenosis) until the facets have substantially hypertrophied.

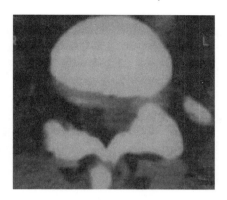

Figure 4: CT scan demonstrating a herniated lumbar disc in a 21-year-old collegiate football player (linebacker) with acute onset of unrelenting low back and radicular pain associated with weightlifting (squats). Examination revealed mildly positive straight-leg raising test and mild unilateral weakness and numbness in the L5 distribution. Large disc herniation at L4-5, with ipsilateral chronic facet degeneration and enlargement, can be seen. Microdiscectomy confirmed large disc herniation. The athlete was able to resume his collegiate career without restrictions.

Treatment and Return To Play

Since the risks of neurological sequelae following such injuries are low, continued athletic participation, with appropriate alterations in training, can often be allowed. The goal of therapy should be to return the athlete to competition as soon as possible, while maintaining the highest regard for the athlete's safety. Initially, the primary mode of therapy should be conservative, as the acute episode will often resolve and allow the athlete to gradually return to full activity and participation in the sport.[38,40,41]

Disc Herniation. Acute lumbar disc herniations presenting with severe back and radicular pain are initially best treated with bed rest, analgesics, muscle relaxants, and non-steroidal anti-inflammatory medications. Less dramatic presentations can be treated with restriction of heavy exertional activity in combination with mild analgesics and a period of time away from practice or competition. Once symptoms lessen, a program of lumbar and abdominal stretching and strengthening exercises can begin, followed by gradual increases in weight training and other routine practice activities that do not place the spine in extremes of axial loading, flexion, and rotation. Continued emphasis on back strengthening and flexibility should become a routine part of the athlete's training from that time forward to reduce the chance of recurrence.

Unlike the other conditions mentioned in this chapter, surgery is a strong consideration in the management of a ruptured lumbar disc. The decision to surgically treat, however, is a serious one, and the chances of impairing the athlete's ability to compete successfully should be weighed against the time lost pursuing a likely unsuccessful conservative treatment regimen. The amateur athlete is usually urged to discontinue that particular sport indefinitely and to find another type of competition that is less stressful physically. Surgery is generally reserved in this population for patients that remain symptomatic despite cessation of the offending activity.

In the "top-level" athlete, in whom years of training have been invested and in whom great financial or other rewards are active or anticipated, cessation of competition has

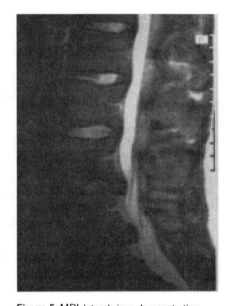

Figure 5: MRI, lateral view, demonstrating disc degeneration, desiccation, and bulging in a 19-year-old football player (offensive lineman) with acute low back pain and bilateral paraspinous spasm. Collapse and desiccation of L4-5 and L5-S1 disc spaces associated with apparent disc herniation can be seen. Symptoms resolved within several weeks after activity restriction and physical therapy. The athlete resumed a successful collegiate and professional career with intermittent tightness episodes; surgical intervention was never required.

much greater consequences and cannot be so easily accepted. Indications for operative intervention are: 1) significant neurological compromise (cauda equina syndrome, foot drop, or other major motor deficit); 2) severe, incapacitating back and radicular pain that does not respond to conservative therapy; and 3) chronically recurring symptoms that persist despite adequate conservative therapy.

Once a decision has been made to operate, the likelihood of the athlete returning to play may be enhanced by selecting a procedure that will relieve the patient's symptoms with minimal disruption of bony, muscular, and ligamentous structures.[7,28,49] In recent times, surgical advances have greatly changed attitudes about the effects of intervention on an athlete's career.[30] In the past, surgery would be considered only as a last alternative, after many weeks, months, or even years of conservative therapy. With minimally invasive techniques, however, most athletes can return to their sport, often during the same season, with no significant loss of flexibility or strength.

The standard intervention is a microdiscectomy, during which the offending fragment is directly extracted.[7,49] Using a small incision and a surgical microscope, the fragment can be removed rapidly and reliably, with minimal disruption of the lumbar paraspinous musculature. Variations of this technique holding future promise include a microendoscopic or percutaneous discectomy.[28,29] Complete bilateral laminectomy and discectomy should generally be discouraged except in patients with large central disc herniations with cauda equina syndrome or a disc rupture in combination with significant spinal canal stenosis. Bilateral laminectomy typically requires a longer incision and more extensive muscle dissection, and may put the athlete at greater risk of postoperative instability or pain syndromes. Accompanying degenerative changes such as spondylosis or spondylolysis, if asymptomatic, should not be disturbed, as a more involved and prophylactic procedure (e.g., lumbar fusion) stands a high likelihood of ending the career of most athletes.[7,49]

Postoperative hospitalization is often not required, and the athlete notes immediate improvement, with only some incisional soreness. After several weeks of rest and restricted activity, a program is begun to re-establish flexibility and strength, after which the athlete is allowed to return to play.[4,18] The exact timing of return should be based on a number of factors, but can be as early as 4 to 6 weeks after the initial surgical procedure. Future training would include the maintenance of strong paraspinous muscular support and flexibility, so as to minimize the chance of recurrence.

Spondylosis. During acute flare-ups of spondylosis, treatment should include rest, restricted activities, physical therapy, and the use of anti-inflammatory drugs. Spondylosis usually becomes a chronic disorder that is overcome by the determination of the athlete and a high endurance for discomfort. As there is no significant risk of neurological injury, the athlete may return to play when symptoms resolve enough to allow comfortable participation.

Advanced cases may ultimately lead to the classic degenerative changes of lumbar stenosis: disc desiccation and collapse, osteophyte formation along the disc spaces, multiple-level facet hypertrophy, and narrowing of the spinal canal. By that time, the athlete's career has invariably ended, so rehabilitation and return to play decisions are not problematic. Surgery should be considered if symptoms suggestive of instability or of typical lumbar stenosis are refractory to conservative measures. An extensive procedure, combined with long-term postoperative inactivity restrictions, make a return to the athletic field unlikely. Modern neurosurgery, however, now includes minimally invasive techniques that produce less disruption of the lumbar paraspinous musculature. Excellent results can be achieved with certain types of athletes, particularly golfers, in returning to play without major restrictions. Whether such procedures would stand up to the rigors of professional weightlifting or contact sports such as football is unclear.

Pars Interarticularis Defects

The pars interarticularis represents the bone isthmus that separates the two facet joints of an individual vertebra. Microtrauma and shear forces placed on the posterior elements during repetitive hyperextension maneuvers can produce a fatigue failure or stress fracture of this area.[5,6,31,33] Early in the clinical course, the region becomes stressed and may remodel, but the integrity of the pars is maintained. With time, however, the inflammatory condition converts to a frank dissolution of the pars (spondylolysis). Once the fracture is firmly established, slippage of the two adjacent vertebrae (spondylolisthesis) may occur.

Incidence, Clinical Features, and Differential Diagnosis

Pars interarticularis defects are believed to occur only in humans, as a consequence of bipedal locomotion in an upright posture. Most evidence indicates that these are acquired defects, in that they are not identified at birth; spondylolisthesis may develop and progress until skeletal maturity, at which point it usually ceases. The period of most rapid slippage occurs between the ages of 9 and 15 years and is rare after this time.[37]

The distribution of structural lesions of the spine in athletes less than 18 years old is divided between pars defects (40%), endplate or growth-plate fractures (40%), spondylolisthesis with instability (10%), and herniated disc (10%).[21] With age, the incidence of disc rupture is progressively higher, while the incidence of pars defects lessens. The incidence of spondylolysis is approximately 6% in the normal population, but in certain athletic populations, the incidence reaches as high as 25%-50% of participants.[20,44] Athletes involved in repetitive hyperextension, such as weightlifters, interior linemen, or gymnasts, are particularly prone to this disorder.

Symptomatic pars defects characteristically cause back pain that occurs during performance or training maneuvers, particularly those that require hyperextension. The onset of symptoms may be acute, subacute, or chronic and may be accompanied by progressive signs of decreased performance. Initially, the diagnosis is difficult to discern from a sprain, strain, or endplate fracture. Symptoms are usually unilateral, with pain in the paraspinous musculature near the midline that often extends into the ipsilateral hip or thigh. Symptoms can often be accentuated by the athlete standing on the affected leg and then leaning backward toward the same side. This test, known as the one-legged hyperextension test, places the spine in a position that stresses the ipsilateral posterior elements.

Once spondylolysis becomes established, spondylolisthesis may develop. The majority of adolescent athletes with grade I spondylolisthesis are relatively asymptomatic.[16,21,25] Those with symptoms often complain of bilateral radicular pain. Hamstring spasm may also be noted as a postural reflex aimed at stabilizing the painfully displaced segment.

Evaluation

Early in the course, plain x-rays may be normal, but bone or SPECT scanning will show increased metabolic activity in the posterior elements in the region of the pars (Figure 6).[1] At this stage, the defect is a stress fracture and may heal with immobilization and rest. With time, the stress fracture frequently progresses to frank dissolution of the pars, at which point it will become evident on an oblique lumbar plain film or CT. When chronic, bone or SPECT scanning may no longer "light up" in the area of the fracture. A lateral plain film will then delineate the degree and progression of any subluxation related to the spondylolysis (Figure 7).

Treatment and Return To Play

For patients with spondylolysis without spondylolisthesis, treatment is conserva-

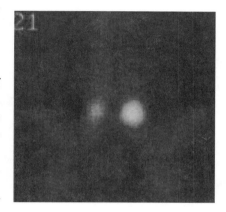

Figure 6: SPECT scan demonstrating a stress fracture of the pars interarticularis (spondylolysis) in a 19-year-old collegiate sprinter who had had recent onset of lower back pain and paraspinous discomfort and tightness. Symptoms were reproduced by hyperextension and rotation of the lumbar spine. Note bilateral "hot spots" at L5 vertebra in the region of the pars interarticularis.

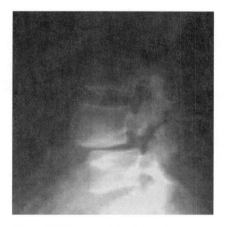

Figure 7: Plain x-rays, lateral view, demonstrating spondylolysis with spondylolisthesis in a 24-year-old former collegiate football player whose career was ended prematurely because of recurrent episodes of lower back pain and spasms. Clear pars interarticularis defects and subluxation of L4 on L5 (grade 1-2 spondylolisthesis) can be seen. The athlete was asymptomatic when not playing or training for football and, therefore, never underwent operative treatment.

tive.[4,18,34,35] Initial treatment regimens should include rest and restricted activities, combined with anti-inflammatory drugs. If pain worsens or continues despite activity restriction, bracing should be considered, particularly in young individuals with stress fractures only. Treatment should continue until symptoms resolve, ideally until SPECT scanning has demonstrated a return to normal.

Treatment for spondylolisthesis is based upon the degree of slippage and the clinical symptoms. In an asymptomatic patient with low-grade subluxation (<25%), the risk of increased displacement from intensive training is minimal and continued activity is not contraindicated.[35] If symptoms develop, conservative measures are instituted and may include withdrawal from competition, restricted activities, and bracing. Athletes with subluxation of greater than 50% are generally advised not to compete in sports that have a high potential for back injury. Surgery is rarely required, and then only when signs of progressive instability are obvious and when conservative measures fail.

Differences in Athletes

The top-level athlete with a lumbar spine problem often has specific physical, motivational, and goals of therapy differences from the general population.[34] Despite the complex movements necessitated by many sports, during which the lumbar spine is subjected to a combination of extreme forces simultaneously, athletes appear to have fewer incidences of serious lower back injuries than expected and a reduced severity of clinical complaints once the injury occurs.[16] These differences may be explained by several factors, including age, natural selection, and training routines.

The age of participation is a substantial factor in both the type and frequency of lumbar region injuries.[21,45] Injuries to the posterior elements comprise most injuries in adolescents, whereas discogenic causes are prominent in adults. The physical demands placed on the young, skeletally immature spine and the growth spurt that produces asynchronous development between bony and musculoligamentous elements make the young athlete vulnerable to specific types of injuries, including spondylolysis, Scheuermann's disease, and hyperlordotic mechanical low back pain.[24,26,32,45] Other contributive age-related factors such as leg length inequality, hypermobile intervertebral joints, and vascular supply to the endplates also contribute to an increased incidence of spinal complaints in the young athlete.

To a large degree, most top-level athletes are pre-selected at an early age according to natural talents, such as flexibility, strength, and coordination, that allow them to excel and advance to higher levels. This enhanced "athleticism" may provide protection to that individual from a variety of injuries, as he/she has more body control and skill to avoid dangerous activities or positions. Strong abdominal and paraspinous musculature, proper warm-up and stretching, and attention-to-precision techniques are qualities particularly well developed and emphasized by the top-level athlete, and may serve as protection from lumbar region injury. Weakness or imbalance in these muscle groups puts abnormal constraints on tendons, ligaments, and bony elements, thus subjecting them to injury.[13] Inflexibility of the hamstring muscles places the axial spine in a hyperlordotic posture, a position that may make the spine less resilient to axial loading and predispose the spine to injuries such as spondylolysis.[5,6,39,44]

It is unclear whether such training can actually strengthen or thicken adjacent ligaments to decrease the propensity to disc rupture. The incidence of free-fragment disc rupture through the posterior longitudinal ligament is significantly less in an "athletic" population than in the general population, a characteristic that could easily be attributable to the differences in disc and ligamentous character associated with age rather than those induced by training.[7]

TABLE 1
LUMBAR REGION ATHLETIC INJURIES: PREDISPOSING ACTIVITIES

Athlete at Risk	Predisposing Activity	Type of Spinal Lesion
Contact sports	field trauma	facet, transverse process fracture, vertebral compression fracture
Weightlifter	squats	vertebral compression fracture
	poor technique	disc degeneration, herniation, endplate fracture, spondylosis, spondylolysis, spondylolisthesis
Gymnast, diver, football lineman	repetitive axial loading in hyperextension	disc degeneration, intraosseous disc herniation, spondylolysis, spondylolisthesis
Golfer	repetitive axial loading	disc degeneration, herniation, spondylosis

Type of Sport and Level of Competition

The type of spinal lesion found and the predisposing activities in certain athletes are described in Table 1. Acute injuries arising as a result of blunt trauma are particularly common in contact sports such as football and rugby, and include soft-tissue contusions, sprains, strains, and fractures. Up to 30% of football players lose playing time from low back pain.[40] In a review of 506 collegiate-level football players, 27% had complaints of low back pain, most commonly a soft-tissue injury from a blow to the low back resulting in some form of a musculoligamentous injury.[42] Spondylolysis defects have been noted in up to one third of all linemen.[12] Weightlifters show a high premature incidence of degenerative disc disease.[36,48] By age 40, 80% of male lifters demonstrate evidence of compression fractures, spondylolysis, and/or disc injuries, presumably from poor lifting techniques and excessive axial loading. Physical size differences and the duration of exposure to high-level training also contribute, with increasing frequency and extent of injury noted in collegiate and professional football players compared to younger groups.

In noncontact sports, most low back injuries are the result of repetitive microtrauma to the lumbar spine and surrounding structures. The extreme and repetitive torsional and flexion-extension motions associated with sports such as gymnastics, running, golf, and diving place unusual demands on certain regions of the lumbar spine not necessarily designed to support such activities. Gymnasts have a particularly high rate of spine injury, with the rate of injury related to the level of competition and the type of event (i.e., floor exercises, balance beam, and parallel bar routines).[19-21] Gymnastics and diving have a very high incidence of spondylolysis compared to other sports and the general population.[5,9,10,16,32,35,39,44,48] Runners show a degree of premature disc degeneration and herniation from repetitive axial loading.

Return To Play

Successful athletes invariably have an intense competitive spirit and desire to win. They are generally not interested in disability, but only in ways to enhance their own physical performance. Dependent on the age of the athlete, other significant motivating factors may include the type of athletic activity, the capability level, and the potential for fame, education, or monetary gain (present or potential). Adolescents may derive substantial personal pleasure from their sport and may gain further support and motivation from their peers or parents. High-school age athletes may view athletics as a way to further their education via a college scholarship. Collegiate athletes may aspire for lucrative professional career opportunities. The financial rewards to some sports professionals are staggering and are obvious goals for many young athletes, worthy of great sacrifice and effort, potentially by both the individual athlete and the treating physicians.

The athlete with a lumbar region injury is anxious to return to competition, and the treating physician must recognize the special goals of therapy and not allow the athlete to return prematurely.[4,10,18,30,38,40,41] The desired end product is a "perfect" result that allows the athlete to have unrestricted flexibility, strength, and agility at former levels; a "good" outcome is not acceptable. The cause of the injury is often expected to continue, especially in traumatic sports such as football, running, and weightlifting, making the decision regarding treatment and return to activity a complicated one, especially in the top-level athlete. In the authors' opinion, a neurological specialist (ideally a neurosurgeon) should be consulted prior to the athlete's return to participation whenever there are neurological deficits or risks of new or further neurological deterioration.

Conclusions

Lumbar spinal injuries in athletes are common. Some are related to training errors, while others are caused by the demands of a specific type of athletic activity. The athlete will invariably be returning to the exact type of activity that precipitated the injury, sometimes making management more complex than for the amateur athlete. Protection and preservation of the nervous system for the remainder of the individual's life is the primary treatment objective. This goal can usually be accomplished even if surgery is required, allowing the athlete to continue his/her career under most circumstances.

References

1. Bellah RD, Summerville DA, Treves ST, et al: Low-back pain in adolescent athletes: detection of stress injury to the pars interarticularis with SPECT. **Radiology 180:**509-512, 1991
2. Blumenthal SL, Roach J, Herring JA: Lumbar Scheuermann's: a clinical series and classification. **Spine 12:**929-932, 1987
3. Cacayorin E, Hochhauser L, Petro GR: Lumbar and thoracic spine pain in the athlete: radiographic evaluation. **Clin Sports Med 6:**767-783, 1987
4. Chilton MD, Nisenfeld FG: Nonoperative treatment of low back injury in athletes. **Clin Sports Med 12:**547-555, 1993
5. Ciullo JV, Jackson DW: Pars interarticularis stress reaction, spondylolysis, and spondylolisthesis in gymnasts. **Clin Sports Med 4:**95-110, 1985
6. Commandre FA, Taillan B, Gagnerie F, et al: Spondylolysis and spondylolisthesis in young athletes: 28 cases. **J Sports Med Phys Fitness 28:**104-107, 1988
7. Day AL, Friedman WA, Indelicato PA: Observations on the treatment of lumbar disk disease in college football players. **Am J Sports Med 15:**72-75, 1987
8. DeOrio JK, Bianco AJ: Lumbar disc excision in children and adolescents. **J Bone Joint Surg (Am) 64:**991-996, 1982
9. Deusinger RH: Biomechanical considerations for clinical application in athletes with low back pain. **Clin Sports Med 8:**703-715, 1989
10. Dreisinger TE, Nelson B: Management of back pain in athletes. **Sports Med 21:**313-320, 1996
11. Epstein JA, Epstein NE, Marc J, et al: Lumbar intervertebral disc herniation in teenage children: recognition and management of associated anomalies. **Spine 9:**427-432, 1984
12. Ferguson RJ, McMaster JH, Stanitski CL: Low back pain in college football linemen. **Am J Sports Med 2:**63, 1974
13. Foster DN, Fulton MN: Back pain and the exercise prescription. **Clin Sports Med 10:**197-209, 1991
14. Ghabrial YAE, Tarrant MJ: Adolescent lumbar disc prolapse. **Acta Orthopaed Scand 60:**174-176, 1989
15. Goldstein JD, Berger PE, Windler GE, et al: Spine injuries in gymnasts and swimmers. An epidemiologic investigation. **Am J Sports Med 19:**463-468, 1991
16. Harvey J, Tanner S: Low back pain in young athletes. A practical approach. **Sports Med 12:**394-406, 1991
17. Hellström M, Jacobsson B, Swärd L, et al: Radiologic abnormalities of the thoraco-lumbar spine in athletes. **Acta Radiol 31:**127-132, 1990
18. Hopkins TJ, White AA III: Rehabilitation of athletes following spine injury. **Clin Sports Med 12:**603-619, 1993
19. Jackson D: Low back pain in young athletes: evaluation of stress reaction and discogenic problems. **Am J Sports Med 7:**364-366, 1979
20. Jackson DS, Furman WK, Benson BL: Patterns of injuries in college athletes: a retrospective study of injuries sustained in intercollegiate athletics in two colleges over a two-year period. **Mt Sinai J Med 47:**423-426, 1980
21. Jackson DW, Wiltse LL, Cirincione RJ: Spondylolysis in the female gymnast. **Clin Orthop 117:**68-73, 1976
22. Keene JS: Low back pain in the athlete. From spondylogenic injury during recreation or competition. **Postgrad Med 74:**209-217, 1983
23. Keene JS, Albert MJ, Springer SL, et al: Back injuries in college athletes. **J Spinal Dis 2:**190-195, 1989
24. Klemp P, Learmonth ID: Hypermobility and injuries in a professional ballet company. **Br J Sports Med 18:**143-148, 1984
25. Kraus DR, Shapiro D: The symptomatic lumbar spine in the athlete. **Clin Sports Med 8:**59-69, 1989
26. Lowe TG: Scheuermann disease. **J Bone Joint Surg (Am) 72:**940-945, 1990
27. Maffulli N: Intensive training in young athletes. The orthopaedic surgeon's viewpoint. **Sports Med 9:**229-243, 1990
28. Maroon JC, Onik G, Day AL: Percutaneous automated discectomy in athletes. **Phys Sports Med 16:**61-73, 1988
29. Mayer HM, Brock M: Percutaneous endoscopic discectomy: surgical technique and preliminary results compared to microsurgical discectomy. **J Neurosurg 78:**216-225, 1993
30. Mazur LJ, Yetman RJ, Risser WL: Weight-training injuries. Common injuries and preventative methods. **Sports Med 16:**57-63, 1993
31. Meeusen R, Borms J: Gymnastic injuries. **Sports Med 13:**337-356, 1992
32. Micheli LJ: Back injuries in dancers. **Clin Sports Med 2:**473-484, 1983
33. Micheli LJ: Back injuries in gymnastics. **Clin Sports Med 4:**85-93, 1985
34. Micheli LJ: Sports following spinal surgery in the young athlete. **Clin Orthop 198:**152-157, 1985

35. Micheli LJ, Wood R: Back pain in young athletes. Significant differences from adults in causes and patterns. **Arch Pediatr Adolesc Med** **149**:15-18, 1995
36. Miller JAA, Schmatz C, Schultz AB: Lumbar disc degeneration: correlation with age, sex, and spine level in 600 autopsy specimens. **Spine** **13**:173-178, 1988
37. Muschik M, Hahnel H, Robinson PN, et al: Competitive sports and the progression of spondylolisthesis. **J Pediatr Orthop** **16**:364-369, 1996
38. Ohnmeiss DD: Non-surgical treatment of sports-related spine injuries, in Hochschuler SH (ed): **The Spine in Sports.** Philadelphia, Pa: Hanley and Belfus, 1990, pp 241-260
39. Rossi F, Dragoni S: Lumbar spondylolysis: occurrence in competitive athletes. Updated achievements in a series of 390 cases. **J Sports Med Phys Fitness** **30**:450-452, 1990
40. Saal JA: Rehabilitation of football players with lumbar spine injury. **Phys Sport Med** **16**:117-127, 1988
41. Saal JA, Saal JS: Nonoperative treatment of herniated lumbar intervertebral disc with radiculopathy. An outcome study. **Spine** **14**:431-437, 1989
42. Semon RL, Spengler D: Significance of lumbar spondylolysis in college football players. **Spine** **6**:172-174, 1981
43. Stinson JT: Spine problems in the athlete. **Md Med J** **45**:655-658, 1996
44. Stinson JT: Spondylolysis and spondylolisthesis in the athlete. **Clin** Sports Med 12:517-528, 1993
45. Swärd L: The thoracolumbar spine in young elite athletes. Current concepts on the effects of physical training. **Sports Med** **13**:357-364, 1992
46. Swärd L, Hellström M, Jacobsson B, et al: Disc degeneration and associated abnormalities of the spine in elite gymnasts. A magnetic resonance imaging study. **Spine** **16**:437-443, 1991
47. Swärd L, Hellström M, Jacobsson B, et al: Vertebral ring apophysis injury in athletes. Is the etiology different in the thoracic and lumbar spine? **Am J Sports Med** **21**:841-845, 1993
48. Tall RL, DeVault W: Spinal injury in sports: epidemiologic considerations. **Clin Sports Med** **12**:441-448, 1993
49. Wang JC, Shapiro MS, Hatch JD, et al: The outcome of lumbar discectomy in elite athletes. **Spine** **24**:570-573, 1999
50. Watkins RG, Campbell DR: The older athlete after lumbar spine surgery. **Clin Sports Med** **10**:391-399, 1991
51. Watkins RG, Dillin WH: Lumbar spine injury in the athlete. **Clin Sports Med** **9**:419-448, 1990
52. Wroble R, Albright JP: Neck and low back injuries in wrestling. **Clin Sports Med** **5**:295-326, 1986
53. Young JL, Press JM, Herring SA: The disc at risk in athletes: perspectives on operative and nonoperative care. **Med Sci Sports Exer** **29** **(Suppl 7)**:S222-S232, 1997

CHAPTER 5

Minimally Invasive Treatment Options for Athletes with Spine Injuries

CRAIG A. VAN DER VEER, MD

The surgical treatment of the athlete with a spine injury represents a unique set of circumstances: the patient is generally youthful and healthy, has a short window of opportunity for surgical intervention, and tends to stress the surgical repair to extremes not seen in the general population. Because of these stresses, the athlete's needs for early stability of the vertebral column predominates even the durability of the surgical repair.

High school and college athletes face challenging situations in terms of their short window of opportunity for eligibility, especially those gifted enough to consider a professional career in sports. A potential All-State or All-American athlete may lose his/her opportunity for a college scholarship or professional contract by the application of what may be the best surgical selection for the general population, requiring time-consuming rehabilitation poorly matched to the athlete's situation. When treating the athlete, special consideration must be given to the age of the athlete, the rigors of the sport involved, the athlete's chronology in the sport, and even the time of the year relative to the athlete's season of competition.

The application of microsurgical techniques to spinal surgery provides treatment options that are minimally invasive, respect the spine's natural stability, and produce less tissue trauma. This satisfies the athlete's need for a more rapid recovery and an earlier return to full activities and, therefore, less loss of conditioning. This also meets the need of the neurosurgeon's quest for elegant focal surgical solutions to what may seem to many to be common but thorny problems.

With increasing salary levels for athletes comes an increase in liability responsibility for the treating physician, the team physician, and those responsible for the financial success of a college or professional team. This places a high level of responsibility on the treating physician to offer the option of less-invasive procedures to effect the same cure as more invasive procedures and longer rehabilitation- and time-intensive solutions of just a year or two ago. The advent of fiberoptics and miniaturized high-resolution endoscopic cameras and monitors offers a new array of options, much less invasive than previously noted. Many are not new procedures, but rather, traditional procedures revisited and reformatted with modern techniques and equipment.

Microinvasive Surgical Principles

Microinvasive spine surgery, whether cervical, thoracic, or lumbar, involves the same principles: 1) less is more, or at least as much; 2) avoid fusion when possible, and 3) preserve the internal tendons of the paraspinous muscles, the long and short rotators. These principles are discussed below.

Less is More, or at Least as Much

A smaller incision does not mean less visualization. The microscopic and endoscopic products now available are designed to enhance the surgeon's field of view. Magnification, either by microscope or microendoscope, provides enhanced, balanced light to the surgical field and, therefore, less risk of injury to nerve and spinal cord distorted by a disc rupture, nerve root injury, or a retained fragment. The array of rigid endoscopes available can provide a range of direct or angled views from a unique vantage point, even actually looking around a nerve root. A smaller incision and less pain postoperatively are simple, welcome byproducts of a minimally invasive technique.

Avoid Fusion If Possible

A fusion is by nature a destructive procedure, altering the biomechanics of the finely balanced machine, the spine. It is to be avoided when another option is available unless there is evidence of spinal instability. Fusion places increased strain on the levels above and below the fusion mass and is believed to accelerate degenerative disease of the adjacent level. The loss of "sagittal balance" is another frequent side effect of fusion, with alteration of the anterior/posterior balance in the muscular and ligamentous support, leading to chronic discomfort.

Preservation of the Internal Tendons of the Paraspinous Muscles, the Long and Short Rotators

Microinvasive surgical techniques share the respect of the muscles that attach to the caudal surface of the lamina and spinous processes. Internal tendons are those shared by a motor unit and which coalesce with other internal tendons into a major tendon. The tendon is readily palpated during a "muscle splitting" approach for microscopic laminotomy. Their detachment from the spinous process and lamina is unnecessary and leads to increased muscle spasm as the detached but innervated muscle contracts and, following contraction, is not restretched to length. The muscle builds up metabolic byproducts and lactic acid, causing spasm and pain. The technique used for the lumbar spine is easily modified to the cervical and thoracic approaches as well.

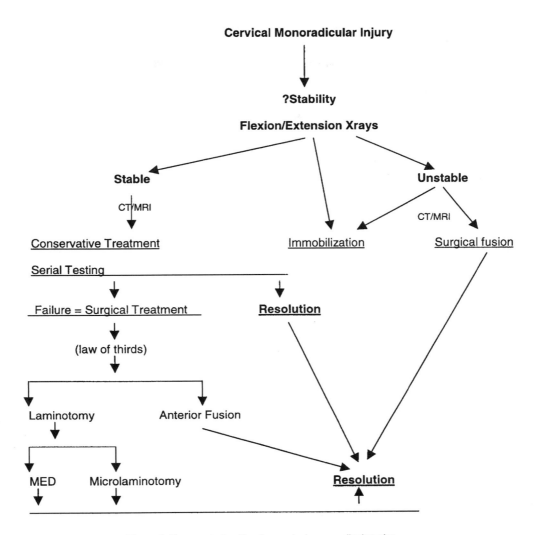

Figure 1: Treatment algorithm for cervical monoradiculopathy.

The Cervical Spine

Cervical spine injuries can present a diagnostic dilemma. Transient stretch injuries of the brachial plexus (especially the upper trunk) can masquerade as a root injury (stinger/burners), and canal dimensions, which appear quite adequate in the static position, may be marginal in flexion or extension. During the initial postinjury phase of conservative treatment, the need for close serial clinical follow-up, maximum muscle power testing, and dynamic flexion-extension radiographs is essential and cannot be overemphasized. Once stability of a cervical segment is assured, the treatment algorithm is simplified drastically (Figure 1).

The primary question to begin the surgical decision-making process is that of stability. Stability is assured on flexion-extension films and, if the patient fails conservative therapy or has a motor deficit, surgical treatment is indicated.

Surgical Decision-making

If the symptoms are monoradicular and stability is assured by adequate testing, it is beneficial to the athlete to avoid an anterior approach with fusion. A microinvasive approach with decompression of the anterior border of the foramen does not compromise flexibility, range of motion, sagittal balance, or the inherent strength of the facet, as long as greater than 50% of the facet surface is intact.[11] If radiographic pathology demonstrates neural compression too medial to be reached via a posterior lateral approach, an anterior fusion procedure may be the best option. This raises other controversies, including the use of autograft vs. allograft and the use of instrumentation to augment the strength and rigidity of the fusion.

A simple construct in the decision-making process is what the author calls "the law of thirds." The anterior border of the spinal canal is divided into thirds from a lateral foramen to contralateral foramen (Figure 2). When pathology is limited to the lateral one third of the spinal canal and the spine is stable, the approach should be posterior. When there is disease of the adjacent two thirds or of all of the spinal canal, the approach should be anterior. When there is pathology of two nonadjacent thirds, the approach may be either anterior or via a bilateral posterior lateral approach. A "tongue" of soft disc material, which extends medially beyond this medial and middle third border can usually be removed posteriorly (Figures 2 and 3). This makes the distinction between hard and soft disc of critical importance. The best test remains thin-cut contrast-enhanced computed tomography scan, as magnetic resonance imaging can be misleading and is poorly predictive of the density of material anterior to the nerve root in the proximal foramen.

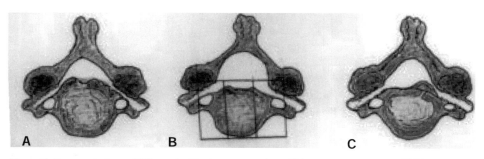

Figure 2: Representations of C6 vertebral body cross-sections. **A)** Lateral disc herniation. **B)** Normal canal with the anterior canal divided into thirds from the lateral vertebral foramen to the contralateral foramen. **C)** Spondylitic disease. Pathology of the lateral one third should be approached posteriorly and that of the adjacent two thirds or all of the spinal canal approached anteriorly.

If the decision has been made to perform an anterior fusion, consideration of autograft vs. allograft and the use of instrumentation must be made. While both have been touted as acceptable alternatives, the match of bone density of a structural tri-cortical autograft with the vertebral body is clearly superior, the rate of uninstrumented fusion is higher,[2,4,5,7] and the rate of late pseudoarthrosis is lower. With the use of microsurgical techniques applied to harvesting autologous bone graft, pain from an autograft is not a limiting factor in the patient's recovery. Allograft is noted to have slower bone formation, delayed vascular ingrowth, delayed incorporation, and a higher rate of rejection.[3]

The placement of instrumentation in the cervical spine is a significant detriment to the college football or basketball player pursuing a professional contract. When an athlete undergoes a medical examination by representatives of the National Football League or National Basketball Association, a well-formed fusion is more likely to be considered a natural segmentation defect (Klippel-Feil syndrome) as long as the spinal canal dimensions are adequate. Multiple-level fusions are usually considered to disqualify the athlete from major contact-sports participation at any level of competition.

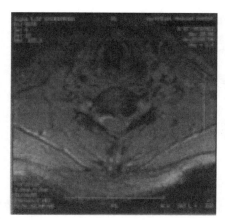

Figure 3: Typical C5-6 lateral disc herniation.

If the decision has been made to operate posteriorly, there are two serviceable and complementary procedures to consider: the microscopic laminotomy/foraminotomy and the microendoscopic laminotomy/foraminotomy, or microendoscopic discectomy. Both are based upon the original key-hole laminotomy procedure for cervical spine pathology popularized by neurosurgeons in the 1940s until the Smith-Robinson anterior approach predominated treatment.[8] The addition of modern microscopic microinvasive techniques and today's ever-shrinking endoscopic fiberoptic cameras provides unique advantages for each procedure. These procedures should not be viewed as alternative techniques, but as complementary solutions to the myriad of individual variations in cervical spine pathology.

Microendoscopic Discectomy vs. Microscopic Laminotomy

While the microendoscopic discectomy (MED) and the microscopic laminotomy/foraminotomy (ML) are both microinvasive, the approach of the MED is less so because muscle fibers or internal tendons are not cut, but are compressed and stretched by a series of dilators. The MED is best suited to soft disc ruptures and proximal foraminal disease because of a smaller arc of dissection and a lack of depth perception. The smaller arc of dissection is limited by the length of the endoscopic tube, which requires a fixed focal length and, therefore, a fixed tube length (Figure 4). The endoscopic technique has no depth of field because there is no stereoscopic image source, but a single 20°-angled fiberoptic camera 1.5 mm in diameter is used (Figure 5).

The ML, because of the additional advantage of depth of field and a greater arc of motion, is better suited to work anteriorly to the nerve root for spondylitic disease and far lateral foraminal nerve root compression. The MED and ML are both performed as outpatient procedures with a minimal complication rate and a high degree of success.[1] Following the MED, the patient averages less than a 5-hour hospital stay and following the ML, there is a 12-24 hour observation period (Table 1).

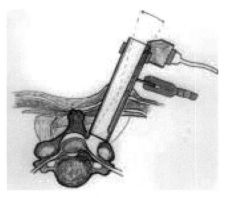

Figure 4: Cross-section representation of the C6 vertebral level with a lateral disc rupture and microendoscopic working channel in place. The arc of instrument movement is limited by the length of the working channel beyond the skin surface.

The Technique of Microendoscopic Discectomy

The microendoscopic discectomy is performed with the patient in a three-point Mayfield headholder (Figure 6A) in the seated position with the back of the neck perpendicular with the floor and distracted mildly. With distraction, the neck is tilted 15°, elevating the mastoid of the symptomatic side. The head tilt slightly opens and unloads the facet joint, allowing greater volume in the foramen, lessening bone removal and the risk of facet weakening. Under C-arm control (Figure 6B), a K-wire is passed through the enveloping fascia 2 cm off the midline through a 1.5-cm skin incision. A four-step Sofamor Danek endoscopic dilator system is used to dilate to a 1.6-cm working channel centered at the inferior edge of the lateral mass (Figure 7A and B). The endoscope is then inserted (Figure 7C), and the laminotomy is begun at the junction of the lamina and lateral mass. The medial third of the lateral mass is removed with a drill or a 2-mm 45° Kerrison rongeur with a flat footplate. The lateral half of the yellow ligament is removed and the rostral

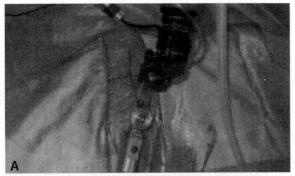
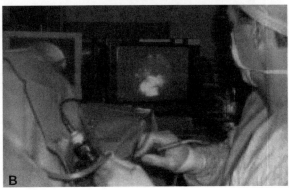

Figure 5: A) Endoscopic camera attached to the working channel. The black depth of field focus is capped with a video coupler. Suction tubing *(left)* and a fiber-optic light source *(right)* are attached. The target level is drawn on the skin. **B)** Positioning of the C-arm x-ray monitor and the endoscopic high-resolution monitor with the endoscopic working channel positioned a comfortable mid-chest height for the surgeon.

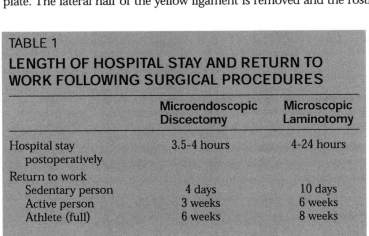

TABLE 1

LENGTH OF HOSPITAL STAY AND RETURN TO WORK FOLLOWING SURGICAL PROCEDURES

	Microendoscopic Discectomy	Microscopic Laminotomy
Hospital stay postoperatively	3.5-4 hours	4-24 hours
Return to work		
Sedentary person	4 days	10 days
Active person	3 weeks	6 weeks
Athlete (full)	6 weeks	8 weeks

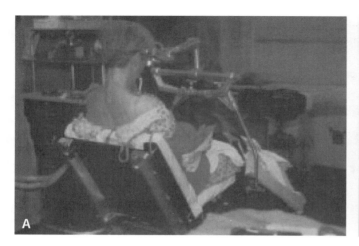
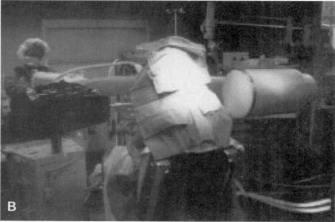

Figure 6: A) The patient is in the sitting position with a three-point Mayfield headholder. The head is mildly distracted, with the head tilted up on the side of surgery. **B)** The C-arm is brought into the field to localize the level and to position the dilators.

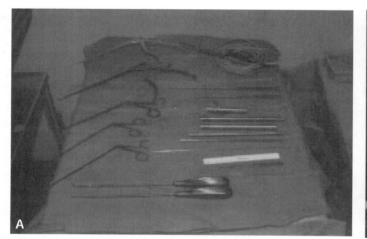
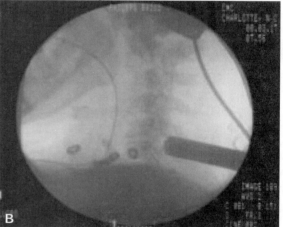

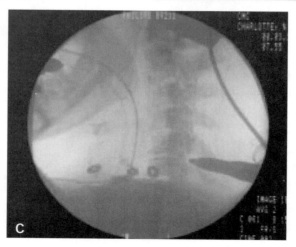

Figure 7: A) The dilators, punches, and curettes for use through the working channel.
B) Lateral view of the cervical spine with four dilators telescoped on insertion centered on the facet junction 2 cm lateral to midline. **C)** Working channel of the endoscope inserted over the dilators.

laminar surface is notched laterally, medial to the edge of the pedicle. A high-speed drill is then used to drill off the superior edge of the pedicle into the proximal foramen, exposing the axilla.

This bony resection is best performed with a 2-mm diamond-tipped drill. The drill can be advanced down the superior pedicle into the base of the spondylitic bar inferior to the disc space and anterior to the anterior division of the nerve root by perforating the bar with the 2-mm drill. The perforated spur can then be crushed with a 45° downpushing Epstein curette and removed piecemeal. The foramen can be further decompressed by amputating the superior tip of the ascending facet, but with some difficulty in larger patients due to the limited range of angles available by "wanding" the endoscopic working channel. All drilling must be done under a layer of irrigation, providing a heat sink to protect the nerve root from thermal damage.

Hemostasis is easily achieved with a small thrombin-saturated Gelfoam pad, and replaced with Medrol-impregnated Gelfoam. The endoscopic working channel is slowly removed with an up-angled bipolar forceps used to coagulate bleeding in the deep muscle layers as the working channel is removed. Closure is effected with two fascial sutures, subcutaneous sutures, and medical adhesive dressing. The musculature is liberally injected with Marcaine.

After a short stay in the postoperative recovery room, the patient is discharged home and is followed as an outpatient in 2-7 days depending on his/her job requirements. Workers whose job does not require heavy lifting usually return to work in less than 4 days; those requiring heavy lifting, return in 3-4 weeks.

The Technique of Microscopic Laminotomy

The microscopic laminotomy in the cervical spine is also performed under general anesthesia with the patient seated in a three-point Mayfield headholder (Figure 6A). The neck is positioned perpendicular to the floor, mildly distracted, and tilted 15°; a spinal needle is placed into the facet 2 cm off the midline, parallel with the floor and confirmed with lateral cervical spine x-ray. Indigo carmine vital dye is then injected as the needle is removed, marking a path through the muscle to the target facet/lateral mass level. (Note: Methylene blue is to be avoided as it has a formalin base and is not suitable for injection, especially around neural structures.)

An incision is made obliquely 2 to 2.5 cm in length, and small "micro Cobb" elevators are used to gently dissect the layers of muscles as in a series of veils, cutting only the skin and the outer layer of the enveloping fascia. Care is taken not to detach the internal tendons from the caudal surface of the lamina and spinous process. Two right-angled, thin-blade, hand-held retractors are placed, one over the other, with one of them rotated 180°. An Aesculap microlaminotomy retractor (Figure 8) is placed down to the facet, exposing only the medial facet and lateral third of the lamina (Figure 9). A microscope, with the field of view perpendicular to the floor, is employed at 10 to 30 times magnification to guide a high-speed drill, with a 2-3 mm diamond bit, to provide a small key-

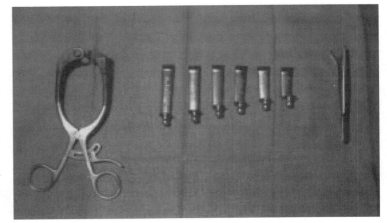

Figure 8: Aesculap microlaminotomy retractor with a variety of blade lengths and a fixed hook on the medial side.

hole laminotomy involving the medial third of the facet and lateral third of the lamina. The lateral half of the ligamentum flavum is removed and, following the nerve root out of the proximal foramen, the epidural venous plexus is coagulated and divided beyond

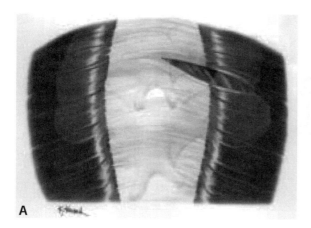
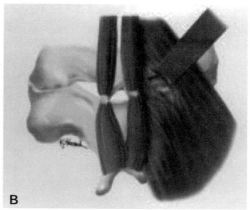

Figure 9: A) The enveloping fascia is incised obliquely, exposing the longitudinal fibers of the splenius capitis and semi-spinalis muscle groups. **B)** The short rotators are separated, exposing the junction of the lamina and overlapping facet.

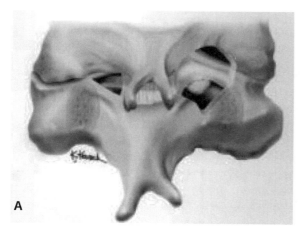
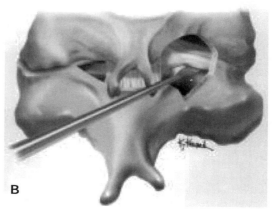

Figure 10: A) A key-hole laminotomy extends one third of the lateral mass width into the inferior pedicle, which makes up the inferior wall of the foramen. Note the notch in the inferior lamina to provide a guide for carving hard disc or spur without compromising the lateral spinal cord. **B)** A Penfield #7 dissector separates the anterior rootlet from the pearl-like disc fragment. The epidural venous veil is cut well beyond the separation of the anterior and posterior rootlets.

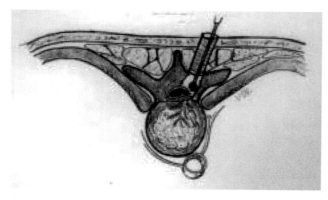

Figure 11: Cross-section of T8 demonstrating the trajectory of the tubular retractor sets. The transpedicular approach offers an excellent view nearly to midline without retraction of the cord or sacrifice of pedicular stability.

the division of the anterior and posterior rootlets. The superior-medial edge of the pedicle is drilled off, traveling down the pedicle to the floor of the spinal canal inferior and then anterior to the root, exposing the axilla (Figure 10). The thin flake of surrounding bone against the axilla is then curetted away. For a soft disc fragment, access is direct and with gentle elevation of the anterior division of the root, the small pearl-like contour of the disc rupture or spondylitic spur is easily identified. Soft disc is incised with a fine blade and removed. The herniation cavity is then probed with a micro-nerve hook, which can be used to probe anterior to the thecal sac as far as the midline. For spondylitic disease, heavily irrigated drill work can be continued with a 2-mm diamond bit anterior to the root, perforating and undermining the uncovertebral spurs and crushing them with a down-pushing Epstein curette (Figure 11). The tip of the ascending facet is then amputated, giving exceptional volume to the foramen without destabilizing the facet or its capsule.

Great care is needed in working anterior to the root and lateral to the pedicle, as a misstep or pressure by curette or probe in this area may damage or dissect the vertebral artery. Hemostasis is controlled with thrombin-soaked Gelfoam, and the root is then covered with a small pledget of Gelfoam impregnated with Depo-Medrol.

Closure is effected with a loose stitch in the deep layers, interrupted sutures in the enveloping fascia, a subcutaneous closure, and a medical adhesive. A long-acting anesthetic is injected into the musculature.

Postoperatively, the patient is discharged home over the next 4-8 hours and followed at 1 week for return to work for office workers and 3-5 weeks for laborers. Athletes are placed in the category of laborers, allowed to work out on a limited basis at 3 weeks and generally released at 6-8 weeks without restriction. This schedule is obviously preferable to a 3-6 month noncontact lay-off following a cervical fusion and does not limit future surgical options. It obviously does not affect the degree of neck motion essential to high-level athletics and requires no bracing or instrumentation.

The Thoracic Spine

The implications of a thoracic disc rupture are frightening for the athlete, both from the standpoint of the loss of function and the potentially highly invasive surgery. Thoracic discs represent a small percentage of the disc ruptures, but because of the limited space in the spinal canal, there is a disproportionate risk of a deficit of anterior spinal cord function. A thoracotomy for a lateral approach to a disc rupture may be a season- or career-ending treatment.

Microinvasive procedures offer a low-risk, short rehabilitation alternative. Thoracoscopic procedures offer the advantage of an intercostal trocar approach with three working channels of 4-8 mm and completely avoid an assault on either the erector spinae musculature or the accessory respiratory muscles such as the serratus posterior inferior, an injury that can hamper a rapid recovery. These procedures offer a time course of recovery similar to the endoscopic cervical discectomy of 6-8 weeks and a return to noncontact conditioning in as little as 2-3 weeks.

Another minimally invasive option providing better stereoscopic vision and tactile feedback is a microscopic transpedicular approach through a microscopic transpedicular laminotomy. With the patient in the supine position, preferably on an Andrews frame for rotational stability, the location of the disc level is established using a spinal needle confirmed by x-ray. The path of the needle is marked with indigo carmine vital dye as the needle is removed. Meticulous attention is needed to assure that the needle is perpendicular to the floor, especially with larger patients, as the needle guides the trajectory to the affected level. A 2-cm incision is then made 2 cm off the midline and is carried down to the thoracodorsal fascia. The facet can be easily palpated beneath the muscle and, working gently with small periosteal dissectors, the muscle fibers are split but not detached, exposing the interlaminar space. Retraction with a small, thin Williams or Aesculap microlaminotomy retractor is adequate, but the use of the Sofamor-Danek dilator system and variable length working channels is optional. A high-power microscope and drill with a 2- to 2.5-mm diamond-tipped burr is then used to form a small laminotomy defect descending into the floor of the spinal canal via the superior medial pedicle margin (Figure 11). Access to the disc space is then easily acquired and, with the angle of vision provided, the surgeon can easily see to midline with minimal or no retraction of the thecal sac.

Thoracic disc ruptures in the youthful tend to be soft and cheese-like in their consistency and are easily removed. The degenerative disc can then be removed, more extensively or not, according to the surgeon's preference, much in the same manner as a lumbar discectomy with cervical downpushing curettes and micropituitary rongeurs. Great care must be exercised to limit the depth of disc removal to less than three fourths the depth of the disc space, especially when working toward the left side of the disc space. The closure is simple, in layers, with subcutaneous sutures and medical adhesive; the musculature is injected with a long-acting anesthetic and the patient is discharged home in 12 hours after bowel and bladder function and ambulation are assumed.

Minimally invasive spinal procedures offer great promise not only for the return of high-level athletes, but also for the middle-aged "weekend warrior." Minimally invasive procedures are also highly applicable to the elderly, as they offer a surgical solution with a minimum of recumbent recovery. The early mobilization not only prevents deconditioning and quadriceps atrophy, but should be very effective in the prevention of deep venous thrombosis and pulmonary embolic phenomena.

The role of micro- and minimally invasive spinal surgery is clearly expanding, driven by both physician expectations and patient/consumer demands. With the rapid expansion of technology, surgeons must continue to expand the limits of small incisions and continue to innovate with new versions of traditional procedures.

References

1. Adamson TE: 100 Consecutive microendoscopic cervical discectomies. **J Neurosurg (In press)**
2. Brown MD, Malinin TL, Davis PB: A roentgenographic evaluation of frozen allografts versus autograft in anterior cervical spine fusions. **Clin Orthopaed 119**:231-236, 1976
3. Dickman CA, Maric Z: The biology of bone healing and techniques of spinal fusion. **BNI Q 10**:2-12, 1994
4. Fernyhough JC, White JL, LaRocca H: Fusion rates in multilevel cervical spondylosis comparing allograft fibula with autograft fibula. **Spine 16**:726-729, 1991
5. Kaufman HH, Jones E: The principles of bony spinal fusion. **Neurosurgery 24**:264-270, 1989
6. Prolo DJ: Biology of bone fusion. **Clin Neurosurg 36**:135-146, 1988
7. Raynor RB, Pugh J, Shapiro I: Cervical facetectomy and its effect on spine strength. **J Neurosurg 63**:278-282, 1985
8. Robinson RA, Smith GW: Anterolateral cervical disc removal and fusion for cervical disc syndrome. **Bull Johns Hopkins Hosp 96**: 223-224, 1955
9. Sach B, Brennen W: Comparison of freeze dried allograft versus autograft in anterior cervical spine fusions. **Cervical Spine Research Society**, 1992, pp 140-141 (Abstract)
10. Young WF, Rosenwasser RH: An early comparative analysis of the use of fibular allograft versus autologous iliac crest graft for interbody fusion after anterior drill in discectomy. **Spine 18**:1123-1124, 1993
11. Zdeblick TA, Sav DD, Warden KE, et al: Cervical stability after foraminotomy. **J Bone Joint Surg (Am) 74**:22-29, 1992
12. Zdeblick TA, Wikson D, Cooke ME, et al: The use of freeze dried allograft bone in anterior cervical fusions. **Spine 16**:726-729, 1991

CHAPTER 6

Peripheral Nerve Injuries in Athletes

ROBERT J. SPINNER, MD, and DAVID G. KLINE, MD

Peripheral nerve injuries occur in the amateur and the professional athlete alike. They may affect the young and the old. Any athlete may develop any type of nerve lesion, and all nerves may be affected. Certain athletes and certain nerves appear to be at higher risk. For example, volleyball players commonly develop suprascapular nerve lesions; baseball players, ulnar nerve lesions at the elbow; and cyclists, median or ulnar nerve lesions at the wrists. Biomechanical studies have identified specific phases of these sports that link the nerve injuries to a sports-related mechanism. Although no prospective studies exist in athletes from the United States, Hirasawa and Sakakida[24] found 66 sports-related cases among a total of 1167 cases (5.7%) of nerve injuries collected over 18 years. In their study, the most frequently injured nerves were the brachial plexus, then the radial, ulnar, peroneal, and axillary nerves (in decreasing frequency); the most common sports responsible for the injury were mountain climbing, gymnastics, and baseball, all popular sports in Japan.

Athletes may develop neural lesions acutely following direct trauma or chronically following repetitive trauma. Neural injuries in athletes typically develop from compression, contusion, stretch, friction, or microtrauma, but in rare instances, may also occur from laceration. For example, the authors treated a basketball player who sustained a radial nerve laceration from a glass bottle when he fell into the crowd trying to retrieve a rebound.

Direct extrinsic compression commonly involves the hands, feet, and perineum and may occur acutely or chronically related to low-grade compression; compression also occurs frequently at sites of potential entrapment and is due to mechanical or vascular causes. Contusion occurs when a nerve that lies superficially or occupies a position of vulnerability (such as the median or ulnar nerve at the wrist, the ulnar nerve at the elbow, and the peroneal nerve at the surgical neck of the fibula) receives direct trauma acutely. Traction occurs when stretch exceeds the elastic and deforming capacity of nerve and soft tissue, and injury relates to the magnitude of traction and rate of nerve deformation. Stretch may occur acutely, if the physiological capacity for stretch is exceeded by a single tensile load, or chronically, if it is delivered more slowly (e.g., tethered by scar). Friction may occur when a hypermobile ulnar nerve dislocates repeatedly over the medial epicondyle. Microtrauma may result in neural injury due to overuse or misuse from cumulative trauma, exacerbated by repetitive motions of the extremity in awkward positions, often against resistance; improper technique or equipment may also play a role. Laceration can occur from sharp (e.g., glass) or blunt cutting (e.g., a propeller) objects.

Underlying anatomic factors may make certain athletes susceptible to developing neural lesions. These factors by themselves may be enough to cause the symptoms; on the other hand, they may incite symptoms in individuals participating in sports that place additional stress on a nerve. These symptoms may only become clinically relevant when the individual participates in a sport for a length of time or one that necessitates holding a limb in a certain position. Anatomic structures may be congenital (e.g., fibrous bands or a small carpal tunnel) or developmental (e.g., hypertrophied musculature). Symptoms may be static or dynamic.

Finally, athletes may also develop nerve lesions totally unrelated to their sport. Older athletes may have subtle long-standing symptoms of carpal tunnel syndrome, which are blamed on the very occasional athletic activity. The authors recently saw a competitive long-distance runner who was treated for presumed exertional compartment syndrome of his leg; he was later found to have a schwannoma of the peroneal nerve.

Physicians must have a broad knowledge of peripheral nerve injuries in order to deal with these athletic injuries, which at times can be serious and potentially career-ending. A thorough understanding of normal and variant anatomy, the type of injury, and the degree of the neural lesion is critical to accurate diagnosis and timely, appropriate treatment.

Mechanisms and the Regenerative Process

Classification

Seddon[46] defined three types of nerve injury to correlate microscopic neural anatomy with prognosis for recovery. Sunderland[54] refined these further into five types of injury. Neurapraxia (Sunderland Grade 1), the mildest form of nerve injury, represents a physiological disruption to the nerve with minimal anatomic distortion. A conduction block across the lesion is present. Mild structural injury can result in segmental demyelination and remyelination. In general, Wallerian degeneration does not occur. Typically, sensory and motor involvement is present transiently. The injury may last from minutes to several months, and complete recovery usually occurs. Surgery is rarely necessary.

Axonotmetic lesions (Sunderland Grade 2 or mild Grade 3) have severe axonal injury, although the connective tissue framework is largely undisturbed. Wallerian degeneration occurs at the point of injury distally, and regeneration follows at a rate of about 1 mm/day until the end organ is reached. Regeneration can occur in an orderly fashion due to the continuity of the connective tissue which serves as a framework for regrowth. However, regeneration may be slowed by retrograde proximal degeneration, scarring due to inflammatory changes at the injury zone, and structural changes near the end organs; these factors may delay clinical or electrical signs of recovery. Recovery is slow and takes many months to occur. During the process of regeneration, atrophy and fibrosis of the end organs also occur. Surgery may be necessary.

Neurotmetic injuries are the most severe, resulting in permanent damage to nerves. There is anatomical discontinuity of the axons and disruption of the internal connective tissue framework. In most cases, however, the nerve is still in continuity (advanced Sunderland Grade 3 or 4) and not transected (Grade 5). Regeneration does not occur spontaneously but may lead to neuroma formation. Recovery is based on surgical repair. Neurotmesis is frequently associated with proximal level injuries, fractures or dislocations, or lacerations.

The vast majority of serious lesions in athletes are stretch/contusion injuries, which are in continuity. Therefore, if left alone the eventual outcome would be unpredictable due to variable injury affecting neural and connective tissue architecture. For example, some lesions in continuity have a predominant amount of neurotmetic change that would not permit functional regeneration. This type of patient would usually benefit from surgery.

Clinical Workup

A detailed history is the most basic element of a clinical examination. A physician must determine if a neurological lesion is present and, if so, its localization and completeness. In acute injuries, the focus should be on delineating the exact mechanism resulting in the injury. In order to do this, it is helpful to recreate the injury in his/her mind. The mechanics of each aspect of the sport must be understood, and the position of the body and the extremity at the time of injury determined. In chronic injuries, one should inquire about risk factors, such as might develop from microtrauma, be it from overuse or misuse. Here, an understanding of the physical training demands of the sport as well as the psychological factors impacting the athlete is necessary.

The physician must methodically analyze the course of events since the onset of symptoms to determine the timing of the neurological deficit and the evolution of the injury in order to understand the severity. If the physician is seeing the patient early, inquiries should be made about related injuries, as these may not have been noticed previously. If seeing the patient in consultation a period of time after the injury, the time of the onset of symptoms and findings and the previous treatment must be tracked. Outside records and studies must be carefully reviewed.

Determining the evolution of a neurological deficit can be critical in a physician's decision making, but may not be easy to ascertain from the patient or from medical records after an injury or after time has elapsed. For example, did the neural deficit occur at the time of the fall when the humerus fracture occurred, after manipulation at the hospital, or after surgical plating? Did the numbness start immediately after the accident when the elbow was dislocated, after it was reduced, or after the elbow was splinted?

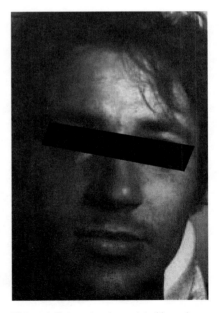

The physician must inquire about associated injuries that may be relevant. For example, was there trauma to the head or spine, or vascular, skeletal, or extensive soft-tissue injury? The presence of these can provide clues as to the mechanism and nature of the injury.

Inquiry must be made about neuritic pain. If present, the medications that the patient has tried in the past and that are currently in use and the various treatment modalities that have been employed must be identified. Pain syndromes are frequent following peripheral nerve injuries or brachial plexus root avulsions.

Performance of an accurate clinical examination is the next step in determining the presence of a neural lesion, localizing it, and ascertaining if it is a complete or partial injury. A complete neurological examination is critical. This includes: grading motor strength; testing sensation in peripheral nerve distributions (especially autonomous zones) and dermatomes and autonomic function, if indicated; evaluating tone and deep tendon reflexes and the presence of pathological reflexes; inspecting for atrophy, Horner's syndrome (Figure 1), or fasciculations; checking for pulses and bruits; evaluating joint range of motion and bone alignment; assessing diaphragmatic excursion; and supplementing other tests when appropriate, including Phalen's test at the wrist for carpal tunnel syndrome, hyperflexion of the elbow for ulnar neuropathy, thoracic outlet maneuvers (e.g., Adson's or Roos) or Tinel's test for regeneration.

Finally, whether seeing the patient early or late, a neurosurgeon remains a generalist

Figure 1: This patient has a right Horner's syndrome and a cervical fracture (collar), suggesting that some neural elements are not candidates for a direct repair.

and must provide a more detailed general examination, consult others as needed, and ensure that all problems are managed appropriately.

Each aspect of the neurological examination has importance. For example, in muscle testing, weakness of proximal muscles (such as the rhomboids or the serratus anterior) or poor diaphragmatic excursion are suggestive of an avulsion injury. Careful muscle testing will help determine if a lesion is partial or complete. In addition, muscle loss may be subtle due to the overall strength of the athlete and Cybex testing is necessary. Individuals can sometimes substitute muscles to compensate for loss. For example, the supraspinatus may result in full abduction of the arm when the deltoid is absent. Elbow flexion may be preserved due to a hypertrophied brachioradialis even when the biceps is absent. Other patients use "trick" movements to substitute for neural loss, especially in the hand; these false actions can make examination difficult if the physician is not astute and experienced.

Careful sensory testing can also help diagnose lesions. For example, a patient suspected of having an ulnar nerve lesion at the wrist should not have sensory abnormality on the dorso-ulnar aspect of the hand since the dorsal cutaneous branch is given off more proximally. This lesion would be more proximal, probably at the elbow. Autonomous zones of peripheral nerves must be distinguished from dermatomes. Examination of sympathetic function might reveal return of sweating. This could represent an early return of neural function.

The presence of percussion tenderness along the nerve often serves to localize the site of injury. The presence of an advancing Tinel's sign suggests regeneration but does not guarantee recovery of useful level(s) of function.

Vascular examination might reveal a dampened pulse in an abducted limb in a patient with thoracic outlet symptoms. A bruit and a palpable thrill might be suggestive of a pseudoaneurysm.

The presence of increased reflexes or abnormal tone in an extremity should indicate an upper motor neuron lesion, from either an associated spinal or intracranial lesion. An abnormal elbow carrying angle from previous supracondylar humeral malunion resulting in a cubitus valgus or cubitus varus deformity might explain an ulnar nerve lesion (tardy ulnar nerve palsy). Severe joint contractures from disuse might limit functional return should neural recovery ensue.

A general examination of a patient (especially one on Coumadin) with a femoral neuropathy might reveal evidence of a retroperitoneal hematoma. The data from the medical history and physical examination help guide the physician in evaluation, interpretation, and management. Detailed knowledge of peripheral nerve anatomy (e.g., neural branching patterns or internal topographic maps) and common variations is necessary for the appropriate care of patients with typical and atypical presentations.

Radiographic/Electrical Workup

Plain radiographs are an important part of the diagnostic evaluation. Patients with brachial plexus injuries should undergo cervical and chest films. The presence of cervical fractures provides useful information regarding the extent and proximity of the injury and predicts avulsion. Chest films will corroborate diaphragmatic function (Figure 2). Review of the chest film will also provide information about the presence of a recent scapula fracture, a recent or old clavicle fracture, or nonunion. In addition, it will provide information about the presence of vascular clips and orthopaedic plates or hardware.

Patients should undergo other films as relevant to their injury. Review of fracture patterns can give an idea about the nature and mechanism of the injury. Certain fractures are associated with high-energy trauma (e.g., a fracture of the scapula). Commin-

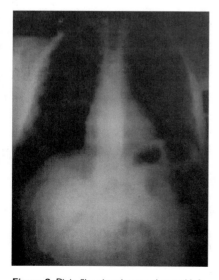

Figure 2: Plain film showing an elevated left hemidiaphragm from a phrenic nerve injury in a patient with a closed stretch injury involving the left brachial plexus.

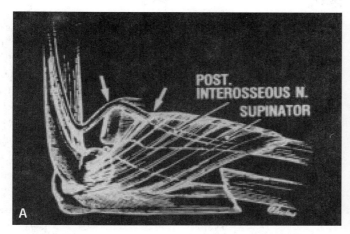

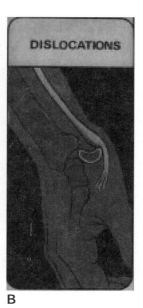

Figure 3: A) A Monteggia (radial head) fracture/dislocation places the posterior interosseous nerve at risk. B) Volar lunate dislocations may be associated with median nerve injury. (Figure 3A reproduced with permission from Siegel DB, Gelberman RH. Nerve injury associated with fractures and dislocations, in Gelberman RH (ed): *Operative Nerve Repair and Reconstruction.* Philadelphia, Pa: JB Lippincott, 1991)

uted fractures also suggest high energy. In addition, certain types of fractures or dislocations are associated with neural injuries (e.g., anterior shoulder dislocations are associated with axillary nerve palsies, humeral shaft fractures with radial nerve, elbow dislocations with ulnar nerve, pediatric humeral supracondylar fractures with anterior interosseous nerve, proximal radius fractures with posterior interosseous nerve (Figure 3A), wrist fractures or dislocations with median nerve (Figure 3B), hip fractures or dislocations with sciatic nerve, and knee dislocations with peroneal nerve injury). Films may show evidence of old deformities that may be relevant to a delayed onset of a neural injury (e.g., a fracture malunion (cubitus varus or valgus) or excessive callous at a fracture site).

The authors do not routinely use computed tomography (CT) or magnetic resonance imaging (MRI) alone as they do not provide enough detail about the roots to prevent the need for myelography when considering brachial plexus avulsion. MRI can be helpful in evaluating peripheral nerve tumors, such as ganglia or nerve sheath tumors, or ruling out associated musculoskeletal pathology, such as rotator cuff tears. MRI is especially helpful in the preoperative evaluation of patients with suprascapular nerve lesions. It also is useful in demonstrating early denervation.

Myelography alone or combined with fine-cut (2 mm) post-CT myelography remains the gold standard for evaluating patients suspected of having avulsion injury to the brachial plexus. Myelography should be performed several weeks after the injury and should not be done acutely so as to avoid arachnoiditis. Myelograms demonstrating a pseudomeningocele (Figure 4) or nonvisualized nerve root sleeve are suggestive of an avulsion. The absence of a pseudomeningocele does not exclude an avulsion and the presence of one does not guarantee an avulsion. Myelograms can show cord edema acutely or atrophy chronically.

Angiography may be necessary early in patients with concomitant vascular injury. It may also be necessary at a later stage if the diagnosis of pseudoaneurysm is being considered, even though it is diagnostic in only one half of cases. Additionally, it can demonstrate vessels that penetrate (and can compress) nerves directly, such as the median nerve in the axilla. Obliteration of the posterior humeral circumflex artery with external rotation and abduction can help establish the diagnosis of quadrilateral space syndrome in an appropriate patient.

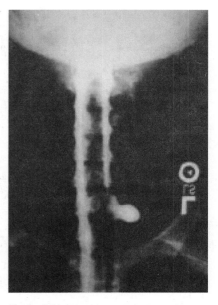

Figure 4: Myelogram showing a pseudomeningocele involving the left C8 nerve root.

The timing and interpretation of electrodiagnostic testing is critical.[57] Electromyography (EMG) obtained during the first week of injury can demonstrate chronic electrical changes that may be important in the future for comparable studies; EMG might also be useful in a patient who has recurrent stingers. EMG is best performed after Wallerian degeneration has occurred, which is at least 2-3 weeks after injury. Studies obtained earlier will not demonstrate evidence of denervation. Fibrillations and positive sharp waves indicate acute denervation, while nascent potentials indicate early reinnervation. EMG evaluation is helpful in confirming a neurological lesion, determining the severity of it, and ruling out other lesions.

Nerve conduction studies (NCS) in a nerve distal to a transected nerve will still stimulate paradoxically for several days, as the nerve has not undergone Wallerian degeneration and still conducts impulses; however, there is no voluntary muscle contraction. In partial neurapraxic lesions, NCS will show slowed conduction across the lesion with normal responses proximal and distal to the lesion. In complete focal neurapraxic lesions, NCS will demonstrate normal responses distal to the lesion but no response across it. In axonotmetic lesions, NCS show no response across the lesion or dorsal to it. These studies give information about fiber count and the condition of the myelin and the site of injury. A loss of fibers can best be identified by decreased amplitude of the sensory nerve action potentials (SNAPs), more so than that for the compound motor action potential. The distal latency and conduction velocity reflect the presence or absence of demyelination.

Electrodiagnostic studies are extremely helpful as an adjunct to clinical examination in confirming a level of localization and in assessing the severity of the lesion. However, they are not a substitute for clinical examination. While an advancing Tinel's sign, improved autonomic or sensory examination, and even improved electrical studies signify some regrowth, it does not guarantee recovery of effective function. If one waits for reinnervation to occur, the window of opportunity may be lost. Therefore, clinical and electrodiagnostic studies must be correlated.

Sensory nerve action potentials can also be useful in differentiating a preganglionic from a postganglionic lesion. A SNAP will be present when the lesion is proximal to the dorsal root ganglion but not when it occurs distal to it. SNAPs are best for assessing C8 and T1 preganglionic lesions and less so for C6 and C7 lesions due to overlap in their dermatomal or innervational zones.

Diagnosis of Brachial Plexus and Peripheral Nerve Lesions

Based on clinical, radiographic, and electrical studies, a diagnosis can be established and a management plan proposed. For brachial plexus lesions, the pattern of injury (e.g., the C5/6 stretch) should be determined. Preganglionic (irreparable) vs. postganglionic (reparable) injury before surgery is then determined. The presence of one or more of the following findings implies a preganglionic lesion (more accurately, indicates intraforaminal lesions) and is a relative stop to direct plexo-plexal repair: weakness of proximally innervated muscles (rhomboids, serratus anterior, diaphragm); the finding of cervical myelopathy or a Horner's syndrome; absent or weak Tinel's sign; radiographic findings of cervical transverse process fractures or a high riding diaphragm; EMG evidence of extensive paraspinal denervation; SNAPs recorded from median and ulnar nerves; or an intact flare component or triple reaction to histamine injection. Unfortunately, a lesion may be both pre- and postganglionic so some studies that demonstrate the preganglionic component such as peripheral SNAP recordings will not be helpful.

For peripheral nerve lesions, it is important to determine if the lesion is partial or complete. Since incomplete lesions frequently improve spontaneously, such a differential has clinical significance.

Indications for and Timing of Operation (Including Brachial Plexus)

Indications for surgery are to improve neurological function or to decrease pain. Acute surgery is rarely indicated for athletic nerve injuries. Sharp, clean lacerations should be treated early to facilitate an end-to-end epineurial repair and diminish retraction of the stumps and the need for interpositional grafts. In these instances, early repair facilitates the determination of fascicular orientation. Vascular complications (hematoma, fistula, pseudoaneurysm, or a compartment syndrome) that result in worsening neurological deficits necessitate early surgery, as does the treatment of causalgia.

Early nerve exploration is indicated in a patient with an associated neural deficit who is undergoing surgery for an open fracture, open reduction internal fixation of a fracture, or a vascular repair. Exploration is also indicated in a patient who loses function after a reduction or who has an irreducible fracture.

Repair of blunt or sharp injuries that also have a contusive element are best performed secondarily, about 1 month after injury. If earlier surgery was performed and revealed stumps that had ragged edges, these should be tacked down to adjacent planes to minimize retraction and allow demarcation to occur.

Delayed surgery is the rule for neural injury from blunt trauma. These nerves are typically in continuity, but have been stretched. Over a period of several months, these lesions define themselves and intraoperative recordings can be used more reliably. During this time, careful surveillance is critical. Serial physical examination and electrical studies should be performed after the injury. Clinical examination may reveal improved motor, sensory, or autonomic function or an advancing Tinel's sign. EMG may show reversal of denervation in proximal muscles. Physical therapy should be instituted during the waiting phase to maintain strength in other muscles and range of motion in involved joints.

For a complete lesion or if there is significant neural deficit, a nonoperative approach can be followed for 3-6 months following injury. Surgery should be considered if there is no clinical or electrical improvement.

The patient and the patient's family should be educated about realistic expectations and outcomes. Relative contraindications for surgery would include patients referred for evaluation late (greater than 1 year since injury) or those with significant comorbidities.

Patients with mild symptoms and an incomplete neurological deficit, such as is seen with chronic peripheral nerve entrapment lesions, should be treated initially with nonoperative measures. These include a trial of relative rest, splinting (if applicable), and nonsteroidal anti-inflammatory agents. Any underlying medical condition or exacerbating activity that could contribute to the neuropathy should be corrected or modified. Sports-related changes relating to equipment, training regimens, or stroke mechanics should also be made. Rehabilitation should include strengthening exercises and conditioning. Surgery should be reserved for those with persistent symptoms or worsening neurological findings who do not respond to these measures.

Surgical Procedures

Surgical Evaluation with Nerve Action Potentials

Clinical inspection and palpation of the nerve do not correlate with the microscopic neural pathology or the potential for regeneration. Electrophysiological recording with nerve action potentials (NAPs) was introduced to augment intraoperative decision making (Figure 5).[29,30,55] The appropriate use of NAPs prevents neurolysis alone in the face of

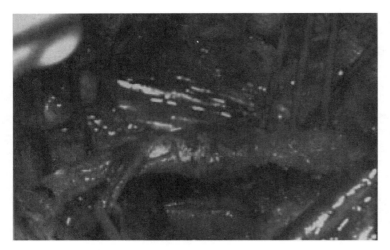

Figure 5: Intraoperative NAPs are being measured. The stimulating electrodes are under the upper trunk and the recording electrodes are under the posterior division. The suprascapular nerve is in a vesi-loop.

a nonregenerating element and likewise spares excision of regenerating elements. With the use of NAPs, a lesion can be judged to see if adequate regeneration is occurring earlier than standard EMG would show recovery. Reliable data about regeneration can be obtained as early as 6-8 weeks after injury. Following neurolysis, NAPs can be obtained on the whole nerve or on larger segments or groups of fascicles. While stimulating the nerve, one can assess for muscle contraction (which might antedate volitional clinical activity). Initially, clinically normal functioning or appearing nerves or other nerve segments (e.g., the proximal nerve or other half of the sciatic nerve) should be tested in order to check equipment. Next, the affected nerve should be tested. If an NAP is obtained, adequate regeneration has occurred across the lesion (the only exception being the preganglionic spinal nerve or root injury); if it is not obtained, this indicates a Sunderland Grade 4 lesion with severe connective tissue proliferation histologically, poor axonal regeneration, and no potential for recovery despite being in continuity. There has been excellent correlation between an absent NAP recording and neurotmetic lesions.

Surgical Technique for Brachial Plexus Lesions

Regardless of their preoperative evaluation, the authors believe that patients with brachial plexus lesions selected for surgery, even those in whom there is a high suspicion for avulsive injury, should undergo formal exploration of the brachial plexus. Certain technical points are helpful in dissecting out the neural elements. The elements can often be identified more distally in healthy tissue planes. The suprascapular nerve can be isolated at the clavicle level and tracked proximally to the upper elements, or fuller infraclavicular exposure can help identify structures and facilitate mobilization of the clavicle. The descending cervical plexus and the phrenic nerve should be preserved and used as guides to the upper plexal elements. Often, the neural elements must be carved out of dense scar and fibrotic scalenes. Foraminal level dissection, which can be technically challenging, is necessary to assess possible proximal but still postganglionic lesions involving spinal nerves.

NAPs are utilized in the surgical decision making (i.e., whether to perform neurolysis, plexo-plexal repair, or extraplexal reconstruction). Neurolysis alone is performed when regenerative NAPs (slower conducting, lower amplitude) are obtained (Figure 6). When NAPs are absent, the lesion is either postganglionic or a combined pre- and postganglionic lesion. In this situation, the lesion is resected and the stumps are trimmed back to healthy fascicles. If good fascicular structure is seen proximally, nerve grafts (sural or antebrachial cutaneous nerves) can be used for a plexo-plexal repair (Figure 7). If preganglionic injury is suspected based on the presence of preganglionic NAPs (rapidly conducting 60-80 m/sec and large amplitude), then nerve transfers can be used for extraplexal reconstruction. First-line potential donors for nerve transfers that are used commonly by the senior author (D.G.K.) include the distal accessory,[1,48] medial or lateral pectoral,[4] descending cervical plexus, and intercostal nerves.[36] Other investigators[9] have reported their experiences with other nerves, including the phrenic,[22] contralateral C7,[21] hypoglossal, and long thoracic nerves. Priorities for reconstruction include shoulder abduction, elbow flexion, and sensation in the hand. Other procedures that may be combined with neural procedures include arthrodeses to stabilize joints (e.g., shoulder or wrist) and muscle/tendon transfers to augment or balance motor function. Recently, free vascularized as well as neurotized muscle transfers have been employed in patients whose prior neural procedures failed or in those presenting for reconstruction after 1 year.[13]

Surgical Technique for Peripheral Nerves

Using loupe magnification, surgeons should obtain wide exposure through internervous planes, when applicable. Major cutaneous branches should be preserved. The affected nerve should be identified in normal tissues, both proximally and distally. One can then work in both directions through the scar to perform circumferential external neurolysis. Dissection through scar can be facilitated using anatomic relationships, such as following the superficial radial nerve proximally, to find the radial nerve. Potential areas of compression should be released. The nerve bed is prepared by excising scar widely.

Once the epineurial scar is carved out, NAP recordings can be obtained. If a regenerative NAP is obtained, external neurolysis alone can be performed with excellent results.[29] However, if no NAP is obtained 2 or more months following injury, there is no potential for recovery and the lesion is resected and repaired. It is infrequent that the neuroma can be resected to enable direct end-to-end repair by suture. In the majority of these cases, interpositional grafting is necessary. The lesion is transected in the middle and both the proximal and distal stumps are cut back to healthy epineurium and fascicular structure. The stumps can be divided into fascicular groups for small-caliber nerve grafting. A tension-free neurorrhaphy should be planned. The gap should be made as minimal as possible using neurolysis and transposition (such as for the ulnar or radial nerve) as applicable. Gentle flexion of a joint can also shorten the nerve gap. Despite these measures at shortening the gap, a tension-free suture is critical. The gap is then measured.

Grafts can be obtained using sural or medial antebrachial cutaneous nerves. The

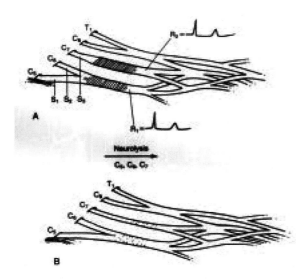

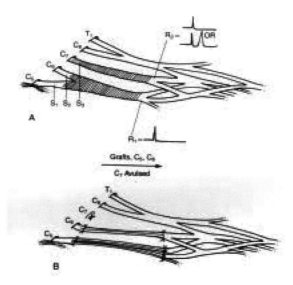

Figure 6: Neurolysis alone was performed on this patient with C5, C6, and C7 injuries and positive NAPs. (Reproduced with permission from Kline DG, Hudson AR (eds): *Nerve Injuries. Operative Results for Major Nerve Injuries, Entrapments, and Tumors.* Philadelphia, Pa: WB Saunders, 1995, 15-4, p 404)

Figure 7: Postganglionic injuries to C5 and C6 (absent NAPs) and a combined pre/postganglionic lesion of C7 can be seen in this patient. Sural grafts were used from C5 and C6 to upper trunk and middle trunk divisions. (Reproduced with permission from Kline DG, Hudson AR (eds): *Nerve Injuries. Operative Results for Major Nerve Injuries, Entrapments, and Tumors.* Philadelphia, Pa: WB Saunders, 1995, 15-5, p 405)

grafts are then fishmouthed to the stumps in an effort to maximize cross-sectional area. Several fascicular sutures with 7-0 Prolene coapt the ends. Failure of grafting is often due to inadequate resection of scar or distraction at the repair site.

If an NAP is obtained in the presence of a severe injury to a portion of the cross-section of a nerve, internal neurolysis of the nerve is performed; the nerve is then split up into "healthy" and "unhealthy" appearing fascicular segments. NAPs can be checked again: the "healthy" appearing fascicles should conduct an NAP, while the "unhealthy" ones may not. In this case, a split repair can be performed by resecting and grafting only the portion of the nerve that did not show regenerative potential.

Internal neurolysis can also be performed in cases of neuritic pain that did not respond to nonoperative measures supervised by a "pain service," including maximal medications, a transcutaneous electrical nerve stimulation unit, and sympathetic blocks, when indicated.

The senior author does not splint the extremity following nerve repairs. Immediately postoperatively, early motion of the extremity is begun so as to prevent stiffness and to facilitate nerve gliding. Serial clinical examinations are performed every 3 to 6 months to monitor for pain control and proximal reinnervation. Electrical studies are used postoperatively to confirm that reinnervation is occurring in an orderly fashion. Inter.sive physical and occupational therapy is encouraged throughout the rehabilitation.

Outcomes

Detailed results for specific patterns of brachial plexus injury and individual nerves have been reported by the senior author.[30] For brachial plexus lesions, recovery rates in patients with C5, C6, and upper trunk lesions are best and those with C8, T1, and lower trunk lesions are extremely poor (because of this, these lesions are generally not operated upon when these are the only elements injured). Approximately 30% of patients with C5/6 lesions regain significant function spontaneously; C5/6 lesions are also the most favorable group to repair/reconstruct. Recovery of the biceps and supraspinatus muscles is better than the deltoid muscles, and good motor function can be achieved in these muscles in more than 50% of cases. Lesions of C5, C6, and C7 fare surprisingly well, even though fewer patients recover spontaneously and root(s) are more likely to be avulsed. In C5-T1 lesions with flail arms, the spontaneous recovery of function is poor and rarely occurs. These patients can be helped with salvage procedures, usually involving nerve transfers, which may restore shoulder abduction and elbow flexion. In addition, protective sensation can be obtained in over 50% of cases.

Infraclavicular lesions occur less frequently than supraclavicular lesions, but as a whole, have a better outcome. Favorable infraclavicular lesions include lateral cord to musculocutaneous and median nerves, posterior cord to axillary and radial nerves,[19] and even medial cord to median nerve. The most unfavorable infraclavicular lesion is medial cord to ulnar nerve (unless neurolysis alone is performed because of a regenerative NAP).

For peripheral nerve lesions, the following generalizations can be made. Neurolysis alone after positive NAPs produces good or better results in over 90% of cases, and is the usual procedure for entrapments. Direct end-to-end repairs do better than graft repairs when there is no tension. Graft repair, however, can produce good results in such cases. Good predictors are based on the age of the patient, the length of repair, repair less than 1 year after injury, and a shorter length of regeneration necessary to the end organ with more distal lesions. The best results have been obtained with grafting the radial, femoral, and tibial nerves. Poor results have been obtained with grafting proximal ulnar nerves, peroneal nerve grafts (especially grafts greater than 3 inches for stretch injuries), and the peroneal division of the sciatic nerve.

Specific Athletic Injuries

Spinal Accessory Nerve

The spinal accessory nerve (cranial nerve XI) is a pure motor nerve that innervates both the sternocleidomastoid and trapezius muscles. After exiting the jugular foramen, it innervates the sternomastoid muscle. The nerve crosses obliquely in the posterior triangle to innervate the trapezius. It runs superficially and is especially susceptible to injury about 1 inch above the clavicle (just distal to its sternomastoid innervation).

Sports-related injuries typically occur as a result of direct trauma (such as from a stick in lacrosse or hockey, or from a helmet in football). Wrestlers may sustain traction or compression to the accessory nerve by the cross-face or neck maneuver. Patients present with shoulder pain and difficulty with shoulder abduction. Examination reveals a drooping shoulder and weakness of shoulder elevation. Weakness of shoulder abduction is due to lack of scapular stability rather than muscle weakness per se. Lateral winging of the scapula is also present. The winging of the scapula from spinal accessory nerve lesions differs from the more typical winging from long thoracic nerve palsies. In accessory nerve lesions, the winging is best brought out with the elbow flexed or the arm adducted; in long thoracic nerve lesions, the winging is manifested with the arm abducted in a forward fashion and the elbow fully extended.

Upper Extremity

Brachial Plexus

The brachial plexus is usually formed from C5-T1 nerve roots, although occasionally there are contributions from C4 or T2. These nerves form the upper, middle, and lower trunks which subsequently subdivide into divisions, then the lateral, posterior, and medial cords, and then the peripheral nerves.

Mechanisms causing brachial plexus injuries are based on traction, compression, or a combination. If the arm is pulled cranially, the lower roots are more vulnerable (Figure 8B). If the arm is pulled in a caudal direction, the upper roots are exposed to increased traction (Figure 8A). Increased force or speed can cause damage to any or all roots in any direction. The weakest point of the plexus is at the level of the rootlets. Compression may occur from fractures, scarring, or edema at a site between the clavicle and first rib. Frequently, some plexal elements are affected more severely and more diffusely than others.

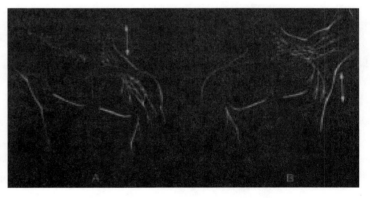

Figure 8: Different patterns of brachial plexus injury are due to the position of the arm to the body. **A)** Traction of the arm in a cranial direction places at risk the lower elements of the brachial plexus. **B)** Traction of the arm in a caudal direction places at risk the upper elements of the brachial plexus. (Reproduced with permission from Kline DG, Lusk MD: Management of athletic brachial plexus injuries, in Schneider RC, Kennedy JC, Plant ML (eds): *Sports Injuries. Mechanisms, Prevention, and Treatment*)

Burners or stingers are transient injuries to the shoulder and upper arm that affect the C5 and C6 nerve segments most frequently. They have been reported in over 50% of football players, but are also seen in wrestlers, weightlifters, and boxers. Despite being underreported, they represent one of the most common neurological disorders affecting athletes. The site of the lesion is controversial, occurring either at the level of the spinal cord, the nerve root, or the plexus. Typically, individuals present with burning in the arm lasting several seconds and weakness (primarily the deltoid, spinati, and biceps) lasting minutes before resolving completely. In approximately 10% of cases, symptoms and findings may be prolonged.[49] Burners may result from traction injuries to the plexus or cervical roots, or direct blows to the plexus at Erb's point. Frequently, common mechanisms identified are ipsilateral shoulder depression, neck extension, and contralateral rotation. When full strength and cervical range of motion have returned, the athlete may return to play.

For persistent symptoms, further workup consisting of cervical radiographs, MRI, and electrodiagnostic studies may be necessary. Individuals with repeated burners should also be evaluated for cervical stenosis. All affected athletes should use neck rolls and elevated shoulder pads. They should undergo neck and shoulder strengthening exercises and learn proper techniques for blocking and tackling.

The vast majority of athletic brachial plexus injuries are of a contusive/stretch type. The senior author has treated a variety of athletes with serious brachial plexus injuries including football players, sledders, snow and water skiers, and bicyclists or dirt bike riders. Typically, injuries involved C5, C6, and C7, although other patterns have been treated, including C8, T1, or flail arms. Supraclavicular injuries are associated with cervical or clavicle fractures and infraclavicular injuries with shoulder dislocations and vascular injuries.

Brachial neuritis (acute brachial neuropathy, neuralgic amyotrophy, or Parsonage-Turner syndrome) is an idiopathic form of brachial plexopathy that can affect athletes.[23] It may occur after a viral illness, an immunization, or trauma. Individuals usually present with shoulder pain followed several days later by shoulder or extremity weakness unilaterally or bilaterally. The brachial plexus is diffusely but disparately affected, and the long thoracic, suprascapular, axillary, and anterior interosseous nerves are commonly involved. The phrenic nerve and trapezius may also be involved. Electrodiagnostic studies can help diagnose this entity and rule out other sites of involvement. Improvement occurs over months, but recovery may not be complete. Scapular winging may persist. Treatment is initially based on pain control and then on rehabilitation.

Thoracic outlet syndrome can occur in athletes and give rise to chronic symptoms of lower trunk brachial plexus compression or irritation.[26,42,53] This syndrome is controversial and refers to a spectrum of neurovascular compressive or irritative syndromes. In particular, the brachial plexus or the subclavian artery or vein may be compressed at the interscalene triangle, the costoclavicular interval, or near the subcoracoid space. In the majority of patients, thoracic outlet syndrome is subjective rather than true (neurological) or vascular.

Symptomatic thoracic outlet syndrome is a clinical diagnosis based on subjective complaints without objective findings. Patients typically present with neck and shoulder pain, upper limb paresthesias, hand weakness, and fatigability. These patients characteristically have normal neurological, radiographic, and electrodiagnostic examinations. The presence of a positive thoracic outlet maneuver (e.g., Roos, Adson's, Wright's, costoclavicular tests, or Tinel's sign) is not especially helpful since they occur in over 50% of the normal population. Symptoms may be due to a depressed shoulder girdle or hypertrophied muscles and may be seen in swimmers, baseball pitchers, tennis players, quarterbacks, wrestlers, and weightlifters.

The diagnosis of true thoracic outlet syndrome is rare but can be made when objective findings (and electrical studies) of a neurological deficit support the subjective complaints and can be localized to the plexus, typically the lower trunk. Radiographs often reveal bony abnormalities such as a cervical rib or an elongated cervical transverse process, although these may not be present in many (Figure 9). Cervical ribs can be found in about 1% of the population, but only 10% of these individuals will develop symptoms of thoracic outlet syndrome. A variety of fibrous bands have also been implicated. The senior author has treated weightlifters, wrestlers, tennis players, and golfers with neurological thoracic outlet syndrome.

Patients with vascular thoracic outlet syndrome have vascular complaints. Depending on whether arterial or venous compression is present, individuals may have ischemic

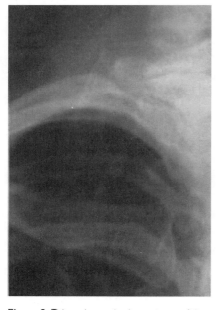

Figure 9: This swimmer had symptoms of thoracic outlet syndrome. Plain film shows a large cervical rib. (Reproduced with permission from Kline DG, Hudson AR (eds): *Nerve Injuries. Operative Results for Major Nerve Injuries, Entrapments, and Tumors.* Philadelphia, Pa: WB Saunders, 1995)

pain that is exercise- or position-related, coolness or pallor of the hands, cyanosis, or edema. Although rare, when it occurs, cervical ribs are commonly identified. Arteriography or venography may be helpful. Some patients may have mixed symptoms of neurovascular compression.

Suprascapular Nerve

The suprascapular nerve is derived predominantly from C5 fibers, with a lesser contribution from C6 and sometimes C4. It originates from the distal portion of the upper trunk. The nerve runs in the posterior triangle of the neck and beneath the trapezius. It follows the omohyoid muscle to the scapula where it typically passes under the transverse scapular ligament. Approximately 1 cm distal to this ligament, it innervates the supraspinatus muscle. It continues around the lateral border of the scapular spine and passes through the spinoglenoid notch, often under a spinoglenoid ligament. It then innervates the infraspinatus muscle. The suprascapular nerve is primarily a motor nerve, but also innervates the shoulder joint.

Suprascapular nerve injury occurs from traction, repetitive trauma, or compression (by ganglia). Traction may cause injury by the "sling effect."[43] Acute trauma, such as from a direct blow to it near Erb's point or following an anterior shoulder dislocation, may also occur. Anatomic variations such as anomalous transverse scapular ligaments may be predisposing factors, especially in those in whom there is bilateral involvement.

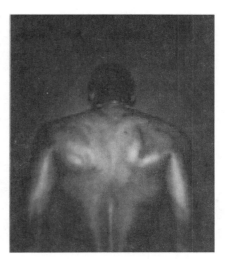

The most common levels of injury are at the transverse scapular ligament or more distally at the spinoglenoid notch. Patients present with posterior shoulder pain and shoulder weakness. Injury at the transverse scapular ligament typically results in combined supraspinatus and infraspinatus weakness and atrophy, and patients have weakness in initiating shoulder abduction and external rotation of the arm. Injury at the spinoglenoid notch results in isolated infraspinatus weakness and atrophy; patients have normal abduction but weak external rotation, and may not have pain. Cutaneous sensation is normal in patients with suprascapular nerve lesions.

Suprascapular nerve lesions have been found in up to 30% of volleyball players.[16,25] In these players, lesions are frequently at the distal site,[17] and some have linked the selective vulnerability to a "floating serve." Suprascapular nerve lesions have also been described in weightlifters and baseball pitchers (Figure 10); other athletes with these injuries include football players, swimmers, boxers, wrestlers, handball players, backpackers, fencers, and parasailors.

Figure 10: This professional baseball pitcher had a suprascapular palsy involving the dominant right throwing arm. Atrophy of the spinati muscles can be seen.

Long Thoracic Nerve

The long thoracic nerve is a pure motor nerve, derived from branches from C5, C6, and C7 and sometimes the C4 and C8 nerve roots that are given off just distal to the neural foramina. The nerve passes deep to the brachial plexus, through the medial scalene muscle, and then runs deep to upper trunk divisions and beneath the clavicle. It courses to the anterolateral aspect of the chest wall where it innervates the serratus anterior muscle and helps stabilize the scapula.

Injury to the long thoracic nerve may occur in athletes, particularly backpackers, weightlifters,[51] and rapellers. Reports also exist of these injuries in tennis, volleyball, and football players, wrestlers, golfers, bowlers, archers, and gymnasts.

Patients with a long thoracic nerve paralysis have shoulder pain and difficulty with scapular movement. Weakness of the serratus anterior results in scapular winging. Injuries may occur after acute trauma (such as after missing a golf ball) or a direct blow to the chest wall. It may also occur from exertion during prolonged exercise or microtrauma from repeated upward movements of the arm, possibly in combination with shoulder girdle fatigue.[56] When a specific mechanism does not exist or more widespread neurological deficit is manifested clinically or electrically, neuralgic amyotrophy must be considered.

Axillary Nerve

The axillary nerve is derived from C5 and C6 nerve roots. It originates from the posterior cord and is the last branch from it before the radial nerve continues. It passes through the quadrilateral space and supplies motor innervation to the deltoid and teres minor and sensory innervation to a small (variable) area of skin in the proximal, lateral arm. Patients with axillary nerve lesions present with shoulder pain and weakness of arm abduction. Some athletes have little functional loss due to compensation by other muscles of the rotator cuff.

Athletes may develop axillary nerve lesions following direct trauma,[27,39,40] typically a direct blow to the posterior shoulder such as in football, wrestling, or hockey. It is also the most common nerve to be affected in anterior shoulder dislocations. Axillary nerve lesions may also occur in association with other shoulder peripheral nerve lesions (such as the suprascapular nerve).

A quadrilateral space syndrome has been popularized by Cahill and Palmer[7] in overhead throwers, but is also described in volleyball players.[38] It is due to compression of the posterior humeral circumflex artery and axillary nerve within the quadrilateral space. Patients may present with aching pain and vague paresthesias in the area of the shoulder. These symptoms typically are worse with overhead activities. Examination reveals point tenderness posteriorly in the quadrilateral space.[34] Neurological examination and electrodiagnostic studies are commonly normal. Arteriography performed with the arm abducted and externally rotated demonstrates an occluded posterior humeral circumflex artery. When surgery is performed in symptomatic patients who failed conservative treatment, fibrous bands within the quadrilateral space or a hypertrophied teres minor are revealed.

Musculocutaneous Nerve

The musculocutaneous nerve is derived primarily from C6 with contributions from C5 and C7. It branches from the lateral cord of the brachial plexus and enters the arm beneath or distal to the coracoid process. It penetrates the coracobrachialis (which it innervates), and then innervates the biceps and brachialis muscles. At the elbow level, it continues as the lateral antebrachial cutaneous nerve that provides sensation to the lateral aspect of the forearm. Patients with musculocutaneous nerve lesions present with elbow flexion weakness and forearm numbness.

Athletes may develop musculocutaneous nerve lesions following direct trauma such as from blows to the proximal arm or after shoulder dislocations.[28] Weightlifters may develop these lesions following strenuous exercise, possibly related to muscle hypertrophy.[3]

Athletes may also develop isolated lesions of the lateral cutaneous branch.[2] The nerve may be compressed by the lateral edge of the biceps tendon. Patients with this lesion present with elbow pain and dysesthesias in the lateral forearm. Symptoms may be exacerbated with elbow extension and forearm pronation. It has been described in tennis and racquetball players as well as swimmers and weightlifters and is possibly related to repetitive forearm rotation.

Radial Nerve

The radial nerve is a continuation of the posterior cord (C5-T1). In the arm, the radial nerve is vulnerable to injury where it emerges between the long and lateral heads of the triceps in the proximal arm and at the spiral groove of the humerus. Just distal to the level of the elbow joint, it bifurcates into the posterior interosseous nerve (motor) and the superficial radial nerve (sensory). The posterior interosseous nerve passes between the two heads of the supinator and then arborizes into smaller muscle branches. The superficial radial nerve continues distally beneath the brachioradialis muscle toward the wrist.

Injury to the radial nerve in the axilla is rare. It produces a complete palsy resulting in paralysis of the triceps, brachioradialis, wrist extensors, supinator, finger and thumb extensors, and the abductor pollicis longus as well as sensory abnormalities in the arm, forearm, and dorsal hand.

Injury to the radial nerve in the arm occurs more commonly. A lesion at this level results in wrist and finger drop with complete radial sensory loss but with normal triceps strength (these oblique branches are given off in the axilla). High radial nerve palsy may result from humeral shaft fractures following falls, direct trauma, or muscle contraction (as in arm wrestling). It may also occur due to a fibrous arch of the lateral[33] or long head of the triceps associated with heavy exercise.[32,35,52] Those affected include tennis players,[41] weightlifters, and discus throwers. Sinson et al[47] reported their experience with "windmill" softball pitchers.

Injury to the posterior interosseous nerve may occur due to the following: fibrous bands from the radiocapitellar joint; recurrent vascular leash; the extensor carpi radialis brevis; the leading edge of the supinator (arcade of Frohse); or within or at the distal edge of the supinator. Patients present with proximal forearm pain and finger drop. There is no sensory abnormality. Wrist extension occurs in a radial direction due to weakness of the extensor carpi ulnaris; the extensor carpi radialis longus is innervated more proximally. Among those treated for posterior interosseous nerve paralysis is a Frisbee player.[18] The senior author has treated tennis players with this lesion.

Compression of the posterior interosseous nerve occurring by the same structures may give rise to the clinical entity of the radial tunnel syndrome or refractory tennis elbow syndrome.[31,44] Examination reveals maximal tenderness over the supinator in the proximal forearm rather than at the lateral epicondyle. Resisted extension of the long finger with the elbow extended or resisted supination of the forearm with the elbow flexed may reproduce symptoms. Electrodiagnostic studies are typically normal. Repetitive forearm pronation and supination or eccentric contraction of the forearm musculature have been proposed as causes of the compression. It has been described in racquet players, weightlifters, and throwing athletes.

Injury to the superficial radial nerve can occur in athletes. Individuals present with dysesthesias near the anatomic snuffbox and the dorsoradial aspect of the hand and thumb. The nerve may be compressed as it emerges from the extensor carpi radialis longus and brachioradialis tendons in the distal third of the forearm.[11] These patients may have percussion tenderness at the site of irritation. The Finkelstein test was described initially for first compartment extensor tendinitis but can also be positive in patients with superficial radial nerve compression. The patient grabs one's flexed thumb and ulnar deviates and palmar flexes one's wrist; pain is produced along the course of the superficial radial nerve. This lesion may occur in athletes who perform pronation/supination activities. The nerve may also be compressed where it runs superficially near the radial styloid process. This is typically due to extrinsic compression, such as from a wristband or a racquetball strap. Some believe that dorsal wrist pain may be due to posterior interosseous nerve innervation of the wrist capsule. The nerve may be irritated locally or compressed by a ganglion. This has been described in gymnasts and weightlifters.

Median Nerve

The median nerve (C6-T1) receives contribution from both the lateral and medial cords. It courses down the medial arm near the brachial artery. Just above the arm, it may pass under the ligament of Struthers, an anomalous ligament associated with a bony supracondylar spur. This anatomic complex has been identified in less than 1% of the population. Typically, it presents as an incidental finding, although rare reports of median (or sometimes even ulnar) nerve compression exist. At the elbow and proximal forearm level, it passes beneath the following structures, which may compress it: the lacertus fibrosus (bicipital aponeurosis), the superficial head of the pronator teres, and the flexor digitorum superficialis arch.

Compression of the median nerve at the elbow region may result in a controversial pain syndrome called the "pronator syndrome." Patients present with pain localized to the proximal volar forearm. They may complain of numbness in the radial 3½ digits. Neurological examination is typically normal, but there may be altered sensation in the median nerve distribution. Tenderness over the pronator teres muscle is characteristic. Provocative tests may help to further localize the compression site: resisted elbow flexion and forearm supination (lacertus fibrosus); resisted pronation with the elbow extended (pronator teres); or resisted flexion of the middle finger proximal interphalangeal joint (flexor digitorum superficialis). Electrodiagnostic studies are usually normal. Athletes including baseball pitchers and weightlifters with hypertrophied muscles or those involved in repetitive forearm movements have developed this syndrome.

The anterior interosseous nerve branch may be compressed by fibrous bands of the deep head of the pronator teres and, on occasion, the flexor digitorum superficialis. Patients with anterior interosseous nerve compression have weakness of the flexor pollicis longus, the flexor digitorum to the index and sometimes the long fingers, and the pronator quadratus. They are unable to make an "O" sign and instead have a "square" pinch due to weakness of the terminal phalanges of the thumb and index finger. They have normal sensation. This has been reported in tennis players, possibly related to intermittent strenuous resisted forearm rotation as well as by a forearm tennis elbow band.[15]

The median nerve is commonly compressed at the wrist at the level of the transverse carpal ligament. This nerve traverses the carpal tunnel with the nine flexor tendons. Patients may present with localized wrist or forearm pain, paresthesias in the radial 3½ digits, and weakness in the hand. Symptoms may be exacerbated at night or following activity or dependency. Examination commonly reveals a positive compression, percussion, and Phalen's test at the wrist. Sensibility in the radial 3½ digits may be altered, and there may be weakness in the median innervated lumbricals, opponens pollicis, and abductor pollicis brevis. Thenar atrophy is a late finding.

Carpal tunnel syndrome has been reported in athletes who are involved in repetitive sustained gripping, those who maintain their wrists hyperflexed or hyperextended, or those exposed to vibration. It may also occur due to direct trauma to the wrist, in association with wrist fractures or dislocations, or with tenosynovitis. It is especially common in cyclists,[5] but has been reported in a variety of athletes including rowers, bodybuilders, golfers, swimmers, climbers, and wheelchair athletes.[6,14]

The ulnar digital nerve of the thumb may be compressed in bowlers[12] and in baseball or tennis players. Patients present with tenderness at the ulnar aspect of the thumb, metacarpophalangeal joint crease, and a sensory disturbance in the distribution of the nerve. Examination may also reveal percussion tenderness over the nerve. Neural irritation is due to repetitive trauma against the bowling-ball thumb hole ("bowler's thumb") or the bat or racquet handle. Other digital nerves may also be affected by extrinsic pressure in athletes participating in sports, such as the radial digital nerve to the index finger in racquetball players.

Ulnar Nerve

The ulnar nerve (C7, C8, and T1) is the terminal branch of the medial cord of the brachial plexus. This nerve courses down the arm near the median nerve, posterior to the intermuscular septum. In the distal arm, it commonly passes through the arcade of Struthers, then continues distally in the ulnar groove. The nerve passes through the cubital tunnel and between the two heads of the flexor carpi ulnaris. At the elbow, the ulnar nerve is most especially susceptible to direct injury where it lies relatively exposed in the notch region, although it may become compressed within the cubital tunnel. Additional compression sites have been described and play an important role in cases of failed ulnar nerve transposition, namely the arcade of Struthers, the medial intermuscular septum, the flexor carpi ulnaris aponeurosis, and the deep flexor-pronator aponeurosis.

Anatomic variations or pathological processes can affect the ulnar nerve. Ulnar nerve instability is present in 16% of normal individuals.[8] More commonly, it results in subluxation (movement of the nerve out of the groove but not over the epicondyle) than in dislocation (movement anterior to the medial epicondyle). However, Childress[8] maintained that ulnar nerve subluxation places the ulnar nerve in a more vulnerable location than an ulnar nerve that has dislocated. Pathology of neighboring structures, including the medial collateral ligament and the medial epicondyle, are important in athletes and can result in ulnar nerve compression. Secondary deformities such as arthritis, loose bodies, calcifications, or cubitus varus/valgus may result in ulnar nerve lesions. Muscle variations such as an anconeus epitrochlear or a hypertrophied triceps muscle[50] (Figure 11) can cause dynamic ulnar nerve compression.

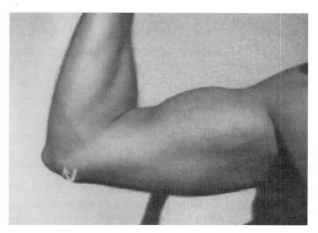

Figure 11: This Olympic swimmer has had snapping, medial elbow pain, and intermittent ulnar nerve symptoms due to coexisting snapping of the medial triceps and dislocating ulnar nerves over the medial epicondyle. More recently, those symptoms interfered with training despite periods of rest. Surgery in this instance must address the dislocating ulnar nerve, the snapping (dislocating) medial portion of the hypertrophied triceps, and the ulnar nerve irritation. Failure to treat the triceps *(arrow)* can result in persistent snapping after an otherwise successful ulnar nerve transposition.

Patients with ulnar nerve lesions at the elbow typically present with elbow pain, sensory abnormalities in the ulnar 1½ digits, and hand weakness. Examination commonly reveals tenderness over the nerve in the notch area, abnormal sensibility in the ulnar 1½ digits and the dorso-ulnar aspect of the hand, as well as intrinsic weakness in the hand and mild clawing of the ulnar 2 digits. Hypothenar and first web space atrophy may be a late presentation. A positive Froment's sign and elbow flexion test are frequently present.

Ulnar nerve lesions at the elbow commonly occur in baseball players, possibly due to compression secondary to inflammation, scarring, or bony irregularities within the ulnar groove, stretch from dynamic valgus forces, or friction from ulnar nerve instability. Javelin throwers, weightlifters,[10] and tennis players also develop ulnar nerve lesions at the elbow. Repetitive flexion/extension activities have been implicated in wheelchair athletes as well.[6,14]

The ulnar nerve is also vulnerable at the wrist. The nerve passes between the pisiform and the hook of the hamate in Guyon's canal. Within Guyon's canal, the ulnar nerve divides into a superficial branch that supplies sensation to the ulnar palm and ulnar 1½ digits and the deep branch which innervates the ulnar intrinsics.

Patients with ulnar nerve lesions at the wrist present with wrist pain, sensory abnormalities in the ulnar 1½ digits, and hand weakness, especially grip or pinch. Findings on examination vary depending on whether the ulnar nerve and/or its branches are involved. Wrist-level lesions could have a combination of the following: tenderness over the ulnar nerve at the wrist, sensory abnormalities in the ulnar 1½ digits but not on the dorsal aspect of the hand, weakness of the ulnar intrinsics, atrophy of the hypothenar and interossei, and clawing of the ulnar 2 digits (clawing is typically more prominent in patients with ulnar nerve lesions at the wrist than it is with elbow-level lesions).

Ulnar nerve lesions at the wrist are common in cyclists ("handlebar neuropathy") due to prolonged wrist position with a sustained grip and pressure on the palm. Martial arts participants, handball players, and gymnasts experience repetitive trauma to the wrist or palms and are at risk of developing these lesions, as are athletes who perform push-ups. Ulnar nerve compression may occur as a result of surgery for ulnar artery aneurysms or wrist fractures.

Lower Extremity

Pudendal Nerve

The pudendal nerve is derived from the S2, S3, and S4 roots. It passes through the greater sciatic notch below the piriformis and through the lesser sciatic notch to enter the perineum. The pudendal nerve supplies sensation to the anal and genital regions. Prolonged cycling has resulted in pudendal nerve compression.

Lateral Femoral Cutaneous Nerve

The lateral femoral cutaneous nerve is a pure sensory nerve derived from the L2 and L3 roots. It emerges from the abdomen by passing approximately 1 cm medial to the anterior superior iliac spine. The nerve then crosses the sartorius and takes on a more superficial position after it has pierced the fascia lata. It provides sensation to the antero-lateral thigh.

Patients with "meralgia paresthetica" have dysesthetic pain in the anterolateral thigh. The nerve is vulnerable to injury near the bony prominence of the anterior superior iliac spine or distally where the nerve is subcutaneous. Athletes may sustain injury to this nerve from a tightfitting weightlifting belt, from hip pointers, or from repetitive flexion/extension of the hip as described in gymnastics or rope skipping.

Femoral Nerve

The femoral nerve forms from the ventral rami of the L2, L3, and L4 nerves. It passes between the psoas and iliacus muscles and exits the abdomen after innervating the ilio-psoas, passing beneath the inguinal ligament through the femoral canal. At this point, it arborizes to innervate the quadriceps and sartorius muscles and supply sensation to the anterior thigh and the medial leg (saphenous nerve).

Patients with complete femoral nerve lesions present with hip flexion and knee extensor weakness and anterior thigh and medial leg numbness. Their knees buckle when they walk. The quadriceps reflex is diminished. These lesions occur following retroperitoneal hematomas or after hyperextension injuries of the hip in dancers, gymnasts, long jumpers, or football players, and are sometimes related to partial iliopsoas ruptures.

Athletes may also injure their femoral nerve at the thigh level, presenting with weak knee extension but normal hip flexion. This type of injury might occur following an anterior thigh hematoma, a compartment syndrome, or a femur fracture.

Sciatic Nerve

The sciatic nerve is the largest nerve in the body. It is derived from the L4, L5, S1, S2, and S3 nerves. It exits the pelvis through the sciatic notch. It typically passes beneath the piriformis and traverses the gluteal region. It then continues down the posteromedial aspect of the thigh. The sciatic nerve is composed of two trunks or anatomically distinct divisions: the peroneal division is more lateral and the tibial is medial. These two divisions become separate in the distal thigh. The peroneal division is more susceptible to injury for unknown reasons.

At the buttock level, sciatic nerve lesions may occur following direct blunt trauma from falls, hip fractures, or posterior hip dislocations. In addition, it has been described following prolonged cycling.[20] Patients may have buttock pain that radiates distally, sensory abnormalities in the entire foot and leg, motor weakness affecting the hamstrings as well as those muscles below the knee, and a diminished ankle jerk. In the thigh, sciatic nerve lesions may occur following femur fractures. Hamstring weakness would be less affected at this level.

Common Peroneal Nerve and Its Branches

The common peroneal nerve is the continuation of the lateral division of the sciatic nerve and is derived from the L4 to S2 roots. It passes laterally through the popliteal fossa, behind the surgical neck of the fibula, and winds around the fibular neck, where it is susceptible to injury. It then passes through an arcade of the peroneus longus and trifurcates into the deep peroneal, superficial peroneal nerve, and an articular branch. The deep peroneal nerve passes into the anterior compartment of the leg, supplies the muscles for foot dorsiflexion and toe extension, and provides sensation to the dorsal first web space. The superficial peroneal nerve descends in the lateral compartment of the leg, innervates the foot everter, and provides sensation to the dorsolateral foot.

Patients with peroneal nerve lesions present with proximal leg or knee pain, dysesthesias, and weakness in the foot. Examination reveals tenderness on percussion over the fibular neck. Depending on the branch or branches involved, weakness may be present in dorsiflexion, foot eversion, or toe extension, with decreased sensation in the dorsal foot.

The peroneal nerve may be injured by direct blunt trauma, stretch, or compression. Direct blows to the fibular neck may result from hockey sticks or pucks, football helmets, or soccer kicks. Stretch injuries commonly occur to the knee, especially the posterolateral corner. These may result from knee dislocation and ligament disruption (Figure 12) or superior tibiofibular dislocation. These injuries are common in football and soccer players. Injuries may extend along a wide segment of the peroneal nerve proximally to the distal sciatic nerve (and occasionally affect the tibial division as well). Swelling by edema or hematoma may compress the nerve especially near the fibular tunnel or at the intermuscular septum. Hematoma may track upward to cause peroneal nerve compression in the proximal leg after inversion ankle sprains.[37]

Compartment syndromes may occur in athletes from trauma involving the anterior and/or lateral compartments. They may occur acutely following direct blows or be associated with fractures. Chronic injuries in runners are typically exercise-induced, presenting with tightness, pain, and paresthesias, although rarely motor loss. The diagnosis of a compartment syndrome is established by measuring compartment pressures.

The deep peroneal ("anterior tarsal tunnel syndrome") and superficial peroneal nerves may be compressed on the dorsal aspect of the foot and give rise to localized foot pain and dysesthesias in their areas of innervation. These are typically related to footwear and may be due to tight ski boots or ice skates.

Tibial Nerve

The tibial nerve is the continuation of the medial portion of the sciatic nerve and is derived from the L4 to S3 nerve roots. It passes in the popliteal fossa near the popliteal artery, through the soleus arch, and descends in the posterior compartment protected by muscles. At this level, the tibial nerve gives off branches for foot plantar flexion, toe flexion and inversion (posterior tibialis), and sensation to the posterior calf. At the ankle, the tibial nerve passes through the tarsal tunnel (a fibro-osseous tunnel posterior to the medial malleolus) along with the posterior tibialis, flexor digitorum, tibial artery, and flexor hallucis. At the distal end of the tarsal tunnel, the tibial nerve divides into medial and lateral plantar nerves, which provide sensation to the plantar aspect of the foot and toes and innervate the foot intrinsics.

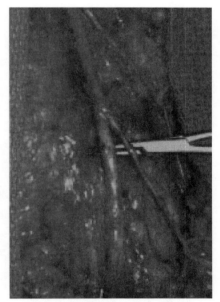

Figure 12: This skier sustained ligamentous disruption and complete peroneal nerve lesion during a high-speed fall. Stretch lesions of the peroneal nerve typically involve a long segment of the nerve and require grafts several inches in length. At times, the injury extends proximal enough to involve the distal sciatic nerve. Recovery in these lesions repaired with lengthy grafts is poor. The sural nerve is in vesi-loops.

Injuries of the tibial nerve at the knee level are relatively rare and, when they do occur, usually involve stretch injuries to the tibial nerve from knee injuries (e.g., dislocations with concomitant posterior cruciate ligament or popliteal artery injury). Hematomas can also compress the nerve, especially in the vicinity of the soleus arch. Tibial nerve injuries can also occur following fractures. Patients present with weakness in plantar flexion and toe flexion and dysesthesias in the plantar foot.

Foot and ankle neurological lesions of the tibial nerve are well described in runners,[45] with many of the syndromes related to shoe wear. Patients with tarsal tunnel syndrome present with plantar surface paresthesias or dysesthesias. Intrinsic foot weakness may also occur but is difficult to detect clinically. It may follow ankle sprains or be related to tenosynovitis or fractures, or dislocations of the ankle. Tarsal tunnel syndrome has also been associated with repetitive dorsi/plantar flexion in athletes. Heel pain in athletes is relatively common and is mostly due to musculoskeletal disorders (e.g., plantar fasciitis or bursitis). The differential diagnosis in athletes should include lesions of the medial plantar nerve (jogger's foot), medial calcaneal branch, or the lateral plantar nerve. Finally, lesions of the interdigital nerves (Morton's neuromas) can occur at the level of the intermetatarsal ligament at the metatarsal head. The third interspace is the most frequently affected. Patients present with burning pain radiating to the toe, and symptoms are worse with standing or walking. Morton's neuromas have been described in cross-country skiers, stair-steppers, and dancers, and commonly respond to local measures such as a change of shoes or the use of inserts.

Conclusion

Nerve injuries in the athlete occur relatively frequently and are often associated directly or indirectly to the added stresses of the sport(s). The causes of these neural lesions are commonly acute trauma or more chronic "microtrauma." While any nerve can be involved at any site, certain nerves at certain sites appear to be predisposed to injury in specific sports. Accurate diagnosis and appropriate management of these disorders can only be made if the physician has a thorough understanding of peripheral nerve anatomy, pathoanatomy, and physiology and a knowledge of sports-related injuries. The diagnosis should be established by correlating the detailed medical history and clinical examination with the electrical studies and imaging. Treatment is determined by the mechanism of the injury, the level of the lesion, the nerve involved, and the completeness of the injury.

For the majority of injuries, a period of nonoperative care is suggested. The physician should evaluate the patient for signs of proximal reinnervation based on serial clinical and electrical studies during the 3-6 months after the injury. For patients without timely evidence of reinnervation or those with persistent symptoms or worsening examination, surgery is indicated. The use of nerve action potentials is an important component in intraoperative decision making as to whether to perform neurolysis, resection and repair, or, with plexus lesion, nerve transfers. Outcomes of surgery are variable but are commonly quite gratifying. In general, athletes are extremely motivated individuals and are eager to return not only to their sport (Figure 13) but also to work.

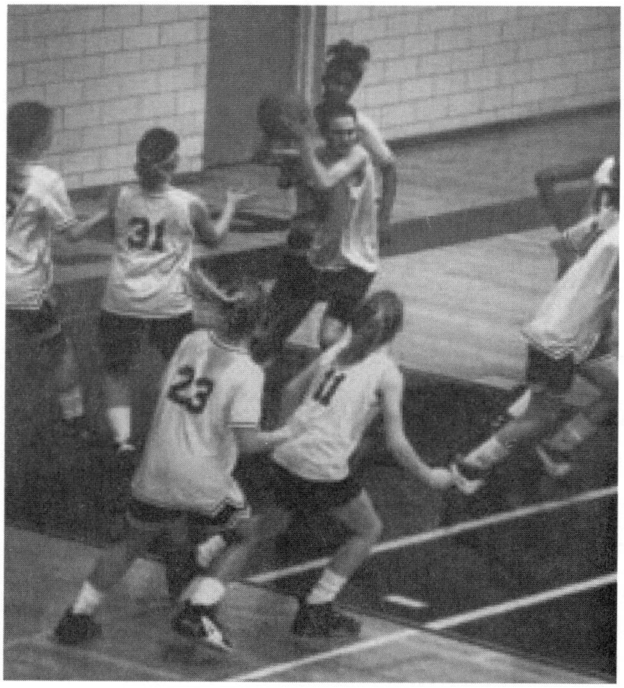

Figure 13: This player has returned to basketball 1¹/2 years after a complete median nerve lesion was treated surgically following a radius and ulnar forearm fracture.

References

1. Allieu Y, Cenac P: Neurotization via the spinal accessory nerve in complete paralysis due to multiple avulsion injuries of the brachial plexus. **Clin Orthop** 237:67-74, 1988
2. Bassett FH, Nunley JA: Compression of the musculocutaneous nerve at the elbow. **J Bone Joint Surg (Am)** 64:1050-1052, 1982
3. Braddom RL, Wolfe C: Musculocutaneous nerve injury after heavy exercise. **Arch Phys Med Rehabil** 59:290-293, 1978
4. Brandt KE, Mackinnon SE: A technique for maximizing biceps recovery in brachial plexus reconstruction. **J Hand Surg** 18A:726-733, 1993
5. Burke ER: Ulnar neuropathy in bicyclists. **Phys Sports Med** 9:53-56, 1981
6. Burnham RS, Steadward R: Upper extremity peripheral nerve entrapments among wheelchair athletes: prevalence, location and risk factor. **Arch Phys Med Rehabil** 75:519-524, 1994
7. Cahill BR, Palmer RE: Quadrilateral space syndrome. **J Hand Surg** 8:65-69, 1983
8. Childress HM: Recurrent ulnar-nerve dislocation at the elbow. **J Bone Joint Surg (Am)** 38:978-984, 1956
9. Chuang DCC: Neurotization procedures for brachial plexus injuries. **Hand Clin** 4:633-645, 1995
10. Dangles CJ, Bilos ZJ: Ulnar neuritis in a world champion weightlifter. **Am J Sports Med** 8:443-445, 1980
11. Dellon AL, Mackinnon SE: Radial sensory nerve entrapment in the forearm. **J Hand Surg** 11A:199-205, 1986
12. Dobyns JH, O'Brien ET, Linscheid RL, et al: Bowler's thumb—diagnosis and treatment: a review of seventeen cases. **J Bone Joint Surg (Am)** 54:751-755, 1972
13. Doi K, Sakai K, Kuwata N, et al: Double free-muscle transfer to restore prehension following a complete brachial plexus avulsion. **J Hand Surg** 20A:408-414, 1995
14. Dozono K, Hachisuka K, Hatada K, et al: Peripheral neuropathies in the upper extremities of paraplegic wheelchair marathon racers. **Paraplegia** 33:208-211, 1995
15. Enzenauer RJ, Nordstrom DM: Anterior interosseous nerve syndrome associated with forearm band treatment of lateral epicondylitis. **Orthopedics** 14:788-790, 1991
16. Ferretti A, Cerullo G, Russo G: Suprascapular neuropathy in volleyball players. **J Bone Joint Surg (Am)** 69:260-263, 1987
17. Ferretti A, De Carli A, Fontana M: Injury of the suprascapular nerve at the spinoglenoid notch. The natural history of infraspinatus atrophy in volleyball players. **Am J Sports Med** 26:759-763, 1998
18. Fraim CJ, Peters BH: Unusual cause of nerve entrapment. **JAMA** 242:2557-2558, 1979
19. Friedman A, Nunley JA, Urbaniak JR, et al: Repair of isolated nerve injuries after infraclavicular brachial plexus injuries: case reports. **Neurosurgery** 27:403-407, 1990
20. Gold S: Unicyclist's sciatica: a case report. **N Engl J Med** 305:231, 1981
21. Gu UD, Zhang GM, Chen DS, et al: Seventh cervical nerve transfer from the contralateral healthy side for treatment of brachial plexus root avulsion. **J Hand Surg** 17B:518-521, 1992
22. Gu Y, Ma M: Use of the phrenic nerve for brachial plexus reconstruction. **Clin Orthop** 323:119-121, 1996
23. Hershman E, Wilbourn AJ, Bergfeld JA: Acute brachial neuropathy in athletes. **Am J Sports Med** 17:655-659, 1989
24. Hirasawa Y, Sakakida K: Sports and peripheral nerve injury. **Am J Sports Med** 11:420-426, 1983
25. Holzgraefe M, Kukowski B, Eggert S: Prevalence of latent and manifest suprascapular neuropathy in high-performance volleyball players. **Br J Sports Med** 28:177-179, 1994
26. Karas SE: Thoracic outlet syndrome. **Clin Sports Med** 9:297-310, 1990
27. Kessler KJ, Uribe JW: Complete isolated axillary nerve palsy in college and professional football players: a report of six cases. **Clin J Sports Med** 4:272-274, 1994
28. Kim SM, Goodrich JA: Isolated proximal musculocutaneous nerve palsy: case report. **Arch Phys Med Rehabil** 65:735-736, 1984
29. Kline DG, Happel LT: A quarter century's experience with intraoperative nerve action potential recording. **Can J Neurol Sci** 20:3-10, 1992
30. Kline DG, Hudson AR: **Nerve Injuries. Operative Results for Major Nerve Injuries, Entrapments, and Tumors.** Philadelphia, Pa: WB Saunders, 1995
31. Lister GD, Belsole RB, Kleinert HE: The radial tunnel syndrome. **J Hand Surg** 4:52-59, 1979
32. Lotem M, Fried A, Levy M, et al: Radial palsy following muscular effort. **J Bone Joint Surg (Br)** 53:500-506, 1971
33. Manske PR: Compression of the radial nerve by the triceps muscle. **J Bone Joint Surg (Am)** 59:835-836, 1977
34. McKowen HC, Voorhies RM: Axillary nerve entrapment in the quadrilateral space: a case report. **J Neurosurg** 66:932-934, 1987
35. Mitsunaga NM, Nakano K: High radial nerve palsy following strenuous muscular activity. A case report. **Clin Orthop** 234:39-42, 1988
36. Nagano A, Tsuyama N, Ochiai N, et al: Direct nerve crossing with the intercostal nerve to treat avulsion injuries of the brachial plexus. **J Hand Surg** 14A:980-985, 1989
37. Nobel W: Peroneal palsy due to hematoma in the common peroneal nerve sheath after distal torsional fractures and inversion ankle sprains. **J Bone Joint Surg (Am)** 48:1484-1495, 1966
38. Paladini D, Dellantonio R, Cinti A, et al: Axillary neuropathy in volleyball players: report of two cases and literature review. **Neurol Neurosurg Psychiatry** 60:345-347, 1996
39. Perlmutter GS, Apruzzese W: Axillary nerve injuries in contact sports. **Sports Med** 26:351-361, 1998
40. Perlmutter GS, Leffert RD, Zarins B: Direct injury to the axillary nerve in athletes playing contact sports. **Am J Sports Med** 25:65-68, 1997
41. Prochaska V, Crosby LA, Murphy RP: High radial nerve palsy in a tennis player. **Orthop Rev** 22:90-92, 1993
42. Rayan GM: Lower trunk brachial plexus compression neuropathy due to cervical rib in young athletes. **Am J Sports Med** 16:77-79, 1988
43. Rengachary SS, Burr D, Lucas S, et al: Suprascapular entrapment neuropathy: a clinical, anatomical and comparative study. Part 2: Anatomical study. **Neurosurgery** 5:447-451, 1979
44. Roles NC, Maudsley RH: Radial tunnel syndrome: resistant tennis elbow as a nerve entrapment. **J Bone Joint Surg (Br)** 54:499-508, 1972
45. Schon LC, Baxter DE: Neuropathies of the foot and ankle in athletes. **Clin Sports Med** 9:489-509, 1990
46. Seddon HJ: Three types of nerve injury. **Brain** 66:238-288, 1943
47. Sinson G, Zager EL, Kline DG: Windmill pitcher's radial neuropathy. **Neurosurgery** 34:1087-1089, 1994
48. Songcharoen P, Mahaisavariya B, Chotigavanich C: Spinal accessory neurotization for restoration of elbow flexion in avulsion injuries of the brachial plexus. **J Hand Surg** 21A:387-390, 1996
49. Speer KP, Bassett FH: The prolonged burner syndrome. **Am J Sports Med** 18:591-594, 1990
50. Spinner RJ, Goldner RD: Snapping of the medial head of the triceps and recurrent dislocation of the ulnar nerve: anatomic and dynamic factors. **J Bone Joint Surg (Am)** 80:239-247, 1998
51. Stanish WD, Lamb H: Isolated paralysis of the serratus anterior muscle: a weight training injury: case report. **Am J Sports Med** 6:385-386, 1978
52. Streib E: Upper radial nerve palsy after muscular effort: report of three cases. **Neurology** 42:1632-1634, 1992
53. Strukel R, Garrick J: Thoracic outlet compression in athletes. **Am J Sports Med** 6:35-39, 1978
54. Sunderland S: **Nerves and Nerve Injuries, 2nd ed.** Edinburgh: Churchill Livingstone, 1978
55. Tiel RL, Happel LT, Kline DG: Nerve action potential recording, method, and equipment. **Neurosurgery** 31:103-109, 1996
56. Vastamaki M, Kauppila LI: Etiologic factors in isolated paralysis of the serratus anterior muscle: a report of 197 cases. **J Shoulder Elbow Surg** 2:240-243, 1993
57. Wilbourn AJ: Electrodiagnostic testing of neurologic injuries in athletes. **Clin Sports Med** 9:229-245, 1990

CHAPTER 7

The Epidemiology of Athletic Injuries

JOHN W. POWELL, PHD, ATC

I n today's secondary school athletic programs, large numbers of boys and girls participate in a wide variety of sports. While sports such as football and basketball maintain
a fairly consistent number of participants, participation is increasing in soccer and
some other sports. These athletic programs provide an environment in which students
can grow and develop physical, mental, and social skills. Student-athletes have numerous
opportunities to develop skills in one or more sports. As these programs continue to
grow, it is the responsibility of school authorities to provide an environment that mini-
mizes the risk of injury.

The risk of injury in physical activity and sports is derived primarily from the nature
of the sport and the specific activities associated with participation. For example, collision sports such as football and ice hockey characteristically have more acute injuries
than sports such as swimming and track, where the injuries are more often associated
with conditions of overuse. Most sports present a general pattern that shows a higher
risk of injury during the game or competition than during the practice session. Additionally, each sport is associated with specific types of injury (e.g., a cauliflower ear in
wrestling and shoulder inflammation in baseball). One injury often associated with collision sports is the concussion or mild traumatic brain injury. This injury often results
from a direct blow to the head or from an acceleration/deceleration force that produces
damage to the tissue of the brain. In sports, the direct blow to the head is generally considered the mechanism that causes the injury. This direct blow may produce focal damage at the site of the impact, damage opposite to the site of impact (counter coup), or
damage to the individual axons in the brain. Detailed discussion of these topics is covered elsewhere in this text.

Historically, "concussion" has been defined by the Committee on Head Injury
Nomenclature of the Congress of Neurological Surgeons as "a clinical syndrome characterized by immediate and transient posttraumatic impairment of neural function, such
as alteration of consciousness and disturbance of vision or equilibrium due to brainstem involvement."[8] In more recent literature, concussion has been described as a
trauma-induced alteration in mental status that may or may not involve a loss of consciousness.[1,12] These injuries may result from a rotational or linear force applied to the
brain from a direct impact or indirect force (i.e., acceleration or deceleration). This

approach includes the classic "ding" associated with a minimal injury to the brain as well as those that may cause permanent disability. In recent literature, the term "mild traumatic brain injury" (MTBI) has been introduced and used to describe a condition of altered mental status that is represented by a wide variety of signs and symptoms. These findings are similar to those described for a concussion and include headache, neck pain, dizziness, nausea, confusion, a feeling of "fogginess," loss of concentration, retrograde amnesia, and tinnitus. This type of definition is useful in research programs regarding MTBI because it allows for a consistent recording of these events across multiple sites. The injury becomes an observable "reportable" incident rather than an incident based on subjective judgment of a variable definition. It is important to remember that the MTBI may result in short- or long-term unconsciousness or no loss of consciousness. The signs and symptoms present at the time of injury may disappear very quickly or may linger for long periods of time. In some rare cases, the initial signs and symptoms may disappear and then reappear with dramatic consequences. To be consistent within discussions in this chapter, the term concussion is considered synonymous with MTBI.

The most challenging issues facing medical and paramedical professionals are the identification of MTBI and the care and management of the injured patient. Once the MTBI has been identified and appropriate medical care made available, the clinician turns to the question of return to participation. How long should the athlete wait to return to collision sports? What is the potential for the player to sustain a second MTBI? Does this second injury create more significant damage than the first one? How can the player be sure that the brain has truly "returned to normal"? The neuroscience and sports medicine communities have identified all of these areas as issues for research. Currently, there are projects that focus on the biological aspects of MTBI, the neuropsychological effects of MTBI from baseline to postinjury and recovery, the natural history of the MTBI and protocols for clinical management of the injured player, and the role of balance in identifying and managing MTBI.[*9,10,13]

The administrators of sports programs also have challenges. They must design and maintain programs that minimize the risk of injury, including MTBI. These administrators must take into consideration the nature of the sport and the activities of the players as they make decisions that will affect the injury risk pattern. Specific areas that require attention are facilities and equipment, player protective equipment, and competition rules and regulations.

The final decisions regarding the player's care and return to participation must combine information from sports medicine clinicians, the coaches, the parents, and the players. In order to evaluate injury-prevention decisions, the sports program administrators must identify and evaluate the current injury pattern and compare it to the pattern that existed prior to the intervention. To provide a foundation for these comparisons, let us examine the historical data regarding the frequency of MTBI in sports, the current knowledge available and information needed to improve the knowledge of prevention, and the care and management of persons with MTBI in the future.

Historical Perspective

Mild traumatic brain injuries have always been a part of competitive athletics. During the 1970s, little attention was paid to this type of injury. In the early 1980s, discussion took a giant leap forward with research that identified some neuropsychological effects associated with MTBI.[2,18] In 1983, an article by Gerberich et al[6] described the magnitude

---

*Personal communication with Elliot Pellman, MD, of the New York Jets and Chairman of the NFL Subcommittee on Mild Traumatic Brain Injury. Also, personal communication with Charles Burke, MD, of the Pittsburgh Penguins and Chairman of the NHL Concussion Committee.

of concussion at the level of high school football. The article was based on data acquired during the 1977 football season. They found that 20% of the reported injuries were concussions, and 14% of the respondents indicated a history of concussion associated a loss of consciousness with the injury. From this work, other authors have projected an annual frequency of 200,000 concussions in high school football. It is important to consider the era for the data collection in this article. In the early 1970s, there was an emphasis on the use of the head as the initial point of contact for blocking and tackling (i.e., "face into the numbers"). Risks associated with this technique were documented, and in 1976, the National Federation of State High School Associations (NFSHSA) football rules committee banned the teaching of this technique in high school football. The players surveyed by Gerberich's study were participants prior to the ban. In addition, football players in the 1970s wore a variety of helmets that have since been discarded due to a perception on the part of the sports medicine community of a lack of protection. While these data provide evidence of a large number of "concussions," they may not reflect accurately the magnitude of the problem for today's high school football player.

During the decade following Gerberich's work, a great deal of discussion flourished among members of the medical and neuroscience community regarding the description and classification of MTBI, the management of persons who suffered MTBIs, and guidelines for the return to competition following MTBI.[3-6,11,19] Boxing and football contributed most of the cases in these early research efforts. As the medical community learned more about the natural history of MTBI, the importance of the injury (regardless of the sport) began to take precedence. The size and scope of the problem grew gradually until the early 1990s, when the issue exploded on the sports pages of daily newspapers. The media and fans fostered this heightened awareness as they learned of high-profile professional athletes who attributed their retirement to repetitive MTBI. Additionally, players who retired for other reasons were being identified with postconcussion syndrome in the months and years following their retirement. As a result, the research areas that are concerned with identification, management, and the long-term effects of MTBI are adding new and exciting information to the professional body of knowledge required to reduce the risk of injury.

It is important to be able to integrate the new knowledge regarding MTBI into programs for prevention. In order to develop a base on which to evaluate these new data, the incidence of MTBI among athletes in various high school sports is discussed.

MTBI in High School Sports

The National Athletic Trainers' Association (NATA) conducted a study of the frequency, type, and severity of injury in selected high school sports for the 1995 through 1997 seasons. Certified athletic trainers at participating high schools recorded the player data, exposure data, and injury data on a daily basis throughout the three academic years of the study. The study included information on the boys' sports programs of football, basketball, soccer, wrestling, and baseball and the girls' sports programs of basketball, soccer, softball, field hockey, and volleyball. An injury that required the player to be removed from the current session was reported. In addition, all fractures (regardless of time loss) and any head injury for which the athletic trainer or team physician conducted an evaluation for MTBI (regardless of time loss) were reported. The data in Table 1 show the estimated number of schools and players participating in the NATA study, in the NFSHSA, and in the U.S. for each of the study sports.[16]

Among the 23,566 reported injuries in the NATA study were 1219 cases of MTBI. The data in Table 2 show the distribution of these injuries over team-seasons, the proportion of MTBIs among all reported injuries in that sport, and the estimated number of players

TABLE 1
ESTIMATED POPULATION AT RISK OF MTBI BASED ON DATA OBTAINED IN NATA STUDY 1995-1997

	No. NATA Schools	No. NATA Players	No. NFSHSA Schools	No. NFSHSA Players	Total No. U.S. High Schools	Total No. U.S. High School Players
Boys' Sports						
Football	400	21,122	13,122	962,138	14,744	1,081,054
Basketball	406	6831	16,632	544,695	18,687	612,016
Baseball	324	6502	14,264	446,237	16,027	501,390
Soccer	315	7539	8491	296,600	9540	333,258
Wrestling	328	8117	8772	225,978	9856	253,908
Girls' Sports						
Basketball	395	6083	16,317	449,185	18,344	504,703
Volleyball	296	4222	12,891	367,251	14,485	412,641
Softball	311	5435	11,891	317,399	13,361	356,628
Soccer	292	6642	6518	209,091	7324	234,934
Field Hockey	128	2805	1471	56,411	1653	63,383
Totals	3195	75,298		3,874,985		4,353,915

in a sport in the U.S. per year. From these data, it appears that the most common activity associated with MTBI in high school sports is collision, either between players or with objects associated with the sport. The injury rates per 1000 athlete exposures were higher for games than for practices in nine of the sports studied, with the exception being a higher injury rate in practice than games in girls' volleyball. Among the sports studied, nearly 80% of the MTBIs resulted in less than 8 days of lost participation time. Of the 1219 reported MTBIs, 56 (4.6%) resulted in time loss greater than 21 days.[17]

From the NATA study, it is clear that MTBIs are most common in football and that there is a potential for players to sustain an MTBI in every sport. It is important that sports medicine clinicians be aware of the nature of the injury and its potential outcomes. A discussion of the MTBIs associated with football serves as an example of one aspect of the difficulties in preventing and managing an MTBI.

What Causes MTBI?

A discussion of MTBIs begins with the mechanism of the injury and the relative opportunities of the injury to occur. The most important sports-related mechanism of MTBI is a direct blow to the head that produces movements of the brain inside the skull. The effect of these impact forces on the brain tissue involves consideration of both linear and rotational forces. Other key components of the brain that influence the extent of the tissue damage from impact are the internal stresses and strains and the material properties of the tissue. There has been a great deal of research regarding the interaction of these forces, as they are relevant to traumatic brain injuries in traffic safety and high-risk sports such as automobile racing. While much is known about the behavior of the brain tissue under these conditions, little is known about the tissue behavior and potential for injury from milder forces.

To evaluate the potential for injury, it is necessary to have a general understanding of the amount of opportunity that exists for an injury to occur. In the case of MTBI, the opportunity for injury can be considered as a function of the nature of the activities of

TABLE 2
REPORTED MTBIs IN HIGH SCHOOL PLAYERS IN NATA STUDY 1995-1997

	No. of Reported MTBIs	Percent of MTBIs*	U.S. Estimate of Total Players
Boys' Sports			
Football	773	7.3%	39,566
Basketball	51	2.6%	4590
Baseball	15	1.7%	1153
Soccer	69	3.9%	3068
Wrestling	128	4.4%	4012
Girls' Sports			
Basketball	63	3.6%	5250
Volleyball	6	1.0%	578
Softball	25	2.7%	1548
Soccer	76	4.3%	3799
Field Hockey	13	2.5%	292
Totals	1219	5.2%	63,856

*Percent MTBIs among all reported injuries.

the players and the potential number of times that the head may sustain a direct impact or indirect force within the context of sports participation. The impact forces may be incidental (unintentional) and occur as a result of the nature of the game or, in some cases, may come from intentional acts such as fighting. There may be impacts from objects associated with the game (e.g., sticks, surfaces, or boundary obstructions) or from game operations equipment. The impacts are sometimes a part of the game as in football or very unusual as in tennis. The important consideration is that an MTBI can occur in any activity regardless of the nature of the activity and that, when the injury occurs, it has a significant potential for lasting effects on the player. Since high school football has the largest number of participants and is most often associated with MTBI, an estimate of the number of head impacts in this sport would provide perspective on the risk of injury.

Head Impacts in High School Football

It is important to have a perspective on the amount of opportunity for an MTBI to occur as we analyze the frequency of the injury and its outcome. To address this issue, we conducted a small survey designed to estimate a conservative number of head impacts in an average season of high school football. The project reviewed 10 films taken during high school football games and counted the number of times there was clear evidence of an impact to the head. Pile-ups in which the head was intentionally impacted were not included. The impacts were classified as head to head, head to body, or head to surface. The data recorded during the analysis reflect the team (offense, defense, or special teams) and type of play (rushing, passing, or kicking). The data recorders for the project were three experienced high school football coaches.

The data collection was conducted on films of five games from a season in which none of the recorders coached a team that was on the film and five games that occurred under the supervision of the three coaches for one of the teams. The data in Table 3 display the results of this analysis. These data can be used to estimate a conservative number of head impacts for high school football.[15]

TABLE 3

ESTIMATES OF HEAD IMPACTS FOR HIGH SCHOOL FOOTBALL

	Sum	Mean	Standard Deviation
Impact Classification			
Head to head	2688	2.26	1.94
Head to body	5015	4.21	1.89
Head to surface	132	0.11	0.33
Team			
Offense	4247	3.57	1.52
Defense	3588	3.01	1.54
Type of Play			
Passing	1982	6.06	2.31
Rushing	700	7.24	2.28
Punting	417	5.02	2.52
Kick off	304	4.54	2.23
Total Head Impacts	7835	6.58	2.48

TABLE 4

ESTIMATED NUMBER OF PARTICIPANTS IN HIGH SCHOOL FOOTBALL IN THE NATA STUDY AND IN THE U.S.

	NATA Study 1995-1997		U.S. Estimates 1995-1997	
	3-Year Total	Average per Season	3-Year Total	Average Per Season
No. of schools	400	133	44,231	14,744
No. of participants	21,122	7041	3,243,163	1,081,054
No. of MTBIs	773	258	76,561	39,566

TABLE 5

ESTIMATED RATE OF SPORTS-RELATED CONCUSSIONS IN HIGH SCHOOL FOOTBALL BASED ON NATA STUDY 1995-1997 FREQUENCY DATA

	NATA Severity Groups	U.S. Annual Estimated MTBIs	Annual Rate of MTBIs/100,000 Players	Severity Adjusted Rates
Minor injury	78%	30,861	2,855	3 per 100 players
Moderate injury	18%	7,122	659	7 per 1000 players
Major injury	4%	1,583	146	15 per 10,000 players
Total	100%	39,566	3,660	3.7 per 100 players

Another area for consideration is the number of schools and players that participate in football annually. According to the NFSHSA Handbook, between 14,000 and 15,000 U.S. high schools offer football.[13] By combining the participation numbers and the frequency estimates, we can estimate the number of head impacts associated with high school football. To keep the math straightforward, we assumed 15,000 schools with an average of 15 games (all levels) per school. We assume that there is an average of 119 plays per high school football game and an average of 6.6 clear head impacts per play (Table 3). Multiplying the head impact data and the participation data results in a conservative estimate of 177 million head impacts annually in high school football games. If we assume that the practice sessions each week contribute at least an equal number of head impacts, then the estimate for sports-related head impacts (game and practice combined) is in the neighborhood of 354 million.

The data in Table 4 show a summary of participation in high school football in the 3-year NATA study. The 400 team-seasons in high school football monitored over 21,000 players and accumulated data from 4685 games and 24,923 practices. The NATA study recorded 10,557 injuries in high school football, including 773 (7.3%) identified as MTBIs. Using an estimated 1,081,054 players per season from the NFSHSA data, it is estimated that 39,566 MTBIs occur over three seasons.[17] Combining these data creates an estimate of approximately 3660 MTBIs per 100,000 players in high school football. Using the NATA study data, if we divide the estimated number of participants by the number of schools, there would be about 53 players per school. Multiplying the rate per 100,000 players by the average number of players per school illustrates approximately two MTBIs per season per school in high school football.

The NATA study used an operational set of categories to describe the relative severity of the injuries that were recorded. The category of "minor injury" restricted the player for 7 days or less; "moderate injury" restricted the player for 8-21 days, and "major injury" restricted the player for more than 21 days. Among the MTBIs reported, an estimated 78% were minor, 18% were moderate, and 4% were major. The data in Table 5 apply the proportions of MTBIs by severity observed in the NATA study to the estimated 39,566 annual MTBIs. Adjusting the denominator groups shows an estimate of three minor injuries per 100 players, seven moderate injuries per 1000 players, and 15 major injuries per 10,000 players. If we assume 50 as an average number of football players per school, the average school would expect one or two major MTBIs in 10 seasons of participation.

The data in Table 6 display the estimated number of MTBIs per 100,000 head impacts from sports-related (practices and games combined) and game-related conditions. It is interesting to note that the rate per 100,000 head impacts under game conditions is slightly higher than for conditions that combine practices and games. This finding is consistent with the idea that the level of risk for games is higher than that for practices for all injury types. A review of the data would seem to indicate that MTBI, given the tremendous potential for head collisions in football, is a relatively infrequent occurrence.

MTBI Prevention

The data from the NATA study show that MTBIs occur in a variety of high school sports. While the general indication is that the vast majority of these injuries have very little effect on the individual's participation, the effect of multiple injuries, either in the same season or over several seasons, is currently unknown. The MTBIs warrant specific attention in the area of prevention and management because of the unique nature of the injury. The foundation of developing an injury-prevention program for high school sports is that, regardless of the preventive steps taken, a certain number of injuries,

TABLE 6

ESTIMATED RATE OF CONCUSSIONS IN HIGH SCHOOL FOOTBALL BY ESTIMATED OPPORTUNITY FOR INJURY AND FREQUENCY IN NATA STUDY 1995-1997

	U.S. Annual Estimated Concussions	Percent of Concussions In Games	Estimated Concussions In Games	Sports-related MTBIs /100,000 Impacts	Game-related MTBIs /100,000 Impacts
Minor injury	30,594	61.0%	18,662	9	11
Moderate injury	7,135	74.1%	5,287	2	3
Major injury	1,838	72.2%	1,327	1	1
Total	39,567		25,276	12	15

including MTBI, will occur. It becomes the task of the injury-prevention team to work toward controlling the number of injuries by approaching the injury pattern from two angles. The program must first focus on preventing the injury and second on minimizing the risk of re-injury for those players who sustain an injury.

To begin the process of developing prevention- or injury-control programs for MTBI, there are three areas for consideration. The program should look at strategies that address the MTBI before it occurs, at the time it occurs, and the time following an injury.

Pre-event Prevention

The pre-event phase of injury control emphasizes things that can be done to minimize the number of MTBIs. These areas include:

1. Establish the presence of a history of brain injury for each participant.
2. Teach the player about protecting the head during participation.
3. Provide proper instruction in techniques that minimize the risk of injury.
4. For sports that require the use of helmets,
   - players should be informed of the warnings regarding the use of the protective helmets,
   - players must be taught that the helmet cannot protect from all head injuries,
   - players must realize the importance of examining their helmet daily in order to identify potential areas that require maintenance, and
   - the protection afforded by the helmet is based on proper use and proper maintenance.
5. For sports that do not require helmet use but use sticks (e.g., women's lacrosse and field hockey), players must be taught to respect the potential for head injury as a result of impact with the stick.

Event Prevention

The prevention of injury focuses on the association between the injury and the conditions that exist at the time the injury occurs (e.g., games and practices). As in the pre-event phase, the equipment being worn is essential for protection and should be monitored during participation for any defects. It is important to continually evaluate and monitor the participation rules that are designed to protect the head. The enforcement of rules regarding the use of the head as the initial point of contact in football, high sticking rules in field hockey, and tackling techniques in soccer must be maintained in order to minimize the risk of MTBI. In all sports, rule infractions stemming from fighting or intentional collisions must be enforced.

In addition to the protective equipment worn by the player, it is important to examine the general participation facility for potential hazards. For example, is there padding of the corners of the scorer's table next to the basketball court? It is important that fields and courts where participation takes place are evaluated for potential hazards and that the risk of a head injury from competition not be increased because of poor playing conditions.

Post-event Prevention

Regardless of the quality of prevention programs established in the pre-event and event phases, MTBIs will still occur. When they do, a management program must be in place to evaluate and refer players to the proper medical professionals. As the player recovers from the injury, decisions regarding the return to participation must be individualized for each player. The challenge of the medical profession is to be able to return the player to competition with a minimum of risk for a second injury. Recent research being done in the area of baseline neuropsychological testing and standardized sideline evaluation represents a positive step forward in offering objective information for use in the return-to-play decision.

MTBI Prevention Recommendations

In 1994, the NATA Research and Education Foundation conducted the Mild Brain Injury Summit in Sports. This program brought together professionals from neurosurgery, neuropsychology, neurology, medicine, and athletic training. Its objective was to examine the current knowledge regarding the risk of MTBIs and the type of programs designed to provide medical care and management for MTBIs. The Foundation published the proceedings of this summit, and copies can be obtained by contacting the NATA office in Dallas, Texas.

Recommendations were established to improve the care and management of the MTBI patient and to provide stronger information evaluating the natural history of the injury. Since the injuries are relatively few in number, the input of consistent information from various sources will lead to the strongest knowledge regarding return-to-play decisions.

Another important area examined by the summit panel members was the question of the current state of knowledge regarding the MTBI. They focused on the types of research that must be done in order to begin to better understand the risks of MTBI in both the short and long term. The following recommendations serve to provide direction of the research programs associated with MTBI.

1. Research will require a multidisciplinary team of professionals. The team will represent the neuroscience community, the rehabilitation professions, and sports medicine team physicians and athletic trainers.
2. Important areas for consideration are the effects of multiple injuries and the relative risks associated with continued participation.
3. Emphasis should be placed on the development of procedures for acquiring neuropsychological baselines in order to evaluate the effect of MTBIs over time.
4. Research efforts that focus on the pharmacological intervention for prevention and management are encouraged.

Recommendations of the Mild Brain Injury Summit

The panel members of the Mild Brain Injury Summit in Sports discussed a wide variety of issues associated with injury. As a result of their dialog, the following recommendations were made for the care and management of mild traumatic brain injury:

1. The injured player should be managed as an individual case.
2. Clinicians should familiarize themselves with current literature in evaluation of MTBIs on the sideline as well as in the office.
3. Consistent and routine follow-up procedures should be implemented in order to monitor the individual's progress.
4. Clinicians should provide accurate and consistent information to the patient's "supporters" regarding danger signals associated with MTBIs.
5. Clinicians should encourage and maintain accurate documentation of the injury event, evaluation findings, and decisions to return to participation.

5. Specific programs must address the recovery time for MTBI and its relationship to re-injury and the long-term effects.

Summary

The concern of MTBI in sports is one that has moved to the forefront in the past few years. The retirement of high-profile professional athletes following repetitive MTBI and postconcussion syndrome has heightened the awareness of the sports community to the importance of these injuries. The potential for serious outcomes from brain injury on the individual player's physical and mental status is generally accepted. The ability to provide objective information regarding the exact nature of the effects of MTBI, both in the short term and over time, has been lacking. The unpredictability of MTBIs and the inability to identify cases in the general population have made large-scale research projects impossible. Thus, the focus of research and education regarding brain injury has been centered on the more serious cases.

Recently, the research community has begun to implement programs for the in-depth study of MTBI in the sports arena. Under these conditions, the risks of head injury can be identified and players with MTBI can be followed for their long-term effects. Today's computer technology has made the uniform documentation of injuries among multiple institutions a reality. The ability to coordinate information from multiple sites, multiple professions, and a wide variety of athletes will provide the foundation for developing intervention programs for preventing and managing persons with MTBI, both for the athlete and the nonathlete.

References

1. American Academy of Neurology: Practice parameter: the management of concussion in sports (summary statement). **Neurology** **48**:581-585, 1997
2. Barth JT, Macciocchi SN, Giordani B, et al: Neuropsychological sequelae of minor head injury. **Neurosurgery 13**:529-533, 1983
3. Cantu RC: Guidelines for return to contact sports after a cerebral concussion. **Phys Sportsmed 14**(10):75-83, 1986
4. Cantu RC: Minor head injuries in sports, in Dyment PG (ed): **Adolescent Medicine: State of the Art Reviews.** Philadelphia, Pa: Hanley and Belfus, 1991, Vol 2, pp 141-148
5. Colorado Medical Society: **Report of the Sports Medicine Committee: Guidelines for the Management of Concussion in Sports (revised).** Denver, Co: Colorado Medical Society, 1991
6. Gerberich SG, Priest JD, Boen JR, et al: Concussion incidence and severity in secondary school varsity football players. **Am J Publ Health 73**:1370-1375, 1983
7. Gronwall D: Rehabilitation programs for patients with mild head injury: components, problems, and evaluation. **J Head Trauma Rehabil 1**:53-62, 1986
8. Gurdjian ES, Varis HC: Report of *Ad Hoc* Committee to study head injury nomenclature. **Clin Neurosurg 12**:386-394, 1966
9. Guskiewicz KM, Riemann BL, Perrion DH, et al: Alternative approaches to the assessment of mild head injury in athletes. **Med Sci Sports Exerc 29** (Suppl 7):S213-S221, 1997
10. Hovda DA, Le HM, Lifshitz J, et al: Long-term changes in metabolic rates for glucose following mild, moderate and severe concussive head injuries in rats. **Soc Neurosci 20**:845, 1994 (Abstract)
11. Kay T: Neuropsychological treatment of mild traumatic brain injury. **J Head Trauma Rehabil 8**(3):74-85, 1993
12. Kelly JP, Nichols JS, Filley CM, et al: Concussion in sports. Guidelines for the prevention of catastrophic outcome. **JAMA 266**:2867-2869, 1991
13. Lovell MR, Collins MW: Neuropsychological assessment of the college football player. **J Head Trauma Rehabil 13**:9-26, 1998
14. **National Federation of State High School Associations Handbook: 1996 High School Athletic Participation Survey.** Kansas City, Mo: National Federation of State High School Associations, 1997
15. Powell JW: Injury patterns in selected high school sports, in Bailes JE, Lovell MR, Maroon JC (eds): **Sports-Related Concussions.** St Louis, Mo: Quality Medical, 1999
16. Powell JW, Barber-Foss K: Injury patterns in selected high school sports: a review of the 1995-1997 seasons. **J Athletic Training 34**: 277-284, 1999
17. Powell JW, Barber-Foss KD: Traumatic brain injuries in high school athletes. **JAMA 282**:958-963, 1999
18. Rimel RW, Giordani B, Barth JT, et al: Disability caused by minor head injury. **Neurosurgery 9**:221-228, 1981
19. Wrightson P: Management of disability and rehabilitation services after mild head injury, in Levin HS, Eisenberg HM, Benton AL (eds): **Mild Head Injury.** New York, NY: Oxford University Press, 1989, pp 245-256

CHAPTER 8

Sideline Assessment of Concussion

MICHAEL McCREA, PhD

Concussion has historically been a common injury in all contact and collision sports,[62] but only in recent years has it garnered increasing interest from sports medicine clinicians, brain injury researchers, the media, and governing bodies within organized sports.[52] This shift is perhaps most clearly illustrated by the volume of research publications, continuing education workshops, and features by the print and electronic media on sports-related concussion relative to 10 years ago. Recurrent injuries to high-profile professional athletes have fueled the exposure, but it is also well established that concussion injuries occur much more frequently at the high school[58] and collegiate[20] levels than we read about in the national headlines. An estimated 300,000 cases of traumatic brain injury (TBI) occur in sports and recreation each year in the United States,[63,68] with nearly 40,000 concussions annually in high school football alone.[58] Public health concerns about the potential effects of sports-related concussion have recently prompted an increase in research funding to support studies on the assessment and management of these injuries.

Since the Mild Brain Injury Summit in Sports sponsored by the National Athletic Trainers' Association (NATA) Research and Education Foundation in 1994,[56] advancements have been made on the assessment of concussion in athletes. Multiple reccent studies have highlighted the value of standardized mental status testing on the sideline immediately following concussion to clarify the acute neurocognitive effects of injury and establish an index of severity against which to track recovery.[50,52] Researchers have also discovered the importance of assessing for subtle deficits in balance and postural stability that may be indicative of concussion.[32,33] Standardized mental status and postural stability testing on the sideline immediately after injury are designed to reduce the amount of "guess work" often encountered by sports medicine clinicians in assessing concussion during the acute stage. Numerous studies have also demonstrated the benefits of more extensive neuropsychological testing to clarify the persistent effects of concussion, track recovery, and make more-informed decisions regarding the eventual return to play.[7,18,34,46-48]

This chapter focuses on methods of immediate, sideline mental status evaluation of the athlete following concussion. Other chapters in this text are dedicated to additional means of concussion assessment, including neuropsychological testing, postural stability testing, neurological evaluation, and neurosurgical management. A comprehensive model of concussion assessment and management should incorporate all of these methods to varying degrees depending on the nature and severity of the injury in question. Ideally, advancements in sports-related concussion will also improve the assessment and management of mild TBI outside of sports, including the hospital emergency department and field assessments by emergency medical service professionals. These implications and future directions for concussion research are also reviewed.

Recognizing Injury: Signs of Concussion and Traumatic Brain Injury

Although universal consensus on the full characterization of concussion has not yet been achieved,[10] changes in sensorium and mental status are central to all contemporary definitions.[4,30] Concussion is typically defined as a clinical syndrome characterized by the immediate and transient alteration of mental status and level of consciousness resulting from mechanical force or trauma.[30,36,38] Injury classification systems within sports also refer to mental status changes as essential and defining features of concussion.[3,11,19,33,59] The clinician must be alert, however, to *all* possible indicators of brain injury and its severity, including neurological deficits, mental status abnormalities, and postconcussion symptoms.

The highest percentage of concussion patients exhibit no focal neurological abnormalities on physical examination,[10] but recognition of these findings is critical to detecting underlying intracranial pathology or complications requiring emergent neurosurgical intervention. Intracranial bleeding can occur even with a relatively mild TBI, with the most common underlying pathology being a subdural hematoma. Epidural hematomas, intracranial hematomas, and cerebral contusions can also occur.[36] Intracranial injury can present with a multitude of findings on neurological examination, including headache, dizziness, lightheadedness, gait ataxia, discoordination, impaired reflexes, motor dysfunction, lateralized weakness, sensory deficits, pupil asymmetry, and perceptual abnormalities. The presence of focal neurological deficits may indicate a more severe form of TBI or possible underlying intracranial pathology requiring more immediate medical attention.

Catastrophic neurological injury can also occur from repeated concussions spaced closely in time. Second-impact syndrome results in severe, diffuse brain swelling after a second concussion[61] while an individual is still symptomatic from an earlier injury.[36] The pathophysiology of this syndrome is believed to involve a loss of autoregulation of the brain's blood supply. This disruption causes diffuse vascular engorgement, markedly increased intracranial pressure, and eventual brain herniation and brain stem compromise.[14] Ocular involvement and respiratory failure typically ensue within minutes of this often fatal traumatic injury. Recognizing the signs and symptoms of the initial injury and closely monitoring a subject's recovery following the initial trauma are critical to the prevention of the second-impact syndrome.

Mental status changes and subtle neurocognitive deficits are the most frequently observed signs following concussion. Confusion has long been considered the hallmark of concussion.[25,38] Unfortunately, the concept of confusion has not always been clearly operationalized. The term is often generically applied to describe a clinician's subjective impression that "something's just not right" with respect to the injured subject's mental status. The field of behavioral neurology has pointed to three principal features of confusion, including a disturbance of vigilance with heightened distractibility, the inability to maintain a coherent stream of thought, and the inability to carry out a sequence of goal-directed movements.[54] Although disorientation may be present during a confusional state, subtle mental status abnormalities are more common.[39,52] For example, memory problems and concentration difficulties are often not obvious on gross interaction with the injured subject, but may be detected on a more sensitive mental status examination.[50,52]

The occurrence and duration of loss of consciousness (LOC) and posttraumatic amnesia (PTA) have traditionally been used by clinicians to determine the presence and severity of TBI. It is now well established, however, that mental status changes and other abnormalities resulting from milder forms of TBI or concussion may or may not involve LOC.[36-39] In most cases, concussion involves no observed LOC.[12] In some instances, only a brief period of "dazed" consciousness is reported or observed.[1,22] Animal research has empirically demonstrated the occurrence of concussion without LOC, including an elegant model of concussion described by Ommaya and Gennarelli[57] in which three of six grades of concussion involved no measurable LOC. Human concussion studies also characterize an array of neuropsychological deficits and other symptoms following concussion without LOC.[44,60,66,73]

Several classic studies have documented the presence of amnesia either instantaneously following a concussion[25] or delayed by several minutes.[72] As with LOC, however, concussion often occurs in the absence of measurable PTA.[52] Several issues complicate the assessment of amnesia following concussion. Measuring the duration of PTA is often subjective, unreliable, and difficult to validate,[8,21,29] especially if there have been repeated briefings by family members and others (e.g., teammates) regarding the circumstances surrounding the injury. Some have suggested that a more standardized means of assessment is likely to improve reliability and validity of PTA as an index of brain injury severity.[45]

Unfortunately, there remains a common misconception that no injury has occurred if no LOC or amnesia is documented. As a result, the possibility of concussion is frequently dismissed if the examining medical professional finds no report of LOC or measurable amnesia. It is now well established that concussion in sports most often occurs without observable LOC or measurable PTA,[12] thereby dismissing the commonly held myth that no injury has occurred if the subject was not "knocked out." Although documenting the occurrence and duration of LOC and PTA are critical to determining the overall severity of concussion and predicting outcome, the possibility of head injury should not be automatically dismissed by the clinician if neither of these phenomena was observed or reported.

Deficits in higher-level cognition are defining features of concussion.[70] Recent research suggests that neurocognitive skills are the domain of neurological functioning most sensitive to change after concussion or mild TBI.[52] It is not uncommon for cognitive deficits to be detected in the absence of LOC or amnesia, gross disorientation, or focal neurological abnormalities, thereby indicating the need for sensitive mental status testing of the injured subject. New learning and memory, attention and concentration, reaction time, cognitive processing speed, and more complex operations related to working memory (i.e., the ability to manipulate information "online" or simultaneously conduct multiple mental tasks) are considered the neurocognitive domains most sensitive to change following concussion.[23]

With respect to memory deficits, it is important to distinguish classic posttraumatic and retrograde amnesia (i.e., the inability to recall events preceding or immediately following injury) from anterograde memory dysfunction (i.e., a deficit in learning new information), as detected on formal mental status testing following concussion. Recent studies indicate that subtle impairment of anterograde memory function is indeed detectable in subjects without any noticeable posttraumatic or ret-

TABLE 1

FREQUENTLY OBSERVED SIGNS AND SYMPTOMS FOLLOWING CONCUSSION*

Frequently Observed Signs of Concussion

Vacant stare (befuddled facial expression)

Delayed verbal and motor responses

Inability to focus attention (easily distracted and unable to follow through with normal activities)

Disorientation

Slurred or incoherent speech (making disjointed or incomprehensible statements)

Gross observable discoordination

Emotionality out of proportion to circumstances (appearing distraught, crying for no apparent reason)

Memory deficits (repeatedly asking same questions or inability to remember new information)

Any period of loss of consciousness (paralytic coma, unresponsiveness to stimuli)

Easy fatigability

Feeling more emotional

Irritability

Lack of awareness of surroundings

Lightheadedness

Memory problems

Sadness

Symptoms Often Reported by the Athlete

Headache

Nausea

Balance problems or dizziness

Double or fuzzy vision

Sensitivity to light or noise

Feeling slowed down

Feeling "foggy" or "not sharp"

Change in sleep pattern (too much or not enough)

Concentration difficulties

* Table adapted from Kelly and Rosenberg.[3,39]

rograde amnesia (i.e., the player may have adequate recall of all events surrounding the injury, but deficits in learning new information).[50,52] Similarly, the injured subject may be able to attend adequately during routine neurological examination, but reveal signs of concentration difficulties, delayed processing speed, slower reaction time, increased distractibility, and other subtle abnormalities on more cognitively demanding mental status testing.

Postconcussion symptoms are often categorized into the physical, cognitive, and emotional domains. Common symptoms include headache, dizziness, fatigue, memory problems, poor concentration, irritability, anxiety, frustration, insomnia, and heightened sensitivity to noise.[23] A summary of signs commonly observed and symptoms frequently reported by injured subjects following concussion, both in sports and in the general clinical setting, is seen in Table 1.[3,39] Postconcussion symptoms can occur alone or in combination after mild head injury, and the severity and duration of symptoms may vary from person to person.[23] Some patients experience essentially no symptoms, and others experience severe symptoms for a few days, followed by gradual improvement and full recovery within a couple of weeks. A small but significant number of patients may complain of persistent symptoms for up to several months postinjury,[8,9,23] the cause of which remains incompletely understood. A combination of injury-related (e.g., neurophysiological changes) and noninjury-related factors (e.g., psychosocial variables, motivation, and litigation) likely contributes to ongoing postconcussion disability.[2,43]

The clinician should be aware that concussion is a syndrome that manifests in a variety of symptoms. Patients may present with a varied combination of physical, cognitive, and emotional symptoms after concussion. Therefore, basic understanding and accurate assessment of all domains of postconcussion symptomatology is critical to injury recognition and proper medical management.

Injury Assessment: Sideline Evaluation of Concussion

Accurate and rapid evaluation of the injured patient is crucial to any form of urgent or emergency care,[65] but often creates a somewhat unique challenge in the case of concussion. This is due in part to the fact that the effects of concussion are usually not dramatic and obviously physical, but more typically are evidenced by subtle changes in cognitive or behavioral functioning.[27] Injury detection is straightforward when the subject loses consciousness, but more than 90% of sports-related concussions result in no observable LOC and minimal or no PTA.[12] As a result, many have reported that the recognition and management of concussion is one of the most challenging problems faced by athletic trainers, team physicians, and other medical personnel responsible for the care of athletes.[42,56]

Early detection and specific documentation of the injury are the most important initial steps in the assessment and management of concussion. An objective, quantifiable initial assessment of the injury is essential to evaluating a player's readiness to return to competition and the potential risks when the player eventually does return to play.[56] Close observation and reliable clinical assessment of the injured athlete could also be critical to the prevention of more serious or catastrophic brain injury,[38,53,61] second-impact syndrome,[15,61] or cumulative neuropsychological impairment.[28,35]

Evaluation of the athlete suspected of TBI should begin with basic life support. The clinician must first determine that the injured subject is breathing spontaneously, has an unobstructed airway, and is registering a pulse.[70] Any unconscious player should be treated as having a possible cervical spine injury, with meticulous attention paid to spinal alignment during on-field examination and transport.[5] A decision should be made relatively quickly as to whether or not further evaluation on the sideline is appropriate or emergency transport to a hospital is indicated. Most current guidelines recommend that any player sustaining measurable LOC or exhibiting focal neurological abnormalities should be transported immediately to the nearest hospital emergency department.[3,13]

Once it is established that no cervical spine injury has occurred, the player should be moved to the sideline for further evaluation. An orderly and systematic process of evaluating the athlete for serious signs and symptoms should be undertaken. In fact, all sports medicine clinicians should have a well-understood protocol for concussion assessment and management to prevent the need for decision making in the midst of serious injury. Any worrisome signs or symptoms identified quickly, and evidence of intracranial pathology must be recognized and dealt with emergently. Prolonged unconsciousness, persistent mental status alterations, worsening postconcussion symptoms, or abnormalities on neurological examination should be carefully documented and may require urgent neurosurgical consultation or transfer to a trauma center.[3] Decisions regarding the need for neuroimaging of the injured athlete should be made by a physician at the hospital emergency department.

Continued evaluation of the injured athlete not requiring emergency transport should consist of a thorough neurological examination, mental status testing, and symptom assessment. The neurological examination should begin with an assessment of the level of consciousness. The Glasgow Coma Scale[67] allows for a quantifiable rating of the level of consciousness by registering the patient's degree of response to verbal, tactile, and painful stimulation. Examination of cranial nerves should be conducted, including pupils (size, position, reactivity to light), visual acuity, facial movements and sensation, hearing, and tongue movement. A brief assessment of coordination, sensation, strength, and motor function should be completed on the sideline. A detailed neurological evaluation should be conducted by a physician at the emergency room for serious injuries requiring immediate transport.

In most instances of sports-related concussion, a precise mental status evaluation is the most sensitive and clinically informative component of injury assessment. When a player suspected of having a concussion is brought to the sideline, a thorough mental status examination should be conducted to determine the severity of injury by assessing for deficits in orientation, concentration, and memory, as well as the presence of retrograde or posttraumatic amnesia.[70] It is also recommended that the injured athlete be examined under conditions of exertion in order to elevate the intracranial pressure and increase the likelihood of detecting postconcussion symptoms. Exertional maneuvers are not necessary in instances where the athlete is already exhibiting signs or reporting symptoms after injury.

The classic line of questioning is typically used to assess for any gross deficits in orientation. The player is often required to provide his/her name, the day of the week, the exact date, and the approximate time, place, and current circumstances. Standardized measures of orientation are also available, the most popular of which is the Galveston Orientation and Amnesia Test (see Chapter 2, Table 11).[45] The clinician should be aware that transient loss of orientation often occurs as a result of concussion and TBI, but that most cases of sports-related concussion do not manifest in profound disorientation. Therefore, assessment of orientation (e.g., "where are we?") alone does not represent a sensitive or sufficient mental status examination following concussion.[49]

Many different methods have traditionally been used to assess attention and concentration, both within and outside sports medicine. The Digit Span Test[69] is perhaps the most common method of assessing attention skills and requires the subject to repeat a string of digits of increasing length in the same order recited by the examiner. The reverse Digit Span Test,[69] which requires the subject to repeat the same line of digits in reverse order, is considered more cognitively demanding and perhaps more sensitive to subtle postconcussion deficits. The routine method for both digits forward and in reverse is to begin with a string of three digits and increase the length to six or seven digits. Serial 7's (counting backward from 100 by intervals of 7 (i.e., 100, 93, 86 . . .)),[26] reciting the days of the week or months of the year in reverse order,[51] spelling words in reverse order,[26] and computing mental arithmetic problems also are methods used to assess for postconcussion attention deficits during the acute injury phase.

It is especially important to properly assess memory function following concussion, both in terms of memory loss for events preceding (retrograde amnesia) or following (PTA) the injury and the inability to retain new information.[3,39] Questions used to assess retrograde or posttraumatic amnesia typically involve the injured subject's recollection of circumstances surrounding the contest or injury, such as identifying the other team, the current quarter or period of the contest, which team scored last, the player's description of the play on which he/she was injured, what ensued immediately following the injury, or significant events occurring earlier in the contest.[41,49,71,72] Questions on more remote memory may also be administered, such as naming the team played against in the previous game, the outcome and score of that game, or recent newsworthy events.[19] Empirical data on the sensitivity and specificity of certain questions in the detection of concussion are very limited.[49,71] Because amnesia following concussion may manifest immediately or be delayed by several minutes,[71] the clinician is advised to monitor for any changes in memory function exhibited by the injured athlete over the course of postinjury recovery.

In addition to assessing for the presence of retrograde or posttraumatic amnesia, it is imperative to evaluate the injured subject's ability to learn new information (i.e., anterograde memory function). Recent research indicates that subtle anterograde memory deficits are often detectable in the absence of classically defined retrograde or posttraumatic amnesia.[50,52] Methods used to assess anterograde memory typically involve the examiner presenting new information to the injured subject once or repeatedly and assessing the subject's recall of the information several minutes later. A repeated word-list learning paradigm is the most common memory measure used during the acute phase of injury. The player is read a list of three to five words and is asked to repeat back to the examiner as many words from the list as he/she can remember immediately. Some methods repeat this procedure for multiple trials,[50,52] while others consist of just one trial.[19,39] Following the immediate memory trial(s), the subject is typically *not* forewarned that their recall for the word list will be tested later. Approximately 6-8 minutes later and following other segments of the neurological or mental status examination, the examiner will inquire to the injured subject, "Do you remember that list of words I read to you a few minutes ago? Tell me as many words as you can remember from that list."

A couple of issues are of interest with respect to memory assessment. First, a five-word list is recommended over a three-word list to increase the cognitive demands of the task and enhance the sensitivity in detecting more subtle memory deficits.[50] Second, initially presenting the information on repeated trials rather than a single trial is recommended to separate memory dysfunction from poor attention and concentration, both of which are common after concussion.

Other methods for assessing new learning follow a similar protocol but substitute visual objects (e.g., pencil, apple, or glove) rather than a word list, while some methods include both words and objects.[19]

The clinician is strongly encouraged to adopt a standardized checklist to assess and quantify postconcussion symptoms. Several scales have been established for this purpose (see Chapter 2) and include between 15 and 30 common postconcussion symptoms.[24,40,46] Some scales simply indicate the presence or absence of symptoms via a yes-no format, while others allow the injured subject to rate the severity of symptoms as mild, moderate, or severe.[46]

It is often difficult to precisely assess mental status following concussion without objective test measures because of the subtlety of postconcussion deficits, sometimes complicated by the injured player's attempt to mask symptoms in order to continue to play. Although ratings from the Glasgow Coma Scale[67] and similar systems for grading mental status following TBI correlate highly with neuropsychological and psychosocial outcome following more severe injuries,[64] these grading systems may not be sensitive to subtle neurocognitive changes that present risks for more severe underlying neurological complications after concussion.[65] The sensitivity of routine neurological examination in detecting underlying cognitive abnormalities after concussion is also limited, as subtle neurological deficits may be missed and there is often little emphasis on a sensitive neurocognitive examination. Neuropsychological testing is considered a sophisticated and sensitive method for detecting subtle cognitive and behavioral abnormalities after concussion, but is not typically feasible immediately after injury in most acute-care situations such as sideline examination of the injured athlete during a sporting event.

There has been a recent movement toward standardizing mental status, neurological, and postural stability testing of the injured subject following concussion. The Quality Standards Committee of the American Academy of Neurology specifically called for the development of a valid, standardized, systematic sideline evaluation designed for the immediate assessment of concussion in athletes.[3] The Standardized Assessment of Concussion was developed by the author and colleagues to provide sports medicine clinicians with a brief, objective tool for assessing an injured subject's mental status on the sidelines during sporting events.[51] Other researchers[32,33] have taken a similar approach to standardizing postural stability testing. The goal of these methods is to create more objective quantifiable indices of injury severity, against which recovery can be tracked over time in order for the clinician to make a more informed, empirically based decision regarding the athlete's readiness to return to play after injury.

Standardized Assessment of Concussion

The Standardized Assessment of Concussion (SAC)[51] was developed in 1995 in response to and in accordance with the recommendation of the American Academy of Neurology practice parameter[3] and the earlier Colorado guidelines.[19] The SAC was also designed to be in line with what the neuropsychological literature demonstrates to be the domains of function most sensitive to the effects of mild TBI and concussion,[16] and the tests best suited to measuring those functions in brain injury patients.[17] The SAC was intended to be a standardized means of objectively documenting the presence and severity of neurocognitive impairment associated with concussion, thereby immediately providing additional information to athletic trainers and other medical personnel responsible for clinical decision making in the care of athletes. The content and length of the SAC were constrained by the conditions of rapid sideline evaluation and the parameter that it be designed for use by clinicians with no prior expertise in psychometric testing.

The SAC is not intended as a substitute for formal neurological or neuropsychological evaluation of the injured athletes. The SAC is also not meant as a stand-alone return-to-play measure, but provides objective data on mental status abnormalities that should be correlated with other clinical information in the assessment of an athlete following concussion.

Because impaired attention and concentration, disorientation, and memory difficulties are among the characteristic cognitive deficits often associated with concussion, the SAC includes measures of Orientation, Immediate Memory, Concentration, and Delayed

NAME: _____

AGE: ___ SEX: ____ EXAMINER: _____

Nature of Injury: _____

Date of Exam: _____ Time: _____ No. _____

1) ORIENTATION:

Month: _____	0	1
Date: _____	0	1
Day of Week: _____	0	1
Year: _____	0	1
Time (within 1 hour): _____	0	1
Orientation Total Score _____		/ 5

2) IMMEDIATE MEMORY:

(All 3 trials are completed regardless of score on trials 1 and 2; score equals sum across all 3 trials)

LIST	TRIAL 1	TRIAL 2	TRIAL 3
Word 1	0 1	0 1	0 1
Word 2	0 1	0 1	0 1
Word 3	0 1	0 1	0 1
Word 4	0 1	0 1	0 1
Word 5	0 1	0 1	0 1
TOTAL			

Immediate Memory Score _____   / 15

NEUROLOGICAL SCREENING

Loss of Consciousness (occurrence, duration)

Posttraumatic Amnesia (poor recall of events after injury)

Retrograde Amnesia (poor recall before injury)

Strength (upper and lower extremities)

Sensation (finger to nose) (Romberg)

Coordination (tandem walk/finger-nose-finger)

3) CONCENTRATION:

DIGITS BACKWARD: (If correct, go to next string length. If incorrect, read trial 2. Stop after incorrect on both trials.)

4-9-3	6-2-9	0	1
3-8-1-4	3-2-7-9	0	1
6-2-9-7-1	1-5-2-8-6	0	1
7-1-8-4-6-2	5-3-9-1-4-8	0	1

MONTHS IN REVERSE ORDER: (entire reverse sequence correct for 1 point)

DEC-NOV-OCT-SEP-AUG-JUL
JUN-MAY-APR-MAR-FEB-JAN   0   1

Concentration Total Score _____   / 5

EXERTIONAL MANEUVERS
(When appropriate):

5 jumping jacks	5 push-ups
5 sit-ups	5 knee-bends

4) DELAYED RECALL

Word 1	0	1
Word 2	0	1
Word 3	0	1
Word 4	0	1
Word 5	0	1
Delayed Recall Score _____		/ 5

SUMMARY OF TOTAL SCORES:

Orientation	_____	/ 5
Immediate Memory	_____	/ 15
Concentration	_____	/ 5
Delayed Recall	_____	/ 5
OVERALL TOTAL SCORE	_____	/ 30

Figure 1: Standardized Assessment of Concussion. (Reproduced with permission[19])

Recall (Figure 1). The maximum total score on the SAC is 30 points. The SAC requires approximately 5 minutes to administer and is designed for use by a non-neuropsychologist with no prior expertise in psychometric testing. Alternate Forms A, B, and C of the SAC were designed to allow follow-up testing of injured players with minimal practice effects in order to track postconcussion recovery. The three forms differ only in the stimulus selection of digits in the Concentration section and the words used to test Immediate Memory and Delayed Recall.

The SAC is printed on pocket-sized cards for convenient use by athletic trainers and other medical personnel examining athletes on the sideline. All instructions for administering and scoring the SAC are printed on the record forms, while a comprehensive manual provides the clinician with more detailed background, research data, and instructions for the instrument.

A standard line of questioning is used to assess Orientation on the SAC. The subject is asked to provide the day of the week, month, date, year, and time of day within 1 hour. A five-word list is used to measure Immediate Memory. The word list is read to the subject for immediate recall and the procedure is repeated for three trials. Concentration is tested by having the subject repeat in reverse order strings of digits that increase in length from three to six numbers. Reciting the months of the year in reverse order is also utilized to assess Concentration. Delayed Recall of the original five-word list is also ascertained. The SAC Total Score (maximum 30) is computed in order to derive a composite index of the subject's overall level of impairment following concussion.

A standard brief neurological screening is embedded in the SAC and includes an assessment of strength, sensation, and coordination. The occurrence and length of LOC, retrograde amnesia, and PTA are also documented on the SAC. As prescribed by the American Academy of Neurology[3] and Colorado guidelines,[19] exertional maneuvers are also performed during the mental status exam in order to create conditions of increased intracranial pressure under which postconcussion symptoms such as headache, nausea, and dizziness are most likely to be observed.

Research efforts initially focused on use of the SAC with football players due to the relatively high incidence rate of concussion,[58] but have now expanded to other male and female contact sports with risk for concussion (e.g., soccer, hockey, and lacrosse). In many ways, the ideal neuropsychological laboratory for the study of concussion was created when studying athletes at risk for head injury.[6] That is, we can identify and have access to a large sample of subjects, of whom epidemiological data indicate that approximately 5% are likely to suffer concussion, and mechanisms can be put in place to examine the subject immediately after injury and at various follow-up points. Multiple studies have yielded normative data on non-injured athletes administered the SAC, as well as data on the clinical validity of the instrument in detecting concussion and tracking postinjury recovery.[50,52]

A normative database of more than 2000 male and female junior high, high school, collegiate, and professional athletes who have undergone the SAC has established the psychometric properties of the instrument,[50-52] including:

- Forms A, B, and C of the SAC are equivalent for clinical use, with no clinically significant differences between total score or domain scores on any of the three forms.

- The SAC is acceptable for use at the junior high, high school, college, and professional levels. Athletes at these levels perform similarly on the SAC. Separate normative data are available for use with junior high athletes.

- There are no significant differences in SAC performance by males and females.

- The SAC is reliable over repeated administrations. A slight practice effect is evident over shorter test-retest intervals (e.g., 48 hours), but diminishes with longer intervals.

- There is no significant difference between the scores of normal subjects examined during practice and on the sideline during actual games. Therefore, extraneous factors such as emotionality, distraction, or fatigue experienced during games do not appear to confound test performance on the SAC. The implication is that baseline testing can be conducted during preseason practice or off-season drills and provide a valid and reliable marker against which to detect change in the event of injury during practice or games.

- The SAC normative database approximates a normal distribution, with only a slight ceiling effect evidenced by approximately 6% of normal control subjects achieving a perfect score of 30 points.

Clinical research has demonstrated that the SAC is a sensitive and specific means to immediately detect even the mildest grade of concussion in the absence of observable

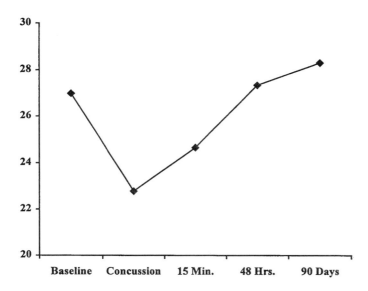

Figure 2: Mean SAC total score for all injured subjects at preseason baseline, time of injury, 15 minutes, 48 hours, and 90 days postinjury. Maximum score is 30.

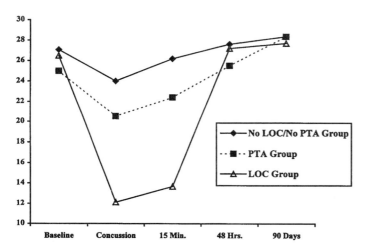

Figure 3: Mean SAC total score at preseason baseline, time of injury, 15 minutes, 48 hours, and 90 days postinjury for subjects with and without LOC or PTA. Maximum score is 30.

neurological signs of injury, and is a gross indicator of post-concussion recovery.[50,52] A clinical database now contains SAC data on more than 130 injured subjects, most of whom are high school and collegiate football players. The vast majority of injuries meet the classification criteria for Grade 1 or 2 concussion,[3,39] while a very small minority sustained any LOC resulting from injury. Most research on the SAC has incorporated a model of baseline-injury-recovery assessment. That is, a large pool of subjects undergo preseason baseline testing on the SAC and any subject suspected of having sustained a concussion during the course of the sports season is administered an alternate form of the SAC immediately after injury and at various postinjury follow-up points. Previous studies have assessed injured subjects at 15 minutes, 48 hours, and 90 days after injury. SAC data have most commonly been collected by certified athletic trainers administering the instrument to non-injured and injured athletes.

Figure 2 illustrates the results of a study on high school and collegiate football players (M. McCrea, J.P. Kelly, C. Randolph, unpublished data). Injured subjects immediately after concussion scored significantly below their preseason baseline performance on the SAC, and below the average score for the larger group of normal, non-concussed athletes. The same study also revealed that concussed players scored significantly below normal controls on the Orientation, Immediate Memory, Concentration, and Delayed Recall sections of the SAC. A gradual increase in SAC scores within minutes and at further intervals from injury also indicates a recovery curve. These results are very similar to the findings of two earlier studies[50,52] with smaller samples of injured subjects.

SAC performance immediately after injury also correlates with other established indicators of brain injury severity, including LOC and PTA (M. McCrea, J.P. Kelly, C. Randolph, unpublished data). Figure 3 indicates the difference between SAC performance immediately after injury and at various follow-up assessment points by subjects with neither LOC nor PTA (No LOC/No PTA, n=75), with PTA but no LOC (PTA, n=8), and with both LOC and PTA (LOC, n=7). The mean SAC score for all three clinical groups at time of injury is significantly below their pre-injury baseline performance, with the No LOC/No PTA group least impaired and the LOC group most severely impaired. Only the LOC group remained significantly impaired on the SAC 15 minutes after injury, and none of the three groups was significantly impaired on the SAC 48 hours or 90 days after injury. These findings further illustrate the importance of sensitive mental status testing in order to detect subtle cognitive changes associated with concussion in the absence of other symptoms.

A survey of clinicians (n=61) experienced with the SAC also supports the instrument's utility as a supplement to routine clinical examination following concussion (Ferrara et al, unpublished data). Eighty-five percent of respondents indicated that use of the SAC in addition to their routine clinical exam resulted in a more accurate assessment of the player suspected of having a concussion, while no respondents believed that the instrument hindered their examination. This same survey also refuted the argument made by some regarding the potential misuse of methods such as the SAC by clinicians in order to more rapidly return a player to competition than what is deemed to be "safe" according to current practice standards. Of those clinicians already using the SAC, 63% indicated that information yielded from the SAC resulted in a player being more likely to be withheld longer from competition than would be the case based solely on routine clinical examination alone. Only 6% of respondents thought a player was less likely to be withheld based on SAC data, while 30% indicated that SAC data would not significantly affect their decision making regarding a player's eventual readiness to return to play.

Baseline testing is the recommended model for use of the SAC in sports. Although it requires a fairly substantial time commitment on the front end, the advantages of baseline testing are numerous. Accessibility to pre-injury objective data allows the clinician to compare an injured player to his/her own normal performance on a given measure. This model also affords greater control for variability across subjects, extraneous variables (e.g., learning disability or alcohol or drug abuse), and the effects of earlier concussion. Finally, a comparison between postinjury and pre-injury data is the most accurate indicator of recovery and allows the clinician to assess for cumulative effects of recurrent concussion. Approximately 6 minutes per player is required to complete baseline testing, which most clinicians agree is time well spent for the clinical returns when assessing an injured subject sometime later during the sports season.

Although the SAC has proved very useful and informative in the assessment of concussion on the sports sideline, the clinician must also be aware of certain limitations related to the use of the SAC and similar screening instruments. The SAC serves as a brief, gross measure of cognitive functioning that is appropriate under the situational constraints often faced on the sideline during sporting events. Screening instruments such as the SAC cannot, however, claim the same level of sophistication as a more extensive neuropsychological test battery. Therefore, the SAC is not intended as a substitute for follow-up neuropsychological evaluation of the injured athlete with persistent symptoms. The clinician will also note that the SAC does not include a checklist to assess for the presence and severity of various postconcussion symptoms. It is strongly recommended that the clinician incorporate one of the existing postconcussion symptom checklists into their injury protocol to supplement information yielded by the SAC and other aspects of clinical examination. Given recent research on the effects of concussion on postural stability, it is also recommended that the clinician more thoroughly assess for subtle deficits in balance exhibited by the injured athlete. Innovative, standardized methods of balance assessment are recommended.[31,32]

Most importantly, the clinician should recognize and understand that the SAC and similar screening instruments do not represent stand-alone return-to-play measures. The clinician should avoid the risks of overstating the power of any one measure during concussion assessment and, instead, rely on all clinical information in making decisions regarding the player's fitness to return to play.

Follow-up Assessment of the Injured Athlete

Close observation of the injured athlete over time is necessary to monitor for the evolution of cognitive dysfunction or other indicators of underlying neuropathological changes.[39] Prolonged unconsciousness, persistent mental status alterations, worsening postconcussion symptoms, or abnormalities on neurological examination may indicate the need for emergency transport and immediate medical evaluation of the injured athlete. The clinician should be aware of current guidelines and techniques for emergency management of more severe injuries, as outlined in other chapters included in this vol-

Research on concussion in sports affords many advantages not typically present in traditional studies on the natural history of mild TBI, including:[6]

- access to a large sample at risk of injury within a relatively small window of time during a sports season;

- the ability to conduct pre-injury baseline standardized testing against which to detect change associated with injury;

- eyewitness accounts by medical professionals regarding the mechanism of injury, LOC, PTA, and other circumstances surrounding the injury;

- feasibility of objective assessment within minutes of injury;

- repeated follow-up assessment of injured subjects to track recovery over hours, days, weeks, and months;

- a comparison of objective assessment measures and subjective/symptomatic indicators of injury; and

- access to healthy and injured (e.g., orthopedic) controls matched to injured subjects by age, gender, education, and baseline test performance.

TABLE 2

COMPREHENSIVE MODEL OF CONCUSSION ASSESSMENT

Preseason

Clinical questions:
Level of functioning pre-injury?
Previous history of head injury?

Methods of Assessment:
Health and concussion history
Pre-participation physical exam
Baseline testing- Neurocognitive
Postural stability
Symptom survey

Time of Injury

Clinical questions:
Is there an injury? If so, how severe?
Need for transport, neuroimaging?
Can player return to play?

Methods of Assessment:
First aid assessment
Neurological exam
Mental status evaluation and balance testing
Symptom survey

First 24 Hours Postinjury

Clinical questions:
What is level of recovery?
Is further evaluation, neuroimaging necessary?
Can player return to play?
Symptom survey

Methods of Assessment:
Mental status evaluation and balance testing
Neurological medical evaluation
Neuropsychological testing
Neuroimaging

24-72 Hours Postinjury

Clinical questions:
What is level of recovery?
Is further evaluation, neuroimaging necessary?
Can player return to play?
Symptom survey

Methods of Assessment:
Mental status evaluation
Balance testing
Neurological/medical evaluation
Neuropsychological testing
Neuroimaging

Extended Follow-up

Clinical questions:
What is level of recovery?
Are there persistent symptoms?
When can player return to play?

Methods of Assessment:
Symptom survey
Mental status evaluation and balance testing
Neurological/medical evaluation
Neuropsychological testing
Neuroimaging

ume. Most of the methods outlined as part of the current chapter are meant for the assessment of injuries during the acute phase. Screening instruments such as the SAC are designed based on the situational constraints faced by the sports medicine clinician. Injured athletes continuing to exhibit cognitive dysfunction or reporting persistent postconcussion symptoms should in most cases be referred for further medical evaluation, neurological consultation, and/or formal neuropsychological testing. Neuropsychological testing has proved to be very useful in detecting subtle brain-related difficulties in athletes following concussion.[46] Information yielded by neuropsychological testing also provides the sports medicine clinician with more objective, empirically based data on which to base decisions regarding an athlete's readiness to return to competition after concussion. Please refer to accompanying chapters in this volume for a full review of neuropsychological testing and other concussion assessment methods currently used in sports.

A comprehensive model of concussion assessment has emerged in recent years. Preseason baseline testing of athletes and the implementation of standardized assessment methods represent the greatest advancements relative to those methods historically used by sports medicine clinicians. A comprehensive model of concussion assessment and management ultimately provides the clinician with valuable information predating a concussion, immediately following injury, and at various follow-up points to track a player's postinjury recovery. The model outlined in Table 2 incorporates both standardized methods and serial examination of the injured athlete, utilizing a symptom survey, mental status examination, neuropsychological evaluation, and postural stability testing. This model emphasizes the need for formal neurological consultation, medical evaluation, and neuroimaging of the injured player reporting persistent symptoms, exhibiting continued abnormalities, or demonstrating a worsening course of recovery after injury.

Future Directions for Sports Concussion Research

Continued research is necessary to advance our current methods of concussion assessment. Standardized, objective assessment methods will eventually help clarify the immediate effects of concussion and, ultimately, the early natural history of mild TBI. The integration of existing methods is essential. Research combining procedures to assess mental status, neurological abnormalities, postural stability, and postconcussion symptoms should take a high priority. This model of research will eventually allow us to identify factors that predict outcome following injury, including normal recovery, risk of re-injury, cumulative neurocognitive impairment, and second-impact syndrome. The ultimate goal of sports concussion research should be the development of empirically based, safe, and practical guidelines for clinical decision making on an athlete's readiness to return to play after concussion. Several large-scale studies on the assessment and management of sports concussion in male and female athletes are currently underway at the high school, collegiate, and professional competitive levels. Continuing education offerings and other efforts to increase awareness of sports concussion are also important. Finally, initiatives focused on injury prevention should be undertaken to enhance the safety of young athletes participating in sports.

Implications for Mild Traumatic Brain Injury Assessment Outside of Sports

Researching mild TBI in sports not only creates a venue to make a major contribution to society by enhancing the safety of young participants in organized sports, but also provides a unique laboratory to advance the science of concussion and mild TBI in the general population.

Further research on sports concussion will undoubtedly advance our understanding of the immediate neurocognitive changes following concussion, the timing of symptom onset, the expected rate and trajectory of recovery, and the early predictors of positive and negative outcome following injury. Current research supports the use of standardized methods in the assessment of mild TBI to detect more subtle mental status abnormalities during the acute postinjury phase. More accurate assessment of acute mild TBI is critical to identifying those patients at risk for more severe neurological complications or persistent symptoms and implementing effective treatment strategies soon after injury to decrease disability and improve overall clinical outcome associated with mild TBI. Standardized screening instruments may improve upon existing methods effective for the classification of more severe forms of TBI (e.g., Glasgow Coma Scale,[67] LOC, and PTA) but lacking sensitivity in the assessment of mild TBI.

Further research is underway to examine the application of standardized methods, such as the SAC, to emergency medical settings outside of sports, including studies in which emergency medical service professionals are conducting assessments at the trauma scene, during emergency transport, and as part of the emergency room evaluation for brain trauma. It is hoped that this model will help further clarify the immediate effects and natural history of mild TBI, as well as factors that predict outcome following these injuries. Correlating objective assessment measures, such as the SAC, with more sophisticated methods, such as functional magnetic resonance imaging and more extensive neuropsychological testing, during the acute postinjury period will eventually increase our understanding of the relationship between the underlying pathophysiology and the outward clinical features of mild TBI.

References

1. Alexander MP: Mild traumatic brain injury: pathophysiology, natural history, and clinical management. **Neurology** 45:1253-1260, 1995
2. Alexander MP: Minor traumatic brain injury: a review of physiogenesis and psychogenesis. **Sem Clin Neuropsychiatry** 2:177-187, 1997
3. American Academy of Neurology: Practice parameter. The management of concussion in sports (summary statement). **Neurology** 48: 581-585, 1997
4. American Congress of Rehabilitation Medicine: Report of the Mild Traumatic Brain Injury Committee of the Head Injury Interdisciplinary Special Interest Group. Definition of mild traumatic brain injury. **J Head Trauma Rehabil** 8:86-87, 1993
5. Bailes J: Head injuries in sports, in Jordan B (ed): **Sports Neurology, 2nd ed.** Philadelphia, Pa: Lippincott-Raven, 1998, pp 215-233
6. Barth J: Athletic laboratory. **Recovery** 9:30-31, 1998
7. Barth JT, Alves WM, Ryan TV, et al: Mild head injury in sports: neuropsychological sequelae and recovery of function, in Levin H, Eisenberg H, Benton A (eds): **Mild Head Injury.** New York, NY: Oxford University Press, 1989, pp 257-275
8. Binder LM: A review of mild head trauma: Part II. Clinical implications. **J Clin Exp Neuropsychol** 19:432-457, 1997
9. Binder LM, Rohling MLS, Larrabee J: A review of mild head trauma: Part I. Meta-analytic review of neuropsychological studies. **J Clin Exp Neuropsychol** 19:421-431, 1997
10. Cantu RC: Athletic head injuries. **Clin Sports Med** 16:531-542, 1997
11. Cantu RC: Guidelines for return to contact sports after a cerebral concussion. **Phys Sportsmed** 14:75-83, 1986
12. Cantu RC: Head injuries in sport. **Br J Sports Med** 30:289-296, 1996
13. Cantu RC: Return to play guidelines after a head injury. **Clin Sports Med** 17:45-60, 1998
14. Cantu RC: Second-impact syndrome. **Clin Sports Med** 17:37-44, 1998
15. Cantu RC, Voy R: Second impact syndrome: a risk in any contact sport. **Phys Sportsmed** 23(6):172-177, 1995
16. Capruso DX, Levin HS: Cognitive impairment following closed head injury. **Neurol Clin** 10:879-893, 1992
17. Clifton GL, Hayes RL, Levin HS, et al: Outcome measures for clinical trials involving traumatically brain-injured patients: report of a conference. **Neurosurgery** 31:975-978, 1992
18. Collins MW, Grindel SH, Lovell MR, et al: Relationship between concussion and neuropsychological performance in college football players. **JAMA** 282:964-970, 1999
19. Colorado Medical Society: **Report of the Sports Medicine Committee: Guidelines for the Management of Concussion in Sports (revised).** Denver, Co: Colorado Medical Society, 1991
20. Dick WD: A summary of head and neck injuries in collegiate athletics using the NCAA Injury Surveillance System, in Hoerner EF (ed): **Head and Neck Injuries in Sports.** Philadelphia, Pa: American Society for Testing and Materials, 1994, pp 13-19
21. Dikmen S, McLean A, Temkin N: Neuropsychological and psychosocial consequences of minor head injury. **J Neurol Neurosurg Psychiatry** 49: 1227-1232, 1986
22. Evans RW: The postconcussion syndrome: 130 years of controversy.

Semin Neurol 14:32-39, 1994

23. Evans RW: The postconcussion syndrome and the sequelae of mild head injury. **Neurol Clin 10:**815-847, 1992

24. Ferguson RJ, Mittenberg W, Barone DF, et al: Postconcussion syndrome following sports-related head injury: expectation as etiology. **Neuropsychology 13:**582-589, 1999

25. Fisher CM: Concussion amnesia. **Neurology 16:**826-830, 1966

26. Folstein MF, Folstein SE, McHugh PR: Mini-Mental State: A practical method for grading the cognitive state of patients for the clinician. **J Psychiat Res 12:**189-198, 1975

27. Gordon WA, Brown M, Sliwinski M, et al: The enigma of "hidden" traumatic brain injury. **J Head Trauma Rehabil 13:**39-56, 1998

28. Gronwall D, Wrightson P: Cumulative effects of concussion. **Lancet 2:** 995-997, 1975

29. Gronwall D, Wrightson P: Memory and information processing capacity after closed head injury. **J Neurol Neurosurg Psychiatry 44:**889-895, 1981

30. Gurdjian ES, Voris HC: Report of *Ad Hoc* Committee to Study Head Injury Nomenclature. **Clin Neurosurg 12:**386-394, 1966

31. Guskiewicz KM, Perrin DH, Gansneder BM: Effect of mild head injury on postural stability in athletes. **J Athletic Training 31:**300-306, 1996

32. Guskiewicz KM, Riemann BL, Perrin DH, et al: Alternative approaches to the assessment of mild head injury in athletes. **Med Sci Sports Exerc 29 (Suppl 7):**213-221, 1997

33. Harmon KG: Assessment and management of concussion in sports. **Am Fam Phys 60:**887-892, 1999

34. Hinton-Bayre AD, Geffen G, McFarland K: Mild head injury and speed of information processing: a prospective study of professional rugby league players. **J Clin Exp Neuropsychol 19:**275-289, 1997

35. Jordan BD, Zimmerman RD: Computed tomography and magnetic resonance imaging comparisons in boxers. **JAMA 263:**1670-1674, 1990

36. Kelly JP: Concussion, in Torg JS, Shephard RJ (eds): **Current Therapy in Sports Medicine, 3rd ed.** St Louis, Mo: CV Mosby, 1995, pp 21-24

37. Kelly JP: Traumatic brain injury and concussion in sports. **JAMA 282:** 989-991, 1999

38. Kelly JP, Nichols JS, Filley CM, et al: Concussion in sports. Guidelines for the prevention of catastrophic outcome. **JAMA 266:**2867-2869, 1991

39. Kelly JP, Rosenberg JH: Diagnosis and management of concussion in sports. **Neurology 48:**575-580, 1997

40. King NS, Crawford S, Wenden FJ, et al: The Rivermead Post Concussion Symptoms Questionnaire: a measure of symptoms commonly experienced after head injury and its reliability. **J Neurol 242:**587-592, 1995

41. Kutner KC, Barth JT: Sports related concussion. **The National Academy of Neuropsychology Bulletin,** 1998, pp 19-23

42. Landry G: Mild brain injury in athletes. **National Athletic Trainers' Association (NATA) Research and Education Foundation: Proceedings from Mild Brain Injury Summit.** Washington, DC, April 14-18, 1994

43. Larrabee GJ: Neuropsychological outcome, post-concussion symptoms, and forensic considerations in mild closed head trauma. **Semin Clin Neuropsychiatry 2(3):**196-206, 1997

44. Leininger BE, Gramling SE, Farrell AD, et al: Neuropsychological deficits in symptomatic minor head injury patients after concussion and mild concussion. **J Neurol Neurosurg Psychiatry 53:**293-296, 1990

45. Levin HS, O'Donnell VM, Grossman RG: The Galveston orientation and amnesia test. A practical scale to assess cognition after head injury. **J Nerv Ment Disord 167:**675-684, 1979

46. Lovell MR, Collins MW: Neuropsychological assessment of the college football player. **J Head Trauma Rehabil 13:**9-26, 1998

47. Macciocchi SN, Barth JT, Alves W, et al: Neuropsychological function-

ing and recovery after mild head injury in collegiate athletes. **Neurosurgery 39:**510-514, 1996

48. Maddocks D, Saling M: Neuropsychological deficits following concussion. **Brain Inj 10:**99-103, 1996

49. Maddocks DL, Dicker GD, Saling MM: The assessment of orientation following concussion in athletes. **Clin J Sports Med 5:**32-35, 1995

50. McCrea M, Kelly JP, Kluge J, et al: Standardized assessment of concussion in football players. **Neurology 48:**586-588, 1997

51. McCrea M, Kelly JP, Randolph C: **Standardized Assessment of Concussion (SAC): Manual for Administration, Scoring and Interpretation.** Waukesha, Wisconsin, 1997

52. McCrea M, Kelly JP, Randolph C, et al: Standardized assessment of concussion (SAC): on-site mental status evaluation of the athlete. **J Head Trauma Rehabil 13(2):**27-35, 1998

53. McQuillen JB, McQuillen EN, Morrow P: Trauma, sport, and malignant cerebral edema. **Am J Forensic Med Pathol 9:**12-15, 1988

54. Mesulam MM: **Principles of Behavioral Neurology.** Philadelphia, Pa: FA Davis, 1985

55. Miller JD: Head injury. **J Neurol Neurosurg Psychiatry 56:**440-447, 1993

56. National Athletic Trainers' Association: **Proceedings from Mild Brain Injury Summit, Washington, DC, April 14-18, 1994.** Dallas, Tx: National Athletic Trainers' Association Research and Education Foundation, 1994

57. Ommaya AK, Gennarelli TA: Cerebral concussion and traumatic unconsciousness. Correlation of experimental and clinical observations on blunt head injuries. **Brain 97:**633-654, 1974

58. Powell JW, Barber-Foss KD: Traumatic brain injury in high school athletes. **JAMA 282:**958-963, 1999

59. Roberts WO: Who plays? Who sits? **Phys Sportsmed 20:**66-72, 1992

60. Ruff RM, Crouch JA, Troster AI, et al: Selected cases of poor outcome following a minor brain trauma: comparing neuropsychological and positron emission tomography assessment. **Brain Inj 8:**297-308, 1994

61. Saunders RL, Harbaugh RE: The second impact in catastrophic contact-sports head trauma. **JAMA 252:**538-539, 1984

62. Schneider RC: Football head and neck injuries. **Surg Neurol 27:** 507-508, 1987 (Letter)

63. Sports-related recurrent brain injuries—United States. **MMWR Morbid Mortal Wkly Rep 46:**224-227, 1997

64. Stein SC: Classification of head injury, in Narayan RK, Wilberger JE, Povlishock JT (eds): **Neurotrauma.** New York, NY: McGraw-Hill, 1996

65. Stein SC, Spettell C, Young G, et al: Limitations of neurological assessment in mild head injury. **Brain Inj 7:** 425-430, 1993

66. Strugar J, Sass KJ, Buchanan CP, et al: Long-term consequences of minimal brain injury: loss of consciousness does not predict memory impairment. **J Trauma 34:**555-559, 1993

67. Teasdale G, Jennett B: Assessment of coma and impaired consciousness. A practical scale. **Lancet 2:**81-84, 1974

68. Thurman DJ, Branche CM, Sniezek JE: The epidemiology of sports-related traumatic brain injury in the United States: recent development. **J Head Trauma Rehabil 13:**1-8, 1998

69. Wechsler D: **Wechsler Adult Intelligence Scale– Revised Manual.** San Antonio, Tx: Psychological Corp, 1981

70. Wojtys EM, Hovda D, Landry G, et al: Concussion in sports. **Am J Sports Med 27:**676-687, 1999

71. Yarnell PR, Lynch S: The "ding:" amnestic states in football trauma. **Neurology 23:**196-197, 1973

72. Yarnell PR, Lynch S: Retrograde memory immediately after concussion. **Lancet 1:**863-864, 1970

73. Yarnell PR, Rossie GV: Minor whiplash head injury with major debilitation. **Brain Inj 2:**255-258, 1988

CHAPTER 9

A Comprehensive Approach to Concussion Assessment

KEVIN M. GUSKIEWICZ, PHD, ATC

Unlike most injuries sustained in sports, a cerebral concussion has the potential for catastrophic outcome if managed inappropriately. Sports medicine clinicians responsible for the care of athletes sustaining concussion must therefore be aware of the potential dangers of returning an athlete to competition following such an injury. Despite the seriousness of these injuries, the concussion literature is rather limited in comparson to injuries of the spine and extremities. There have been several notable sports-related concussion articles published over the last 20 years; however, few have provided evidence based on controlled clinical research studies. Several of the documents are review-type articles outlining the various clinical grading scales and return-to-play guidelines,[6,16-20,24,48,76,95] while others focus on epidemiological issues such as incidence-of-injury and exposure rates.[3,15,25,33,40,81]

This chapter focuses on neuropsychological and postural stability testing as contemporary methods for assessing concussion in athletes. A presentation of the justification for a comprehensive approach to concussion assessment as well as a historical perspective of postural stability testing and neurocognitive testing in athletes are presented. Additionally, several techniques and ideas for how to institute alternative testing into the sports medicine setting are presented.

The Limits of Grading Scales and Return-to-play Guidelines

Although the published literature has contributed significantly from an epidemiological perspective, the reports are limited in the ability to help substantiate the recommended concussion grading scales and return-to-play guidelines used by clinicians. Much of the disagreement surrounding the various grading scales and guidelines stems from the lack of empirical data to support them. Most are based on anecdotal information or clinical experience, both of which are important but not likely to provide the most valid criteria. Experts agree that most of the proposed protocols are safe and that athletes are placed at little risk if the guidelines are adhered to closely. The problem remains that none of the grading scales and guidelines are followed with any consistency and none has emerged as the gold standard.

The question raised most often is one of practicality in the sports setting. Many clinicians believe that the return-to-play guidelines are too conservative and they choose to base decisions on clinical judgment of individual patients rather than on a general recommendation. A recent study of 1003 football-related concussions revealed that 30% of all high school and college players sustaining concussion returned to competition on the same day of injury.[40] The remaining 70% averaged 4 days of rest prior to returning to participation. Most grading scales suggest that participation be withheld for at least 7 days following a Grade I or II concussion. Most team physicians and athletic trainers deviate from these recommendations and are more liberal or lenient in making return-to-play decisions. Until guidelines are proposed based on empirical data, it is likely that clinicians will not to adhere to any one protocol.

Another issue is that of subjective versus objective assessment. The complexity of the brain and the few objective signs often manifested at the time of injury make the assessment of concussion uniquely challenging. Clinicians are often solely dependent on subjective symptoms rather than on sound objective data. In addition to being underreported by anxious athletes, subjective signs and symptoms may resolve immediately after injury, a time when underlying pathology may still be undetected.[4,18,20,45,80] Return-to-play decisions in these circumstances are often based on speculation rather than certainty. The result of prematurely returning an athlete to competition following concussion can be catastrophic. The incidence and danger of second-impact syndrome are discussed elsewhere in this book and are well documented in the literature.[19,30,49,64,87] Of less concern, but still worthy of consideration, is the risk of predisposition to other injuries during activities that alter sensory input to either one or more sensory systems.[38,39] Thus, there exists a substantial need for the development of objective measures that can be utilized during both sideline and clinical assessments.

Reports of the cumulative effects of multiple head injuries and head impacts on long-term cognitive functioning are causing clinicians to rethink their approach to managing concussion in sports.[23,59,60,92,93] Alternative methods of concussion assessment are indicated for any athlete at high risk for sustaining a concussion. These techniques should involve the use of objective, quantifiable criteria for assessing the athlete's neurocognitive function and postural stability. The literature has reported deficiencies in neurocognitive functions such as attention span, memory, concentration, and information processing as a result of cerebral concussion.[10,32,35,36,52,56,58,85] Additionally, it has been reported that the areas of the brain that are disrupted as a result of concussion are responsible for the maintenance of equilibrium.[1,7,41,61,65,66,88] As a result of these findings, neurocognitive and postural measures have been proposed as a means through which mild head injury can be objectively assessed.[5,10,23,38,39,46,52,58,62,63,79,82,83] Clinicians traditionally utilized the Romberg test for assessing disequilibrium in head-injured athletes, but recently computerized posturography has become available to offer a more objective and challenging assessment. Likewise, clinicians have used verbal concentration tests, such as "serial 7's," and questions of orientation and amnesia, such as those on the Galveston Orientation and Amnesia Test,[55,56] to assess concussion, yet recently they have begun the more consistent utilization of neuropsychological tests.

To use an analogy of an athlete recovering from a serious knee injury, a clinician would rarely return an athlete to participation unless they were certain that the athlete's flexibility and strength were within normal limits when compared to baseline measurements taken from the contralateral limb. Unfortunately, comparison to a contralateral limb is not an option when assessing cerebral concussion. Therefore, it is imperative to have access to preseason baseline information upon which comparisons can be made. The other unique challenge in returning a concussed player to participation is that, unlike with a knee injury, the clinician is unable to observe the cardinal signs of inflammation such as swelling, redness, warmth, pain, and loss of function.

Traditional Methods of Head Injury Assessment

Many methods of assessing the severity of head and brain injury have been developed. Such evaluation tools are crucial for determining the severity of the injury and predicting outcomes and future rehabilitation needs. Computed tomography (CT) and magnetic resonance imaging (MRI) have enhanced the capability of diagnosticians to identify certain types of brain lesions; however, they are of little value in measuring the potential range of brain injury severity.[89] Two widely accepted methods to assess this are the Glasgow Coma Scale and the Abbreviated Injury Scale; however, their usefulness is questioned in many instances, especially in managing sports-related head injury.

The Glasgow Coma Scale requires observation of the patient's eye opening, verbal performance, and motor response. Total scores range from 3 (no response to any stimulation) to 15 (no abnormalities in the three performance criteria). The scale demonstrates good validity, but in certain cases is limited in its applicability.[89] For example, eye opening may be impossible with facial swelling and verbal response may be compromised by an endotracheal tube.[51]

The Abbreviated Injury Scale is designed to assess overall injury severity along with severity of injury to specific body parts. Under this grading scheme, brain injuries are classified as either anatomic or non-anatomic. Anatomic lesions are confirmed through CT or MRI, while the severity of suspected lesions is assessed through the markers of loss of consciousness, length of unconsciousness, current level of consciousness, response to external stimuli, and neurological deficit. When information is available regarding the level of consciousness and a substantiated anatomic lesion, each parameter is coded and the higher of the two scores is assigned. The scores for brain injury range from 1 (awake on admission, no prior unconsciousness, may have headache or dizziness) to 5 (unconscious on admission, unconscious for more than 24 hours, neurological deficit). Although the Abbreviated Injury Scale avoids some of the problems of the Glasgow Coma Scale, according to Sorenson and Kraus,[89] it has some limitations of its own. This scale depends on a valid physician diagnosis and, barring that, a clear enumeration of symptoms in the medical record to allow assignment of an injury score.

Contemporary Methods of Head Injury Assessment

Postural Control System

The postural control system is responsible for the maintenance of upright posture and balance. The system operates as a feedback control circuit between the brain and the musculoskeletal system. The musculature of the legs, feet, and truncus, through the use of this feedback circuit, allows for erect standing against the forces of gravity.[41,47,69,94] Postural stability is also greatly influenced by a person's physical condition, such as nervous disorders, dysfunction of the optic nerve and vestibular mechanism, fatigue, and mental state.[90] To fully understand how the body maintains its upright posture, we must first understand how the brain processes information from various sources. It is well known that maintaining balance requires the aid of vestibular, visual, and proprioceptive sensations. Feedback obtained from these sensors sends commands to the muscles of the extremities, which then generate an appropriate contraction to maintain postural stability.[43,47,69,88,90]

Vestibular and Visual System

The vestibular apparatus is the organ responsible for detecting sensations concerned with equilibrium. The apparatus is composed of a system of bony tubes and chambers within the temporal bone called the bony labyrinth. It is adjacent to and continuous with the cochlear duct of the inner ear. It also consists of three semicircular canals and two large chambers known as the utricle and the saccule. The utricle, the semicircular canals, and the saccule are the integral parts of the equilibrium mechanism.[41,94]

The macula, however, is considered the sensory organ of the utricle and saccule and is responsible for detecting the orientation of the head with respect to gravity. Specifically, the macula of the semicircular canals detects angular acceleration during rotation of the head, while the macula of the utricle and saccule provides information about linear acceleration and changes in head position relative to the forces of gravity.[94] Each macula is covered by a gelatinous layer, in which many small calcium carbonate crystals ("otoliths") are imbedded. Also, within the macula are thousands of hair cells that synapse with sensory axons of the vestibular system.[41] Information about hair cell stimulation is relayed from the vestibular apparatus to the brainstem by cranial nerve VIII, the same nerve that carries acoustic information to the brain.

Information from the vestibular apparatus can be used in three ways. First, the information is used to control eye muscles so that when the head changes position, the eyes can stay fixed on the same point. Second, vestibular information can be used for reflex mechanisms in maintaining upright posture. The vestibular organs are often referred to as the "sense organs of balance," despite research findings to the contrary. Very few postural reflexes rely primarily on vestibular input.[44,69,73,91] A third use of vestibular information involves conscious awareness of the body's position and acceleration after information has been relayed to the cortex by the thalamus.[94] Most investigators agree that the vestibular system is primarily involved in the stabilization of slow body sway, which is achieved by a much lower level of leg activation. Under normal conditions, most persons rely more on visual and somatosensory inputs to control body sway.[27,44,69,73] However, when sudden changes or perturbations are induced, causing a person to change the direction of movement or head position (i.e., leaning the head sideways, forward, or backward), the automatic control mechanism provided by vestibular input becomes crucial for stabilizing the direction of gaze of the eyes and, ultimately, one's equilibrium.

Vision is obviously very important for maintaining control of balance and this becomes especially important under such conditions of postural perturbation. Moreover, the eyes would be of little use in detecting an image unless they remained fixed on an object long enough to gain a clear image. Therefore, when the head is suddenly tilted, signals from the semicircular canals cause the eyes to rotate in an equal and opposite direction to the rotation of the head.[41] This is a function of the vestibulo-ocular reflex. Thus, when both the support surface and the visual surroundings are moving, the vestibular input automatically takes precedence.[69] In short, the vestibular apparatus mainly contributes to posture by maintaining the reflexes associated with keeping the head and neck in the vertical position and allowing the vestibulo-ocular reflex to control eye movement.

Proprioceptive System

The proprioceptive system is best described through the mechanoreceptive senses of touch, pressure, vibration, and tickle (the tactile senses) and the sense of position, which determines the relative positions and rates of movement of the different parts of the body.[41,94] This discussion focuses on the muscle afferent fibers and their role in sensing body positioning.

Muscle spindles and Golgi tendon sensory receptors (proprioceptors) play a vital role in the nervous system's control of posture. They provide the nervous system with continuous feedback as to the instantaneous status of each muscle. Muscle length and changes in length are monitored by stretch receptors embedded within the muscle. These receptors consist of endings of afferent nerve fibers that are wrapped around modified muscle fibers, several of which are enclosed in a connective-tissue capsule. The entire structure is called a muscle spindle.[41,94] Muscle spindles send information to the nervous system about the muscle length or the rate of its change in length. When afferent fibers from the muscle spindle enter the central nervous system (CNS), they divide into branches that can take several different paths. One path directly stimulates motor neurons going back to the muscle that was stretched, thereby completing a reflex arc known as the stretch, or myotactic, reflex. This reflex causes a muscle contraction in response to a muscle being stretched.[94]

Golgi tendon organs, located in the tendons near their junction with the muscles, serve as a second type of afferent receptor (proprioceptor). They are responsible for sending information about tension or rate of change of tension in the muscle.[41,94] The afferent neuron's firing activity supplies the motor control systems (both locally and in the brain) with continuous information about the muscle's tension. The Golgi tendon organ is designed to serve as a protective mechanism to relax a muscle that is being overstretched. It senses tension within a muscle, transmits the information to the CNS, and, through polysynaptic reflexes, inhibits the motor neurons of the contracting muscle.[94]

Rotation of the ankles is the most probable stimulus of the functional stretch (myotactic) reflex that occurs in many persons. It appears to be the first useful phase of activity in the leg muscles after a change in erect posture.[70] The myotactic reflex can be seen when perturbations of gait or posture automatically evoke functionally directed responses in the leg muscles to compensate for imbalance or increased postural sway.[27,70] Muscle spindles sense a stretching of the agonist, thus sending information along its afferent fibers to the spinal cord. The information is then transferred to alpha and gamma motor neurons that carry information back to the muscle fibers and muscle spindle, respectively, and contract the muscle to prevent or control additional postural sway.[27]

Balance Control: The Hierarchy of Balance

It can be said that "everything is in balance, or that balance is in everything." Balance plays a vital role in the maintenance of fluid dynamic movement common in sports. It is the process of maintaining the center of gravity within the body's base of support and is maintained through a feedback system. The human body is a very tall structure balanced on a relatively small base, and its center of gravity is quite high, being just above the pelvis.[94] Many factors enter into the task of controlling balance within this designated area. The system involves a complex network of neural connections and centers that are related by peripheral and central feedback mechanisms. A hierarchy integrating the cerebral cortex, cerebellum, basal ganglia, brainstem, and spinal cord is primarily responsible for controlling voluntary movements.[41,94]

The highest level of the hierarchy involves areas of the brain responsible for memory and emotion, as well as associated cortex for receiving and correlating input from other brain structures. The middle level involves the sensorimotor cortex, the cerebellum, parts of the basal ganglia, and some brainstem nuclei. The cerebellum is the most important center for coordinating and learning movements and for controlling posture and balance. In order for the cerebellum to carry out these functions, it must receive information from the muscles, joints, skin, eyes, ears, and even the viscera.[41,94] The afferent pathways of the reflex arcs come from three sources: the eyes, the vestibular apparatus, and the proprioceptors, and their actions are referred to as postural reflexes. The efferent pathways are the alpha motor neurons to the skeletal muscles, and the integrating centers are neuron networks in the brainstem and spinal cord. Afferent input from several sources is necessary for effective postural adjustments, yet interfering with any one of these inputs should not cause a person to lose total control of balance.[41,88]

The lowest level of the hierarchy involves the brainstem and the spinal cord from which the motor neurons exit. These structures receive information from the middle level via the descending pathways. Its function is to specify tension of particular muscles and the angle of joints necessary to carry out the programs transmitted from the middle level.

Sensory Organization and Muscle Coordination

From our knowledge of the involvement of the CNS in maintaining upright posture, the processes can be divided into two components. The term "sensory organization" involves those processes that determine the timing, direction, and amplitude of corrective postural actions based upon information obtained from vestibular, visual, and somatosensory (proprioceptive) input. Despite the availability of multiple sensory inputs, the CNS generally relies on only one sense at a time for orientation information. For healthy adults, the preferred sense for balance control comes from somatosensory information (i.e., the feet in contact with the support surface).[69]

The second component, "muscle coordination," describes processes that determine the temporal sequencing and distribution of contractile activity among the muscles of the legs and trunk, which generate supportive reactions for maintaining balance. Balance deficiencies in persons with neurological problems can result from inappropriate interaction among the three sensory inputs that provide orientation information to the postural control system. A patient may be inappropriately dependent on one sense for situations presenting intersensory conflict.[69,88]

Clinical Test of Sensory Interaction and Balance

Studies have attempted to isolate and clarify which sensory inputs are most involved with regulating posture and how the interaction among these inputs affects postural control.[26-28,44,72,77] A technique described by Shumway-Cook and Horak[88] and Ingersoll and Armstrong,[46] called the Clinical Test of Sensory Interaction and Balance has been used to systematically remove or conflict sensory input from one or more of the three senses. The technique uses combinations of three visual and two support-surface conditions during assessment of postural sway.

The visual conditions include: (normal) eyes open (conditions 1 and 4); blindfolded for eliminating visual input (conditions 2 and 5); and a visual-conflict dome for producing inaccurate visual input (conditions 3 and 6) (Figure 1). The visual-conflict dome, when attached to the head, moves in phase with the subject's head movement and restricts peripheral vision from the top, bottom, and

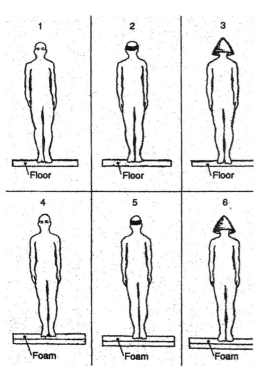

Figure 1: The Clinical Test of Sensory Interaction and Balance using visual conditions. The patient is standing on the floor in conditions 1-3 and on foam in 4-6. In conditions 1 and 4, the patient has eyes open, in conditions 2 and 5, is blindfolded for eliminating visual input, and in conditions 3 and 6, a visual-conflict dome is used for producing inaccurate visual input.

sides. Vertical and horizontal lines on the inside of the dome remain vertical and horizontal in the line of vision regardless of the subject's vertical orientation. Therefore, increased postural instability while wearing the visual-conflict dome (condition 3) suggests abnormal reliance on vision for posture control, which is common with patients having vestibular postconcussion syndrome or benign paroxysmal positional nystagmus.[69]

The support-surface conditions include: 1) the use of any hard, flat surface that ensures accurate orientation information from the somatosensory system; and 2) a compliant 50×50×8-cm section of medium-density foam that reduces the accuracy of the orientation information. Increased postural instability under conditions where proprioceptors of the feet are eliminated (conditions 4-6) suggests that the other sensory modalities (vestibular and/or visual) are not adequately compensating for the loss of proprioception.

Sensory Organization Test

An alternative to the Clinical Test of Sensory Interaction and Balance is the Sensory Organization Test, which was developed by Nashner et al[69,73] and utilizes sophisticated force-plate technology which has a moving visual surround and a tilting base of support. The advantage of this test is that clinicians can easily isolate sensory modalities, providing afferent information to the postural control system. As previously discussed, under normal circumstances a person balances with the aid of information from the visual, vestibular, and somatosensory systems. If one system is deficient, the other systems should compensate for the deficiency.

The Sensory Organization Test is designed to systematically disrupt the sensory selection process by altering the orientation information available to the somatosensory and/or visual inputs while measuring a subject's ability to maintain equilibrium. The test protocol consists of three 20-second trials under three different visual conditions (eyes open, eyes closed, or sway-referenced) and two different surface conditions (fixed or sway-referenced) (Figure 2). Subjects are asked to stand as motionless as possible for each trial, in a normal stance with the feet shoulder-width apart. The term "sway-referenced" involves the tilting of the support surface and/or visual surround to directly follow the athlete's center of gravity sway such that the orientation of the surface remains constant in relation to the center-of-gravity angle. By using this technique, the somatosensory and/or visual systems report that the subject's orientation to gravity is constant when, in fact, it is changing, requiring the subject to ignore the inaccurate information from the sway-referenced sense(s).

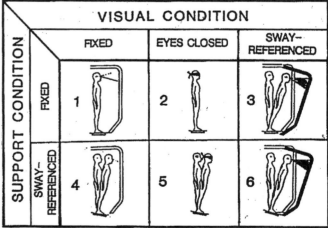

Figure 2: Six testing conditions, using visual and support conditions, for the Sensory Organization Test used with the EquiTest and Smart Balance Master.

A composite equilibrium score describing a person's overall level of performance during all of the trials in the Sensory Organization Test is calculated, with higher scores being indicative of better balance performance. The composite score is the average of the following 14 scores: the condition 1 average score, the condition 2 average score, and three equilibrium scores from each of the trials in conditions 3-6. The equilibrium scores from each of the trials represent a nondimensional percentage, comparing the subject's peak amplitude of an anteroposterior sway to the theoretical anteroposterior limit of stability.

Additionally, relative differences between the equilibrium scores of various conditions are calculated using ratios to reveal specific information about each of the sensory modalities involved with maintaining balance. For example, a vestibular ratio is computed by using scores attained in condition 5 (eyes closed and sway-referenced platform) and condition 1 (eyes open and fixed platform). This ratio indicates the relative reduction in postural stability when visual and somatosensory inputs are simultaneously disrupted. These ratios are useful in identifying sensory integration problems.

In summary, the nervous system is responsible for providing the necessary visual input, vestibular mechanisms, and proprioceptive reflex activities for the maintenance of static and dynamic equilibrium. The consensus is that the reliance on one or more of the three senses for postural control varies depending on periods of life and specific pathological conditions.

Pathological Balance Assessment

Disorders of orientation and balance can be debilitating, especially in an athletic environment. The complexity of the balance system makes localization of the problem difficult, since the abnormality may occur in one or more of the sensory modalities (vision, vestibular, or somatosensory system) or in the motor system involved with carrying out a particular movement.[74] While sensory isolation deficits have been studied at length, other research has focused more on specific pathologies such as cerebral palsy,[75] Parkinson's disease,[90] idiopathic scoliosis,[86] and convergent strabismus,[78] and their effect on postural equilibrium. These studies compared postural actions of subjects with pathology to normal subjects and described the organization of sensory processes as they related to the specific pathologies.

Contrary to clinical belief, studies have demonstrated that motor deficits are present in a mildly head-injured patient 1 year after injury, suggesting that motor skills should be routinely assessed after a concussion.[42,50] Moreover, if motor deficits are present, balance deficits are also likely to be present. Research suggests that the areas of brain damaged as a result of head injury are often the areas responsible for the maintenance of postural equilibrium.[2,9,11,22,66] Symptoms of persons with cerebellar damage generally include the following:[94]

- cannot perform movements smoothly;
- walks awkwardly, with the feet well apart. Difficulty in maintaining balance causes unsteadiness of gait;
- cannot start or stop movements quickly or easily. Motions are slow and irregular; and
- cannot easily combine the movements of several joints into a smooth, coordinated motion (i.e., to move an arm, he/she might first move the shoulder, then the elbow, and finally the wrist).

Severe and Chronic Head Injury

Despite the common dysfunction of cerebral and/or vestibular mechanisms accompanying head injury, few studies have focused on the effects of head injury on postural equilibrium. A study by Arcan et al[7] compared foot-ground pressure patterns of normal subjects to 17 hemiplegics and 15 craniocerebral-injured patients. Tests performed on normal subjects (free of known pathological conditions) indicated that 45%-65% of body weight is carried on their heels, 1%-8% on their midfoot, and 30%-45% on their forefoot. The sagittal stance ratio varied between 0.33 and 0.51, while the lateral stance ratio varied between 0.50 and 0.56, indicating a fairly symmetrical foot-ground pressure pattern.

Hemiplegia is a condition involving paralysis of the upper extremity, trunk, and lower extremity on one side of the body. Hemiplegics tested by Arcan et al[7] at the beginning of their rehabilitation period tended to carry 75%-85% of their weight on one leg; however, a group tested at the end of their rehabilitation period demonstrated a more symmetrical stance. These patients did not exhibit deviations in heel-midfoot-forefoot distribution. Results of the craniocerebral-injured patients tested revealed an interesting characteristic. Nine of the 15 patients carried their weight mostly on the heel of one foot and the forefoot of the other, therefore distributing a large part of the weight along one diagonal of the quadrilateral defined by the four local centers of pressure. The authors named this condition the "diagonal pressure pattern." The other six craniocerebral-injured patients presented a foot-ground pressure pattern similar to the hemiplegics.

These findings suggest a disruption to one or all of the mechanisms responsible for controlling equilibrium. The feedback system responsible for providing the nervous system with proprioceptive cues by way of the stretch reflex exists in both craniocerebral-injured patients and hemiplegics. Moreover, voluntary control is affected in hemiplegics in the same way that it is in craniocerebral patients.[7,41] Thus, the investigators ruled out the stretch reflex and voluntary muscle control as being the sources of the diagonal pattern. Instead, they speculate that subcortical centers affected by trauma might be the cause of poor muscle coordination.

In an attempt to better understand the role of the cerebellum in posture, postural sway was studied in three groups of subjects with restricted cerebellar lesions.[61] Patients with anterior lobe lesions demonstrated a specific tremor in the anteroposterior direction. Mediolateral sway was less characteristic and smaller in amplitude, although patients with uncompensated vestibular lesions showed marked lateral sway and eventually fell, as did patients with vestibulo-cerebellar lesions. Patients with lesions of the hemispheres showed only slight postural instability without directional preference. Their sway parameters with eyes open were within normal ranges and were not significantly different from normal subjects, even with eyes closed. Thus, the investigators concluded they could not distinguish brain-injured patients from normal subjects according to their platform recordings.

A study using a force platform and the six testing conditions previously discussed in the Clinical Test of Sensory Interaction and Balance (Figure 1) monitored translation of the center of pressure in subjects divided into four groups according to level of head injury: 1) no head injury; 2) mild head injury (no loss of consciousness); 3) moderate head injury (unconscious for less than 6 hours); and 4) severe head injury (unconscious for 6 hours or more). All subjects were at least 1 year postinjury, but averaged 8.9 years. Severely head-injured subjects demonstrated greater anteroposterior and mediolateral sway than mildly head-injured or normal subjects. The investigators concluded that, although total sway did not differ between groups, head-injured subjects maintained their center of pressure at greater distances from the center of their base of support. Furthermore, these subjects made fewer postural corrections, especially when one or more of the sensory modalities were conflicted or eliminated.[46] The investigators suggested that sensory modality communication most likely had been lost in these chronically injured individuals.

Mild and Acute Head Injury

Postural control has proved to be an objective measure in the evaluation of acute mild head injury or concussion in athletes. Guskiewicz et al[38] revealed decreased postural stability (in comparison to control subjects) in athletes with acute mild head injury using a modified Clinical Test of Sensory Interaction and Balance protocol on the Chattecx Balance System (Chattanooga Group, Inc., Hixon, TX). The decreases in postural stability in comparison to control subjects persisted for up to 3 days following injury and were most evident when the subjects were standing either on a foam or a moving (tilting) surface.

In similar studies, decreases in postural stability have been reported for up to 3 days postinjury using the Sensory Organization Test on the Smart Balance Master (Neuro-Com International, Clackamas, OR).[39,82] Again, differences between mild head-injured and control subjects became most evident when visual and support surface conditions were altered. The most important finding from these studies, as well as our ongoing work, is that athletes demonstrated sensory interaction problems during the first few days following mild head injury. The overall postural stability results indicated that athletes with acute mild injury demonstrate decreased stability until approximately 3 days following injury. The athletes gradually recovered to mimic the scores of their matched control subjects by Day 10 postinjury (Figure 3). It appears that this deficit is related to a sensory interaction problem, whereby the injured athlete fails to use the visual and vestibular systems effectively (Figures 4 and 5).

The integration of visual and vestibular information is essential for the maintenance of equilibrium under certain altered conditions similar to those performed during the Sensory Organization Test.[69-73] If a subject has difficulty balancing under conditions in which sensory modalities have been altered, it can be hypothesized that he/she is unable to ignore altered environmental conditions and, therefore, selects a motor response based on the altered environmental cues. This has the potential to cause problems and perhaps predispose athletes to further injury when encountered with activities that alter sensory input to one or more systems. An example of an athlete having altered sensory input might be a basketball player during the transitional phases of returning to the ground following a rebound, selecting a visual target, running forward, and passing the ball.

While the aforementioned studies suggest that vertical-ground reaction forces and postural sway measurements provided by force-plate systems are valuable in making return-to-play decisions following concussion, there is still a question of practicality and accessibility for the sports medicine clinician. In an attempt to provide a more cost-effective, yet quantifiable method of assessing balance in athletes, researchers at the University of North Carolina at Chapel Hill developed the "Balance Error Scoring System." This system also utilizes six testing conditions under varying stances and surface conditions, but does not require the use of an expensive force-plate system (Figure 6). Balance performance is judged by totaling the number of errors committed during six 20-second test conditions. The specific errors are described later in this chapter (see Table 2).

Significant correlations between the Balance Error Scoring System and force-platform sway measures using normal subjects have been established for five static balance tests (single leg stance-firm surface, tandem stance-firm surface, double leg stance-foam surface, single leg stance-foam surface, and tandem stance-foam surface), with inter-tester reliability coefficients ranging from 0.78 to 0.96.[84] Another study by the same group then compared balance performances between mild head-injured and control subjects using the Balance Error Scoring System with the intention of identifying test variations that would best elicit postural unsteadiness following mild head injury. Additionally, the Sensory Organization Test was administered to determine whether the results of the clinical balance tests paralleled results attained with a force-plate system.[83] Significant group differences on Day 1 postinjury were revealed using the Balance Error Scoring System with the double leg, single leg, and tandem stances on both the firm and the foam surface (Figure 7). The results of the Sensory Organization Test composite scores paralleled the results revealed with the clinical balance tests and are similar to recovery curves reported in previous investigations.[38,39] Resolution of signs and symptoms recorded across the three postinjury testing sessions appears to coincide with the postural stability recoveries demonstrated by the mild head-injured subjects.

The results of this study revealed greater differences between injured and non-injured subjects when the balance tasks became more challenging (i.e., adding the foam surface

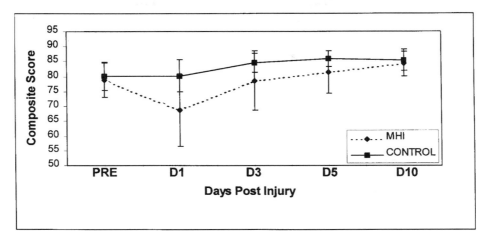

Figure 3: Composite score (mean ± SD) on the Smart Balance Master for 22 mild head-injured (MHI) and 22 control subjects for each testing session (preseason (PRE) and Days 1, 3, 5, and 10 postinjury (D1, 3, 5, and 10)).

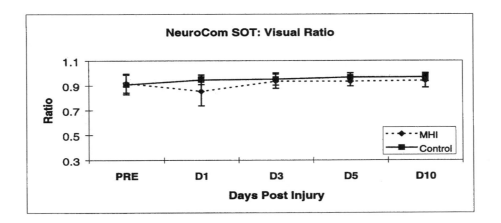

Figure 4: Visual ratio score (mean ± SD) on the Smart Balance Master for 22 mild head-injured (MHI) and 22 control subjects for each testing session (preseason (PRE) and Days 1, 3, 5, and 10 postinjury (D1, 3, 5, and 10)).

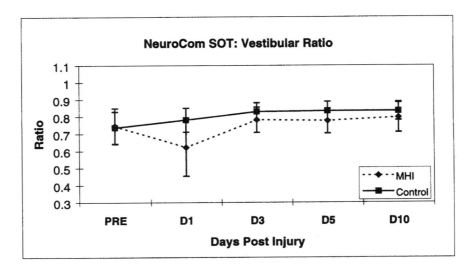

Figure 5: Vestibular ratio score (mean ± SD) on the Smart Balance Master for 22 mild head-injured (MHI) and 22 control subjects for each testing session (preseason (PRE) and Days 1, 3, 5, and 10 postinjury (D1, 3, 5, and 10)).

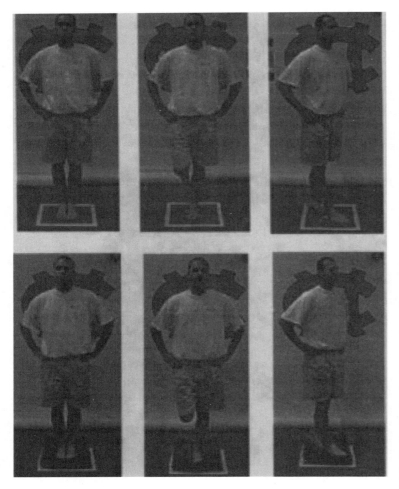

Figure 6: Demonstration of stance positions for the Balance Error Scoring System performed on a firm surface *(top)* and foam surface *(bottom)*.

and narrowing the base of support). Although the standard Romberg test has been advocated for use in mild head injury assessment,[6,8,14] that study failed to reveal significant differences between mild head-injured and control subjects using the double leg, single leg, and tandem stances on a firm surface. Potential reasons for this failure to elicit postural instability following mild head injury may be attributed to an inability of presenting a balance task capable of challenging the postural control system of conditioned athletes. Clinicians should exhibit caution in relying on less challenging tests to elicit postural instability during acute mild head injury assessments.

Techniques of Balance Assessment

Subjective Assessment

The assessment of static balance in athletes has traditionally been performed using the standing Romberg test. This test is performed by having the athlete stand with feet together, arms at the side, and eyes closed (Figure 8). Normally, a person can stand still in this position, but the tendency to sway or fall to one side is considered a positive Romberg's sign or indicates loss of proprioception. Typically, the clinician will make the test progressively more challenging by requiring the person to then perform the test while standing on a single

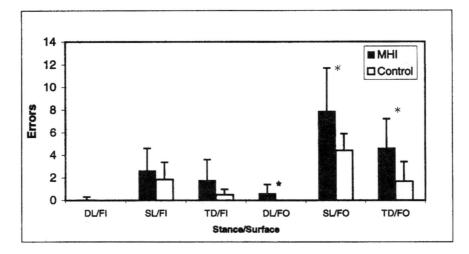

Figure 7: Balance Error Scoring System (mean ± SD) for the three stances on both surfaces for 16 mild head-injured (MHI) and 16 control subjects on Day 1 postinjury. There were no errors committed by the control group for either the DL/FI or DL/FO tests. DL = double-leg stance, SL = single-leg stance, TD = tandem stance, FI = firm surface, FO = foam surface, * = significantly different from other group. (Reproduced from Riemann and Guskiewicz[83] with permission)

leg, followed by a tandem stance (heel to toe), and finally a double-leg stance after completing a series of 360° revolutions (spinning Romberg test). The object in most of these tests is to decrease the size of the base support, in an attempt to determine an athlete's ability to maintain his/her center of gravity within a safe limit of stability. The Romberg test has, however, been criticized for its lack of sensitivity and objectivity. It is considered to be a rather qualitative assessment of static balance because a considerable amount of stress is required to make the subject sway enough for an observer to characterize the sway.[47] Dynamic balance assessment has traditionally been performed through functional reach tests and/or timed agility tests such as the figure-eight test or the carioca or hop test, but are also criticized for lacking objectivity.

Objective Assessment

More recently, advancements in technology have provided the medical community with commercially produced balance systems for quantitatively assessing and training static and dynamic balance. These systems provide easy, practical, and cost-effective methods of quantitatively assessing and training functional balance through analysis of postural stability. Thus, the potential exists to assess injured athletes as follows: 1) identify possible abnormalities that might be associated with injury; 2) isolate various systems that are affected; 3) develop recovery curves based on quantitative measures for determining readiness to return to activity; and 4) train the injured athlete.[37]

Most manufacturers use computer-interfaced force-plate technology consisting of a flat, rigid surface supported on three or more points by independent force-measuring devices (Figure 9). As the athlete stands on the force-plate surface, the position of the center of vertical forces exerted on the force plate over time is calculated. The center of vertical force movements provides an indirect measure of postural sway activity[71] (Figure 10). The Kistler force plate was used for much of the early work in the area of postural stability and balance;[13,29,34,61,68] however, other manufacturers such as the Chattanooga Group, Inc., and NeuroCom International, Inc., have developed systems with expanded diagnostic and training capabilities. Clinicians must be aware that the manufacturers often use conflicting terminology to describe various balance parameters. These inconsistencies have created confusion in the literature (e.g., what some manufacturers classify as dynamic balance, others claim is static balance).

Force platforms ideally evaluate four aspects of postural control: steadiness, symmetry, dynamic stability, and dynamic balance. *Steadiness* is the ability to keep the body as

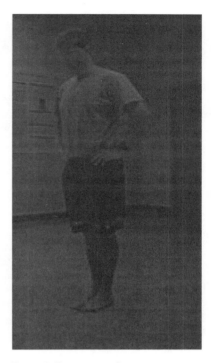

Figure 8: The standard Romberg test.

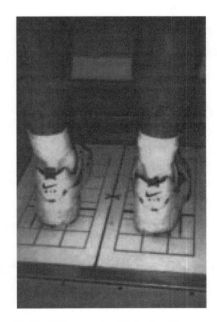

Figure 9: Force plate with double-leg stance.

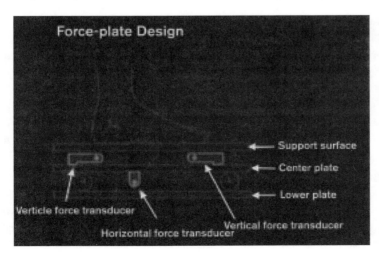

Figure 10: Force-plate design.

motionless as possible. This is a measure of postural sway. *Symmetry* is the ability to distribute weight evenly between the two feet in an upright stance. This is a measure of center of pressure, center of balance, or center of force, depending on the testing system being used.

Although inconsistent with the author's classification system, *dynamic stability* is often defined as the ability to transfer the vertical projection of the center of gravity around a stationary supporting base.[34] This is often referred to as a measure of one's perception of the "safe" limits of stability, as the goal is to lean or reach as far as possible without losing the balance. Assessment of *dynamic balance* is somewhat different, in that postural responses are measured in response to external perturbations from a moving platform in one of four directions: tilting toes up, tilting toes down, shifting mediolaterally, and shifting anteroposteriorly. Platform perturbation on some systems is unpredictable and determined by the positioning and sway movement of the subject (e.g., the NeuroCom Equi-Test and Smart Balance Master). In such cases, a person's reaction can be determined. Other systems have a more predictable sinusoidal waveform that remains constant regardless of subject positioning (e.g., the Chattecx Balance System).

Many of these force-platform systems measure the vertical-ground reaction force and provide a means of computing the center of pressure. The center of pressure represents the center of the distribution of the total force applied to the supporting surface. This is calculated from horizontal moment and vertical force data generated by triaxial force platforms. The center of balance, in the case of the Chattecx Balance System, is the point between the feet where the ball and heel of each foot has 25% of the body weight. This point is referred to as the relative weight positioning over the four load cells as measured only by vertical forces. The center of vertical force on the EquiTest is that center exerted by the feet against the support surface. In any case, the total force applied to the force platform fluctuates because it includes both body weight and the inertial effects of the slightest movement of the body which occurs even when one attempts to stand motionless. The movement of these force-based reference points is theorized to vary according to the movement of the body's center of gravity and the distribution of muscle forces required to control posture. Ideally, healthy athletes should maintain their center of pressure very near the anteroposterior and mediolateral midlines.

Once the center of pressure, center of balance, or center of force is calculated, several other balance parameters can be attained. Deviation from this point in any direction represents a person's postural sway. Postural sway can be measured in various ways, depending on the stability system being used. Mean displacement, length of sway path, length of sway area, amplitude, frequency, and direction with respect to the center of pressure can be calculated on most systems. An equilibrium score, comparing the angular difference between the calculated maximum anteroposterior center of gravity displacements to a theoretical maximum displacement, is unique to the EquiTest. The sway index, representing the degree of scatter of data about the center of balance, is unique to the Chattecx Balance System.

Force-plate technology allows for quantitative analysis and understanding of a subject's postural instability. These systems are fully integrated with hardware/software systems for quickly and quantitatively assessing and rehabilitating balance disorders. Most manufacturers allow for both static and dynamic balance assessment in either double- or single-leg stances, with eyes open or closed. The EquiTest System and Smart Balance Master are both equipped with a moving visual surround (wall) that allows for the most sophisticated technology available for isolating and assessing sensory modality interaction. As previously mentioned, the clinician is able to collect a composite equilibrium score, as well as the ratio scores, for the various sensory systems.

Neurocognitive Functioning

Clinicians evaluating athletes suspected of having suffered a cerebral concussion usually focus first on physical symptomatology such as headache, dizziness, blurred vision, tinnitus, and poor equilibrium. Neurocognitive deficits, despite being less obvious, are also common and should be evaluated in a timely manner following injury. Cognition can be divided into the areas of intellect, language, memory, attention/concentration, information processing, and perceptual and motor function.[21] Intelligence, language functioning, and perceptual and motor functioning remain intact following mild head injury;[21,53,55] however, memory, attention, and information processing are more often affected.[36,53] These represent the so-called "postconcussion symptoms," which are often reported by athletes, especially in cases of recurrent head injury.

Cognitive impairment is one of the most disabling sequelae of closed head injury,[21,53] and memory may be the cognitive domain most prone to impairment following head trauma.[54] Of 42 patients tested at 16 to 42 months following closed head injury (injuries were not all mild), 28% had deficits in memory functioning. Concentration, according to Binder,[12] is the domain of attentional processing most affected following mild head trauma. A study by Gronwall and Wrightson[36] utilizing the Paced Auditory Serial Addition Test (PASAT) revealed deficits in information processing rates among concussed patients. This test is a task involving rapid presentation of auditory numeric material for complex mental manipulation and requires a high level of attention, concentration, and immediate recall memory. In studying several groups of patients according to severity of injury (based on posttraumatic amnesia), they concluded that severity of injury was directly related to the time taken to recover the information processing rate. Furthermore, they concluded that postconcussion symptoms regressed as intellectual function returned. In another study by Gronwall and Wrightson,[35] concussion produced a deficit in the rate of information processing. The rate usually returned to normal within 1 month, but was reduced for an extended period if symptoms of postconcussion syndrome developed. In addition, patients who had been concussed for a second time demonstrated a greater decrease in the rate of information processing and recovered more slowly (7 days longer) than their matched first-concussion group. Therefore, they concluded that the capacity to process information rapidly is reduced immediately after suffering a concussion and that reduction is significantly greater and lasts significantly longer when a patient has previously been concussed.

Leininger et al[52] performed neuropsychological assessment on a group of concussed patients using the Wechsler Adult Intelligence Scale-Revised (WAIS-R) Vocabulary, WAIS-R Digit Span Backward, Category, Trail Making Test Part B, Auditory Verbal Learning, Complex Figure Copy and Memory Trials, Controlled Oral Word Association, and the PASAT-Revised (PASAT-R) tests. Nearly 60% of the subjects had received a concussion strong enough to render them unconscious (<20 minutes), while the other injuries displayed less serious signs and symptoms of a concussion. The results of the neuropsychological testing showed the concussion subjects performing significantly worse on the Category, PASAT-R, and Auditory Verbal Learning tests when compared to a control group of 23 subjects.

Pathological Neurocognitive Assessment

Neuropsychological techniques have been developed to reliably assess the extent of neurocognitive deficits following cerebral concussion in athletes. Due to variations in the neurocognitive abilities of athletes, the acquisition of baseline (pre-injury) measurements for comparison following injury is a necessity when instituting a neuropsychological testing program for athletes. This model is not realistic for use in a clinic or hospital setting, but has endless potential when used in the sports medicine setting where baseline testing is possible for athletes at high risk for injury.

Neuropsychological testing has revealed cognitive declines from preseason levels at 24 hours posttrauma in areas of attention, concentration, and rapid-complex problem solving.[10] These mild deficits were directly correlated with reported symptoms of increased headaches, dizziness, and problems with memory.

Barth et al,[10] considered the pioneers in neuropsychological testing of athletes, used the Trail Making Test Parts A and B, Symbol Digit Modalities Test, and PASAT to evaluate the cognitive function of college football players having sustained concussion. The players were tested during preseason, 24 hours, 5 days, and 10 days postinjury, and at postseason. Results of the PASAT revealed that student controls demonstrated significant improvement between 24 hours and 5 days, but showed no significant changes in the interval from 5 to 10 days and the interval from 10 days to postseason. However, injured athletes demonstrated significant improvement between 24 hours and 5 days and between 5 and 10 days, with no significant improvement in the 10 days to postseason interval. It was concluded that the student controls displayed the normal testing behavior (i.e., there was an initial practice effect), which is expected in the PASAT. The head-injured athletes maintained a preseason baseline score in the preseason to 24-hour postinjury period, and then displayed apparent recovery in the 24-hour to 5-day interval. Recovery continued in the 5- to 10-day interval, and then leveled off throughout the remainder of the season. It was concluded that neuropsychological recovery takes place in healthy, young athletes within 10 days of suffering a mild head injury.[10]

Neuropsychological deficits were similarly found in college football players sustaining a mild head injury in a 1996 report by Macciocchi et al.[57] The authors revealed a significant difference between baseline and postinjury tests administered 24 hours after the injury on the Trail Making Test Parts A and B between injured athletes and control subjects for whom age, gender, and educational levels matched.

In 1997, McCrea et al[62] introduced the Standardized Assessment of Concussion (SAC) to the sports medicine community by reporting that concussed high school football players assessed using the SAC scored significantly below nonconcussed controls and below their own baseline (pre-injury) performance, after having suffered a Grade I concussion (see Chapter 8).[62,63] The SAC, which includes measures of orientation, immediate memory recall, concentration, and delayed recall, was designed to provide athletic trainers and other medical personnel responsible for clinical decision-making in the care of athletes with immediate objective data concerning the presence and severity of neurocognitive impairment associated with concussion. The SAC is gaining popularity among sports medicine clinicians and is considered a useful adjunct to the sideline clinical examination following concussion.

Other studies have attempted to identify a relationship between neurocognitive impairment and the incidence of soccer-related concussion.[59,60,92,93] Tysvaer and Løchen[93] studied "headers" and "nonheaders" using the Trail Making Test Parts A and B, the Halstead-Wepman-Reitan Aphasia Screening Test, motor tests, tests for hemisphere dominance, tests for sensory-perceptual functions, and the Benton Visual Retention Test Part C. The players had ended their careers a mean of 14 years earlier, after playing an average of 359 games. Results revealed that 81% of the players demonstrated some level of neuropsychological impairment compared to 40% of a nonsoccer control group. The authors also stated that the "header" group showed a higher degree (20%) of neuropsychological impairment than the "nonheader" group (8%). This finding, however, was not statistically significant.

Matser et al[59] conducted a similar study comparing professional soccer players paired with nonsoccer athletes who served as control subjects. Players were grouped by position and classified as either "header" or "nonheader." The authors categorized midfielders and goalies as "nonheader," while forwards and defensive players were deemed "headers." The tests utilized for this analysis were the Raven Progressive Matrices Test, Wisconsin Card-Sorting Test, PASAT, Digit Symbol Test, Trail Making Test Parts A and B, Stroop Test, Bourdon-Wiersma Test, subtests of the Wechsler Memory Scale, Complex Figure Test, 15-Word Learning Test, Benton's Facial Recognition Task, Figure Detection Test, Verbal Fluency Test, and Puncture Test. Results revealed significant cognitive impairment in players when compared to the control group. The soccer players demonstrated deficits in verbal and visual memory, planning, and visuoperceptual processing tasks. The significance between the two groups remained even after correcting for confounding variables.

Matser et al[60] again examined the effects of heading a ball by soccer players, this time using amateur players. Utilizing those who played for an average of 17 years, matched with control subjects of swimmers and runners, the authors performed a series of neuropsychological tests that included the Raven Progressive Matrices Test, Wisconsin Card-Sorting Test, PASAT, Digit Symbol Test, Trail Making Test Parts A and B, Stroop Test, Bourdon-Wiersma Test, Wechsler Memory Scale, Complex Figure Test, 15-Word Learning Test, Benton's Facial Recognition Task, Figure Detection Test, Verbal Fluency Test, and Puncture Test. Results of the study revealed planning and memory impairments in the amateur players. Impairments in memory included 27% of the subjects and 7% of the control group; 39% of the amateur players showed moderate to severe impairment on the planning tests compared to 13% of the controls. Soccer players also showed deficits in the Complex Figure, Digit Span, Logical Memory, Visual Reproduction, and Associate Learning tests, and sections of the Wechsler Memory Scale after corrections were made for nonsoccer-related concussions, alcohol intake, education level, and exposure to general anesthesia.

Recommended Protocols for Assessment of Concussion

Symptom resolution should be at the forefront of the clinician's mind when evaluating an athlete who has suffered a concussion. It is important for the clinician to quantify the symptomatology so that comparisons can be made during serial examinations. This can best be accomplished through the use of a symptom checklist, similar to the one presented in Table 1. Using the total symptom score and the total number of symptoms reported takes some of the guesswork out of determining an athlete's readiness to return to activity. The additional use of objective measures, such as postural stability assessment and neuropsychological evaluation, can be invaluable to the sports medicine clinician. These three measures, combined with a thorough clinical examination, provide the best resources for making a sound clinical diagnosis and a safe return to participation.

It is important for the certified athletic trainer and team physician to work together in making the return-to-play decision and to recognize the value of other resources such as neurosurgeons and neuropsychologists. The certified athletic trainer typically has daily contact with the athlete and has an understanding of the athlete's personality, pain tolerance, and motivation to return to activity. The athletic trainer can therefore more easily detect lingering symptomatology such as irritability, sadness, concentration deficits, etc., that might otherwise go unnoticed by the team physician. It is also useful to talk with the athlete's teammates, parents, friends, roommates, coaches, etc., regarding any abnormal behaviors that might be indicative of lingering symptomatology.

The athlete should be referred to a neurosurgeon if postconcussion symptoms worsen within the first few hours postinjury. Neuropsychologists can also play an im-

TABLE 1
POSTCONCUSSION SYMPTOM SCALE

Circle appropriate number for each symptom

Symptom	None	Mild		Moderate		Severe	
1. headache	0	1	2	3	4	5	6
2. nausea	0	1	2	3	4	5	6
3. vomiting	0	1	2	3	4	5	6
4. balance problems/dizziness	0	1	2	3	4	5	6
5. fatigue	0	1	2	3	4	5	6
6. trouble sleeping	0	1	2	3	4	5	6
7. sleeping more than usual	0	1	2	3	4	5	6
8. drowsiness	0	1	2	3	4	5	6
9. sensitivity to light	0	1	2	3	4	5	6
10. blurred vision	0	1	2	3	4	5	6
11. sensitivity to noise	0	1	2	3	4	5	6
12. sadness	0	1	2	3	4	5	6
13. irritability	0	1	2	3	4	5	6
14. numbness/tingling	0	1	2	3	4	5	6
15. feeling like "in a fog"	0	1	2	3	4	5	6
16. difficulty concentrating	0	1	2	3	4	5	6
17. difficulty remembering	0	1	2	3	4	5	6
18. neck pain	0	1	2	3	4	5	6
Column Total Score							
Total No. of Items Endorsed							
Total Symptom Score							

portant role if the symptoms persist during the first several days postinjury. They have advanced training in the administration and interpretation of neuropsychological tests. It is recommended that sports medicine teams include these specialists, at the very least, for referral purposes.

A key component to this alternative method of evaluation involves instituting baseline testing for athletes who are at high risk for sustaining a concussion. Baseline testing should include a combination of the symptom checklist, postural stability tests, and neuropsychological tests (see below). The baseline tests should be conducted during the athlete's preseason, and should be used for comparison against any subsequent postinjury tests. The following testing sequence is recommended: time of injury, postgame, and Days 1, 2, 3, 5, 7, and 10 postinjury.

Based on previous research findings, the majority of injured athletes will be asymptomatic by Day 7 postinjury, and back to participation prior to Day 10 postinjury.[3,10,15,37-40,57] However, the decisions made during the initial few days following injury are the most crucial and potentially the most costly if made without full knowledge of the athlete's condition. The Day 10 assessment provides an important follow-up to determine the athlete's response to exertion and activity.

Sports medicine clinicians should always consider restricted return to participation prior to full return to participation. Close attention must be paid to the results of the symptom checklist and the neuropsychological and postural stability testing before a full return to participation is permitted. Obviously, the clinician should continue testing if the athlete is not asymptomatic within the initial 10 days. A postinjury assessment at Day 60 or 90 is also useful for identifying any lingering postconcussion symptoms. Results from each postinjury test should be compared to the athlete's baseline scores, as well as to the natural recovery curves that have already been established in the literature.[10,23,38,39,62,63,83]

Postural Stability

Postural stability in the mild head-injured athlete is best measured through the use of the Sensory Organization Test on the NeuroCom EquiTest or Neuro-Com Smart Balance Master (Figure 11). These systems, like other force-plate systems, measures vertical-ground reaction forces produced from the body's center of gravity moving around a fixed base of support. As previously mentioned, the NeuroCom systems offer a movable base of support and movable visual surround, allowing for isolation of sensory modalities that may be disrupted following a cerebral concussion.

Other force-plate systems such as the Kistler, Bertec, AMTI, and Chattecx can also be used for assessing a concussed athlete's postural stability; however, the clinician should attempt to isolate the sensory modalities by testing the athlete under various visual and support surface conditions. One means of doing this is through the Clinical Test of Sensory Interaction and Balance protocol. This procedure has been described by Shumway-Cook and Horak[88] using normal subjects and, as previously mentioned, has been used to identify deficits in athletes with acute mild head injury[38] and nonathletes with moderate to severe head injury.[46]

In the absence of sophisticated force-plate technology, the use of a quantifiable clinical test battery such as the Balance Error Scoring System is recommended. The Balance Error Scoring System is especially useful on the sideline, where force-place technology is unlikely to exist. As previously described, three different stances (double leg, single leg, and tandem) are completed twice, once while on a firm surface and once while on a 10-cm thick piece of medium-density foam (45 $cm^2 \times 13$ cm thick, density 60 kg/m^3, load deflection 80-90) for a total of six trials (Figure 6). The athlete is asked to assume the required stance by placing his/her hands on the iliac crests; upon eye closure, the 20-second test begins. During the single-leg stances, the subject is asked to maintain the contralateral limb in 20°-30° of hip flexion and 40°-50° of knee flexion. Additionally, the athlete stands as quietly and as motionless as possible, keeping the hands on the iliac crests and eyes closed. The single-limb stance tests are performed on the nondominant foot. This same foot is placed toward the rear on the tandem stances. Subjects are told that, upon losing their balance, they are to make any necessary adjustments and return to the testing position as quickly as possible. Performance is scored by adding one error point for each error committed (Table 2). Trials are considered incomplete if the athlete is unable to sustain the stance position for longer than 5 seconds during the entire 20-second testing period. These trials are assigned a standard maximum error score of "10." This method of testing has been described elsewhere in detail and has been shown to be both valid and reliable using normal subjects.[84]

Balance test results should be compared to baseline measurements; in the absence of baseline measurements, the clinician can utilize the recovery curves for normal control subjects presented in Figures 3, 4, 5, and 7. Baseline testing should ideally be conducted in a quiet, controlled environment prior to the start of an athlete's season. The athlete should be rested and free from any musculoskeletal injury to the lower extremity for the baseline assessment. Tests such as the Balance Error Scoring System and the Clinical Test of Sensory Interaction and Balance can be performed either on the sideline or in the training room following injury.

Several commercial balance systems with the potential to assess various aspects of the postural control system are available to the medical community (Figures 11-13). While there are reasons to believe that these systems could be useful in quantifying balance deficits in athletes suffering from cerebral concussion, there are no data to support this claim at the present time.

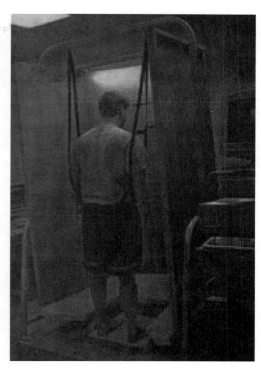

Figure 11: The Smart Balance Master (NeuroCom International, Inc.).

TABLE 2
BALANCE ERROR SCORING SYSTEM*
Errors
• hands lifted off iliac crests
• opening eyes
• step, stumble, or fall
• moving hip into more than 30° of flexion or abduction
• lifting forefoot or heel
• remaining out of testing position for more than 5 seconds

*The score is calculated by adding one error point for each error.

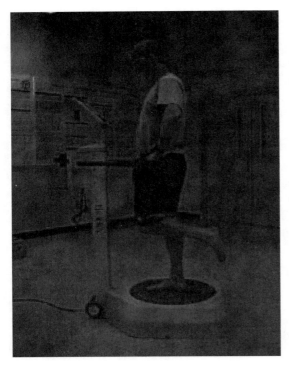

Figure 12: The Biodex Stability System (Biodex Medical Systems, Inc.).

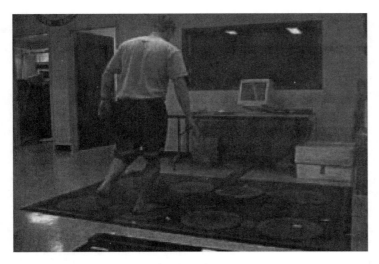

Figure 13: The FASTEX System (Cybex Inc.).

Neuropsychological Testing

Several commercially available tests are available for evaluating neurocognitive function. As previously mentioned, multiple components (abilities) contribute to cognitive functioning, and the clinician should attempt to evaluate as many as possible in a timely fashion. While selected tests are considered by the neuropsychological community to carry a lot of weight, there is currently no battery of tests accepted as the gold standard. When used in the athletic setting, it is recommended that the battery of tests assess a combination of neurocognitive abilities, while not exceeding 30 minutes of test time. Serial neuropsychological testing that exceeds 30 minutes often results in the athlete losing motivation to cooperate.

Testing can be administered by certified athletic trainers, team physicians, neurosurgeons, or neuropsychologists. A neuropsychologist, however, should provide the clinician with initial training using standard administration and scoring procedures. Testing is usually conducted at a table, in a quiet, controlled environment.

Several neuropsychological tests have been successfully utilized as part of the University of North Carolina's Prevention Initiative over the past several years. The following tests were selected because of their ability to assess various aspects of cognitive function often depressed following concussion.

1) The *Hopkins Verbal Learning Test* (Johns Hopkins University, Baltimore, MD), in which each form consists of a 12-item word list composed of four words from three semantic categories used for assessing verbal learning and memory. The athlete is instructed to listen carefully and memorize the word list (HVLT Immediate Memory Recall). The athlete then recalls as many words as possible in any order. The examiner records the number of correct responses, and the same procedure is repeated for two more trials. At the conclusion of all six neuropsychological tests, the athlete is asked to repeat as many of the 12 words he/she can remember from the original list (HVLT Delayed Recall). The athlete is then read 24 words and is asked to identify words contained in the original list. The number of incorrect responses is subtracted from the overall recall score (HVLT Recognition).

2) The *Trail Making Test Parts A and B* (Reitan Neuropsychological Laboratory, Tucson, AZ), in which athletes are asked to sequentially trace a series of 25 numbers (Trail A) or a series of alternating numbers and letters (Trail B) on a piece of paper as fast as possible using a pen. This task assesses visual scanning, attention, and executive functioning. The time required for successful completion is recorded.

3) The *Wechsler Digit Span Test* (Psychological Corp., San Antonio, TX) consists of a two-part protocol and is used to examine a patient's short-term auditory attention and concentration. During both parts of the test, the athlete is presented with a series of numbers and asked to repeat the digits in either the same order (Digits Forward) for the first part or in the reverse order (Digits Backward) for the second part. The number of successful trials for each part is recorded as the total score (Digits Total).

4) The *Stroop Color Word Test* (Stoelting Co., Wood Dale, IL) is designed to assess cognitive flexibility and attention span by examining an athlete's ability to separate

word- and color-naming stimuli through the use of three separate subtests. Each subtest contains 100 items presented in five columns of 20 items. The athlete has 45 seconds to complete each subtest, and the total score is calculated from the sum of each subtest. During the first subtest, athletes are asked to read aloud the words red, green, or blue written in black ink. For the second subtest the athlete is asked to identify aloud the colors red, green, or blue printed in "XXXX." The third subtest involves the words on page 1 blended with the colors on page 2; however, in no case does the word match with the print color. Athletes are asked to read the color of print instead of the actual word.

5) The *Symbol Digit Modalities Test* (Western Psychological Services, Los Angeles, CA) is a complex scanning test that assesses visual tracking and incidental learning. Subjects are asked to view (and memorize) a list of symbols and their corresponding digit for 30 seconds. After a 10-second rest, the subject is asked to recite the symbols in sentence form as they correspond to a 4-digit number. An alternative version of this test requires the subject to write the number that corresponds to a specific symbol found on a key at the top of the page. Subjects are instructed to work as quickly as possible (moving left to right along the paper) until the examiner says "stop." The number of correct responses completed in 90 seconds is recorded.

6) The *Controlled Oral Word Association Test* (Psychological Assessment Resources, Inc., Odessa, FL) assesses verbal fluency. It consists of three word-naming trials. The sets of letters, C-F-L and P-R-W, were chosen on the basis of the frequency of English words beginning with these letters. Subjects are asked to say as many words as they can think of that begin with the given letter of the alphabet (first C, followed by F, and then L), excluding proper nouns, numbers, and the same word with a different suffix. The P-R-W set is used at the next session. The score, which is the sum of all acceptable words produced in the three 1-minute trials, is adjusted for age, sex, and education. The adjusted scores can then be converted to percentiles.

The Standardized Assessment of Concussion is another valuable tool for assessing neurocognitive deficits following concussion in athletes. This tool was developed specifically for athletic trainers in response to the recommendation of the American Academy of Neurology practice parameter[6] and the Colorado Medical Society guidelines.[24] It should be considered a valuable tool for sideline evaluation of a concussed athlete (see Chapter 8).

Conclusions

Regardless of which concussion grading scale is used, sports medicine clinicians should focus on the signs and symptoms associated with concussion. The one guideline that everyone agrees on is that no athlete should be permitted to return to competition while still symptomatic. Unfortunately, many of these signs and symptoms are difficult to assess objectively. Empirical studies involving neurocognitive function and postural stability have emerged in recent years that help validate this comprehensive approach to the assessment of concussion. Controlled clinical studies suggest that concussion can be objectively assessed, especially if baseline data are collected during the preseason.

The information obtained from controlled clinical studies similar to those presented in this chapter will hopefully enable researchers and clinicians to develop a more definitive recovery curve for athletes sustaining concussion. Future research is needed to describe this recovery curve for athletes with varying levels of injury and for those with multiple episodes of concussion. This research will hopefully result in developing better concussion grading scales and return-to-play guidelines that will make it easier to determine when an athlete can safely return to participation.

References

1. Adams J: The neuropathology of head injuries, in Vinken P, Bruyn G (eds): **Handbook of Clinical Neurology: Injuries of the Brain and Skull.** Amsterdam: North-Holland, 1975, pp 35-65
2. Adams J, Mitchell D, Graham D, et al: Diffuse brain damage of immediate impact type. **Brain 100:**489-502, 1977
3. Albright JP, McAuley E, Martin RK, et al: Head and neck injuries in college football: an eight-year analysis. **Am J Sports Med 13:**147-152, 1985
4. Alexander MP: Mild traumatic brain injury: pathophysiology, natural history, and clinical management. **Neurology 45:**1253-1260, 1995
5. Alves WM, Rimel R, Nelson W: University of Virginia prospective study of football induced minor head injury: status report. **Clin Sports Med 6:**211-218, 1987
6. American Academy of Neurology: Practice parameter. The management of concussion in sports (summary statement). **Neurology 48:** 581-585, 1997
7. Arcan M, Brull M, Najenson T, et al: FGP assessment of postural disorders during the process of rehabilitation. **Scand J Rehabil Med 9:** 165-168, 1977
8. Arnheim D, Prentice W: **Principles of Athletic Training. 9th ed.** Madison, Wisc: Brown & Benchmark, 1997
9. Bakay L, Glasauer F: **Head Injury.** Boston: Little, Brown, & Co, 1980
10. Barth JT, Alves WM, Ryan TV, et al: Mild head injury in sports: neuropsychological sequela and recovery of function, in Levin H, Eisenberg H, Benton A (eds): **Mild Head Injury.** New York, NY: Oxford University Press, 1989, pp 257-275
11. Becker D, Gudeman S: **Textbook of Head Injury.** Philadelphia, Pa: WB Saunders, 1989
12. Binder LM: Persisting symptoms after mild head injury: a review of the post-concussive syndrome. **J Clin Exp Neuropsychol 8:**323-346, 1986
13. Black O, Wall C, Rockette H, et al: Normal subject postural sway during the Romberg test. **Am J Otolaryngol 3:**309-318, 1982
14. Booher J, Thibodeau G: **Athletic Injury Assessment.** St Louis, Mo: Mosby-Year Book, 1994
15. Buckley WE: Concussion in college football. A multivariate analysis. **Am J Sports Med 16:**51-56, 1988
16. Cantu RC: Cerebral concussion in sports: management and prevention. **Sports Med 14:**64-74, 1992
17. Cantu RC: Guidelines for return to contact sports after a cerebral concussion. **Phys Sportsmed 14(10):**75-83, 1986
18. Cantu RC: Minor head injuries in sports. **Adolescent Med 2:**141-154, 1992
19. Cantu RC: Second-impact syndrome. **Clin Sports Med 17:**37-44, 1998
20. Cantu RC: When to return to contact sports after a cerebral concussion. **Sports Med Digest 10:**1-2, 1988
21. Capruso DX, Levin HS: Cognitive impairment following closed head injury. **Neurol Clin 10:**879-893, 1992
22. Chason J, Hardy W, Webster J, et al: Alterations in cell structure of the brain associated with experimental concussion. **J Neurosurg 15:** 135-139, 1958
23. Collins MW, Grindel SH, Lovell MR, et al: Relationship between concussion and neuropsychological performance in college football players. **JAMA 282:**964-970, 1999
24. Colorado Medical Society: **Report of Sports Medicine Committee: Guidelines for the Management of Concussion in Sports, in National Athletic Trainers Association: Proceedings of the Mild Brain Injury in Sports Summit,** Washington, DC, April 14-18, 1994. Dallas, Tx: National Athletic Trainers' Association Reserach and Education Foundation, 1994, pp 106-109
25. Dick RW: **Football Injury Report. 1997-98 NCAA Injury Surveillance System.** Mision, Kansas, National Collegiate Athletic Association, 1998
26. Diener H, Dichgans J, Guschlbauer B, et al: The significance of proprioception on postural stabilization as assessed by ischemia. **Brain Res 296:**103-109, 1984
27. Dietz V, Horstmann G, Berger W: Significance of proprioceptive mechanisms in the regulation of stance. **Prog Brain Res 80:**419-423, 1989
28. Dornan J, Fernie G, Holliday P: Visual input: its importance in the control of postural sway. **Arch Phys Med Rehabil 59:**586-591, 1978
29. Ekdahl C, Jarnlo G, Anderson S: Standing balance in healthy subjects: evaluation of a quantitative test battery on a force platform. **Scand J Rehabil Med 21:**187-195, 1989
30. Fekete JF: Severe brain injury and death following minor hockey accidents. The effectiveness of the "safety helmets" of amateur hockey players. **Can Med Assoc J 99:**1234-1239, 1968
31. Fisher A, Wietlisbach S, Wilberger J: Adult performance on three tests of equilibrium. **Am J Occup Ther 42:**30-35, 1988
32. Gentilini M, Nichelli P, Schoenhuber R, et al: Neuropsychological evaluation of mild head injury. **J Clin Exp Neuropsychol 48:**137-140, 1985
33. Gerberich SG, Priest JD, Boen JR, et al: Concussion incidences and severity in secondary school varsity football players. **Am J Publ Health 73:**1370-1375, 1983
34. Goldie P, Bach T, Evans O: Force platform measures for evaluating postural control: reliability and validity. **Arch Phys Med Rehabil 70:** 510-517, 1989
35. Gronwall D, Wrightson P: Cumulative effects of concussion. **Lancet 2:** 995-997, 1975
36. Gronwall D, Wrightson P: Delayed recovery of intellectual function after minor head injury. **Lancet 2:**605-609, 1974
37. Guskiewicz KM, Perrin DH: Research and clinical applications of assessing balance. **J Sport Rehab 5:**45-63, 1996
38. Guskiewicz KM, Perrin DH, Gansneder BM: Effect of mild head injury on postural stability in athletes. **J Athletic Training 31:**300-306, 1996
39. Guskiewicz KM, Riemann BL, Perrin DH, et al: Alternative approaches to the assessment of mild head injury in athletes. **Med Sci Sports Exerc 29 (Suppl 7):**S213-S221, 1997
40. Guskiewicz KM, Weaver N, Padua D, et al: Epidemiology of concussion in collegiate and high school football players. **Am J Sports Med 28:**643-650, 2000
41. Guyton A: **Textbook of Medical Physiology.** Philadelphia, Pa: WB Saunders, 1986, pp 1610-1615
42. Haaland K, Temkin N, Randahl G, et al: Recovery of simple motor skills after head injury. **J Clin Exp Neuropsychol 16:**448-456, 1994
43. Hellebrant F, Braun G: The influence of sex and age on the postural sway of man. **Am J Phys Anthropol 24:**347-359, 1939
44. Horstmann G, Dietz V: The contribution of vestibular input to the stabilization of human posture: a new experimental approach. **Neurosci Lett 95:**179-184, 1988
45. Hough D: Mild brain injury in sports, in: **Proceedings of the Mild Brain Injury in Sports Summit.** Dallas, Tx: National Athletic Trainers' Association, 1994, pp 31-39
46. Ingersoll C, Armstrong C: The effects of closed-head injury on postural sway. **Med Sci Sports Exerc 24:**739-742, 1992
47. Jansen E, Larsen R, Mogens B: Quantitative Romberg's test: measurement and computer calculations of postural stability. **Acta Neurol Scand 66:**93-99, 1982
48. Jordan BD: Sports injuries, in: **Proceedings of the Mild Brain Injury in Sports Summit.** Dallas, Tx: National Athletic Trainers' Association, 1994, pp 43-46
49. Kelly JP, Nichols JS, Filley CM, et al: Concussion in sports. Guidelines for the prevention of catastrophic outcome. **JAMA 266:**2867-2869, 1991
50. Klonoff P, Costa L, Snow W: Predictors and indicators of quality of life in patients with closed-head injury. **J Clin Exp Neuropsychol 8:** 469-485, 1986
51. Kraus J, Arzemanian S: Epidemiologic features of mild and moderate brain injury, in Hoff J, Anderson T, Cole T (eds): **Mild to Moderate Head Injury.** Boston, Mass: Blackwell Scientific, 1989, pp 9-28
52. Leininger BE, Gramling SE, Farrell AD, et al: Neuropsychological deficits in symptomatic minor head injury patients after concussion and mild concussion. **J Neurol Neurosurg Psychiatry 53:**293-296, 1990
53. Levin HS, Benton A, Grossman RG: **Neurobehavioral Consequences of Closed Head Injury.** New York, NY: Oxford University Press, 1982
54. Levin HS, Goldstein F, High W: Disproportionately severe memory deficit in relation to normal intellectual functioning after closed head injury. **J Neurol Neurosurg Psychiatry 51:**1294-1301, 1988
55. Levin HS, Grossman R, Rose J: Long-term neuropsychological outcome of closed head injury. **J Neurosurg 50:**412-422, 1979
56. Levin HS, Williams DD, Eisenberg HW, et al: Serial MRI and neurobehavioural findings after mild to moderate closed head injury. **J Neurol Neurosurg Psychiatry 55:**255-262, 1992

57. Macciocchi S, Barth JT, Alves W, et al: Neuropsychological functioning and recovery after mild head injury in collegiate athletes. **Neurosurgery** 39:510-514, 1996

58. Maddocks D, Saling M: Neuropsychological sequelae following concussion in Australian rules footballers. **J Clin Exp Neuropsychol** 13: 439, 1991

59. Matser EJT, Kessels AG, Jordan BD, et al: Chronic traumatic brain injuries in professional soccer players. **Neurology** 51:791-796, 1998

60. Matser EJT, Kessels AG, Lezak AD: Neuropsychological impairment in amateur soccer players. **JAMA** 282:971-973, 1999

61. Mauritz K, Dichgans J, Hufschmidt A: Quantitative analysis of stance in late cortical cerebellar atrophy of the anterior lobe and other forms of cerebellar ataxia. **Brain** 102:461-482, 1979

62. McCrea M, Kelly JP, Kluge J, et al: Standardized assessment of concussion in football players. **Neurology** 48:586-588, 1997

63. McCrea M, Kelly JP, Randolph C, et al: Standardized assessment of concussion (SAC): on-site mental status evaluation of the athlete. **J Head Trauma Rehabil** 13(2):27-36, 1998

64. McCrory PR, Berkovic SF: Second impact syndrome. **Neurology** 50: 677-683, 1998

65. McIntosh T, Vink R: Biomechanical and pathophysiologic mechanisms in experimental mild to moderate traumatic brain injury, in Hoff J, Anderson T, Cole T (eds): **Mild to Moderate Head Injury.** Boston, Mass: Blackwell Scientific, 1989, pp 135-145

66. Mitchell D, Adams J: Primary focal impact damage to the brainstem in blunt head injuries. **Lancet** 4:215-219, 1973

67. Mitchell S, Lewis M: Tendon-jerk and muscle-jerk in disease and especially in posterior sclerosis. **Am J Med Sci** 92:363-372, 1986

68. Murray MA, Seireg A, Sepic S: Normal postural stability: qualitative assessment. **J Bone Joint Surg (Am)** 57:510-516, 1975

69. Nashner L: Adaptation of human movement to altered environments. **Trends Neurosci** 5:358-361, 1982

70. Nashner L: Adapting reflexes controlling the human posture. **Exp Brain Res** 26:59-72, 1976

71. Nashner L: Computerized dynamic posturography, in Jacobson G, Newman C, Kartush J (eds): **Handbook of Balance Function and Testing.** St Louis, Mo: Mosby-Year Book, 1993, pp 280-307

72. Nashner L, Berthoz A: Visual contribution to rapid motor responses during postural control. **Brain Res** 150:403-407, 1978

73. Nashner L, Black F, Wall C: Adaptation to altered support and visual conditions during stance: patients with vestibular deficits. **J Neurosci** 2:536-544, 1982

74. Nashner L, Peters J: Dynamic posturography in the diagnosis and management of dizziness and balance disorders. **Neurol Clin** 8: 331-349, 1990

75. Nashner L, Shumway-Cook A, Marin O: Stance postural control in select groups of children with cerebral palsy: deficits in sensory organization and muscular coordination. **Exp Brain Res** 49:393-409, 1983

76. Nelson WE, Jane JA, Gieck JH: Minor head injury in sports: a new system of classification and management. **Phys Sportsmed** 12:103-107, 1984

77. Norre M: Sensory interaction testing in platform posturography. **J Laryngol Otol** 107:496-501, 1993

78. Odernick P, Sandstedt P, Lennerstrand G: Postural sway and gait of children with convergent strabismus. **Dev Med Clin Neurol** 26: 495-499, 1984

79. Oliaro S: Establishment of normative data on cognitive tests for comparison with athletes sustaining mild head injury. **J Athletic Training** 33:36-40, 1998

80. Ommaya A, Ommaya A, Salazar A: A spectrum of mild brain injuries in sports, in: **Proceedings of the Mild Brain Injury in Sports Summit.** Dallas, Tx: National Athletic Trainers' Association, 1994, pp 72-80

81. Powell JW, Barber-Foss KD: Traumatic brain injury in high school athletes. **JAMA** 282:958-963, 1999

82. Riemann B, Guskiewicz K: Assessment of mild head injury using measures of balance and cognition: a case study. **J Sport Rehabil** 6:283-289, 1997

83. Riemann B, Guskiewicz K: Effects of mild head injury on postural sway as measured through clinical balance test. **J Athletic Training** 35:19-25, 2000

84. Riemann B, Guskiewicz K, Shields E: Relationship between clinical and forceplate measures of postural stability. **J Sport Rehabil** 8:71-82, 1999

85. Rimel R, Giordani B, Barth J, et al: Disability caused by minor head injury. **Neurosurgery** 9:221-228, 1981

86. Sahlstrand T, Ortengren R, Nachemson A: Postural equilibrium in adolescent idiopathic scoliosis. **Acta Orthop Scand** 49:354-365, 1978

87. Saunders RL, Harbaugh RE: The second impact in catastrophic contact-sports head trauma. **JAMA** 252:538-539, 1984

88. Shumway-Cook A, Horak F: Assessing the influence of sensory interaction on balance. **Phys Ther** 66:1548-1550, 1986

89. Sorenson S, Kraus J: Occurrence, severity, and outcomes of brain injury. **J Head Trauma Rehabil** 6:1-10, 1991

90. Sugano H, Takeya T: Measurement of body movement and its clinical applications. **Jpn J Physiol** 20:296-308, 1970

91. Taguchi K: Relationship between the head's and the body's center of gravity during normal standing. **Acta Otolaryngol** 90:100-105, 1980

92. Tysvaer A, Storli OV, Bachen NI, et al: Soccer injuries to the brain: a neurologic and electroencephalographic study of former players. **Acta Neurol Scand** 80:151-156, 1989

93. Tysvaer A, Løchen E: Soccer injuries to the brain: a neuropsychologic study of former players. **Am J Sports Med** 19:56-60, 1991

94. Vander A, Sherman J, Luciano D: **Human Physiology: The Mechanisms of Body Function,** 5th ed. New York, NY: McGraw-Hill, 1990

95. Wilberger JE: Minor head injuries in American football: prevention of long-term sequela. **Sports Med** 15:338-343, 1993

CHAPTER 10

The Role of the Athletic Trainer in the Care of the Injured Athlete

VINCENT HUDSON, MS, PT, ATC, and JOHN NORWIG, ATC

One of the more fastidious medical decisions in athletics today occurs immediately following an injury to the head or spine. The decision of when and how to transport an athlete is as complex as the on-the-field diagnosis. Precautions must be taken by trained medical professionals who have the expertise to make such decisions. Although axial loading is the most common mechanism of injury of the spine in athletics, other causes of spinal injury include flexion alone, flexion with a rotational component, or hyperflexion/hyperextension.[1] Personnel trained in treating and immobilizing injured athletes must be cautious not to create a secondary complication following the initial trauma.

With approximately 10,000 spinal injuries occurring annually, one would assume that athletics sustains its share of trauma, and approximately 10% are related to athletics.[2,7] In football, there has been a significant decrease in spinal cord injury to less than 10 injuries annually.[2] The reasons for the reduction vary, but education of the athlete and the medical and athletic training staffs, as well as improvements in technology, have certainly contributed to the decreased incidences.

The Role of Athletic Trainers

Since 1950, athletic trainers have been the first responders to athletic injury. Although not viewed as an allied health professional in the early years, the profession of athletic training has made significant advances in attaining the respect of the medical community over the last 15 years. The thousands of certified athletic trainers are currently relied upon by athletes, coaches, parents, and physicians to provide prevention, first aid, rehabilitation, and traumatic-injury care. The training of such individuals is overseen by the National Athletic Trainers' Association (NATA) and its committees on education and accreditation. Prior to qualifying to take a national certifying examination, athletic trainers must have more than 1000 hours of experience.

The primary reason for athletic trainers on a sideline during a sporting event is to be prepared to provide immediate care for injuries sustained, ranging from a sprained ankle to a fractured spine. Recently, there has been an increased awareness of significant head and spinal injuries sustained in athletics. The onsite athletic training staff is usually the initial source of services ranging from immediate first aid to saving the life of an athlete.

Prior to Injury

Prior to a game, the preparation of the athletic training staff should include mock episodes of spinal injuries, with each staff member having specific tasks as well as understanding all responsibilities of each member of the staff. Cross-training of the staff members allows for proper medical care under game and practice conditions in the event of an absent staff member. All staff should be well versed in the application of all equipment associated with on-the-field care of the cervical spine-injured athlete. All specialized equipment for emergency care should be checked on a regular basis for wear, safety, and loss. Typical equipment includes a spine board, scoop stretcher, rigid collar, and support padding for immobilization.

While on the sideline, the athletic trainer uses a keen and experienced eye to assess and recognize any unsafe or potentially hazardous activity on the playing field. During this survey, the trainer often has the opportunity to see an injury occur. Although rare in most healthcare professions, the ability to see the mechanics of an injury as it occurs allows the trainer the opportunity to respond to the athlete's needs without using unnecessary time for an extensive subjective evaluation.

Immediately Following Injury

The Primary Survey

Immediately after an injury, a primary survey is taken which consists of assessment of the level of consciousness and the initial life-threatening complications associated with cervical injury and spinal cord involvement. The conscious athlete has a much easier onfield assessment for obvious reasons. The unconscious athlete poses a variety of additional complications for onfield assessment, with the prone unconscious athlete being the greatest challenge. The team approach is utilized, with one staff member assuring stabilization of the cervical spine by holding the head or helmet and applying inline stabilization, while another staff member assesses the athlete's neurological status, including sensory and motor evaluations. There should always be one person in charge while performing any onfield maneuver regarding the spine-injured athlete. Often, this person is a team physician; however, in the intramural, club, high school, and small college settings, a physician is not always available and the head athletic trainer assumes the role of team leader.

During the actual episode of a spinal injury on the field, NATA has set forth specific guidelines for all first responders. The guidelines stress that any athlete suspected of having a spinal injury should not be moved and should be treated as though there is a spinal injury. Via a battery of tests in a short period of time, the athlete's state of consciousness and the functioning of airway, breathing, and circulation are evaluated.

The first step in treating the "downed" athlete with a suspected cervical spine injury is an assessment of breathing and circulation.[5] The athlete is frequently lying prone or side-lying following a spinal injury. Once the vital signs are present and stable in the prone conscious athlete, there is no significant rush to move the athlete to a supine position until further assessment is completed. Prior to moving the athlete with suspected spinal injury, it is important that the initial assessment of airway, breathing, and circulation be performed with the patient in the position in which he/she is found.

An unconscious athlete must be treated as though there is the possibility of a cervical spine injury and spinal cord involvement. Palpation techniques must be quickly performed to assess airway, breathing, and circulation. The airway must be established and maintained. High-level spinal cord injuries affect the diaphragm, creating a need for artificial respiration. Circulation is rarely a concern with a cervical spine injury, although hypotension may result when there is a high cervical cord lesion.

In an injured conscious athlete, obtaining a medical history provides an immediate appraisal of brain function based upon the athlete's response to specific questions. This provides a baseline measurement of the athlete's mental status, and it must be continuously re-assessed throughout the onfield and sideline evaluation as well as during transportation. With any cervical spine injury, one must take into consideration the potential for a head injury as well. The secondary benefit of a thorough medical history is that it provides a clear mechanism of injury.

If the athlete must be moved, in circumstances where he/she needs to be positioned from prone to supine, the spine must be immobilized during the process. This includes moving the head, neck, and trunk as one unit, avoiding any protracting or retracting of the cervical spine, or any rotation, flexion, or lateral flexion of the entire spine. Watkins[10] suggests using a five-person team headed by a physician (Figure 1). Flexion and extension movements should be particularly avoided, because they are most likely to compromise the circumference of the spinal canal.[4] Securing the patient's head to the trunk in a splint is an acceptable process. A spine board should always be available and placed under the athlete as he/she is rolled into a supine position, avoiding any further movement (including sliding the board under the athlete) after the roll technique is performed (Figure 2).

In 1997, the American Orthopedic Society for Sports Medicine issued similar guidelines and agreed that helmet removal is best performed in the controlled environment of a hospital emergency room.[9] Research has been performed regarding types of spine board immobilization, addressing the classic wooden spine board and the vacuum splint type (Figure 3). The study concluded that the vacuum splint was more easily and quickly applied; however, its efficacy of cervical immobilization required additional padding to support the spine.[6] Improved models are being used today that include winged apparatus to compensate for larger athletes and the equipment that they wear. Transport personnel have been leaders in the development of a more functional spine board design.

Positioning of the cervical spine during transport has also been assessed (Figure 4). Researchers attempted to determine the degree of flexion or extension of the cervical spine that would provide the greatest capacity within the spinal canal. Maximizing the area within the canal can reduce pressure within the spinal column and

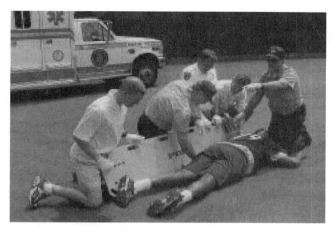

Figure 1: Sufficient personnel and a team approach are used to safely move an injured player. The team leader is responsible for stabilizing the head and neck.

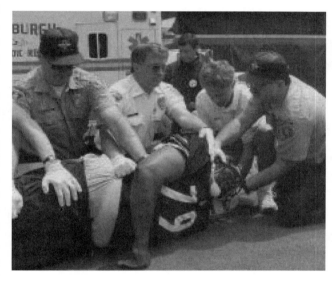

Figure 2: The team uses a spine board to roll the player into a supine position with careful attention given to spine alignment.

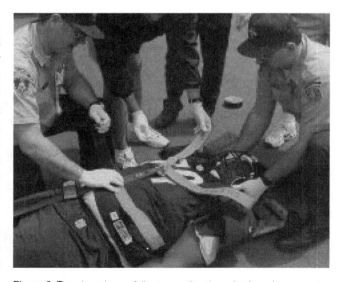

Figure 3: The player is carefully strapped to the spine board to prevent any movement or further injury.

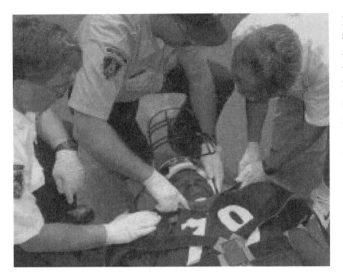

Figure 4: The cervical spine is carefully stabilized and the helmet is ordinarily left in place.

possibly reduce cord damage following an injury. Results demonstrated that a supine adult should have his/her occiput raised approximately 2 cm off the board to effect the most open angle within the spinal canal.[4] This is usually achieved by the typical football, hockey, or lacrosse helmet. In athletes who do not wear helmets, additional posterior padding may be required to maintain neutral spinal positioning.

If the injured athlete is wearing a facemask, it should be removed prior to initiating transport, regardless of the circulatory or respiratory status. Specific tools are available to perform this task. The use of a utility knife is not recommended. The helmet and chin strap should be removed only under the following circumstances:

- if a secure fit effecting immobilization of the head and neck cannot be maintained;
- if the facemask cannot safely be removed in a reasonable time frame;
- if the helmet impedes the ability for ventilation, if necessary, even after the facemask is removed; or
- if the helmet forces the head to rotate or extend/flex, creating unsafe conditions for immobilization during transportation.

Additional equipment, such as shoulder pads, may need to be removed to secure and maintain cervical immobility while transporting. Larger pads have a tendency to create cervical hyperextension in the supine position. Shoulder pads and helmets are usually best removed simultaneously in order to preserve anatomical alignment of the neck.

Unless there is adequate help to assist with movement or assessment, the prudent provider should activate the Emergency Medical Services (EMS) for transport and immediate first aid care on the field. There is always the potential for a scenario where a spinal trauma initially appears stable but becomes unstable within seconds.

Secondary Assessment

Once the airway is secured and access attained, the secondary assessment is initiated. This includes general and specific manual muscle and sensory tests to address and rule out any motor or sensory dysfunction. Table 1 lists the specific tests that athletic trainers use as guidance for evaluating potential cervical spine injury; the assessment begins at the vital extremities and moves proximally to avoid unnecessary movement of the head and neck. Table 2 indicates the tests used for sideline assessment of cranial nerves II-XII

TABLE 1

TESTS USED BY ATHLETIC TRAINERS FOR SIDELINE CERVICAL ASSESSMENT

Nerve Root	Sensory	Motor
C2	occiput	lateral flexion
C3	platysma	cervical flexion
C4	upper trapezius	shoulder elevation
C5	lateral deltoid	shoulder abduction
C6	dorsal thumb and index	wrist extension
C7	palmar surface 3rd finger	wrist flexion
C8	medial 4th and all of the 5th finger	thumb extension
T1	medial forearm	finger abduction

with respect to any head injury to assist in ruling out a concussion.

A general assessment follows or is conducted simultaneously with the neurological assessment; this includes measuring vital signs, particularly blood pressure and heart rate. In a traumatic episode, both are often well elevated from the normative. Maintaining constant readings at specific intervals is important when addressing shock and systemic concerns due to trauma. A general orthopedic assessment should follow to note the presence of secondary noncervical orthopedic involvement in a cervical spine injury. Although not life threatening, these orthopedic conditions may create increased pain when transporting or positioning, causing greater challenges for the onfield assessment team. Head trauma should be continuously monitored throughout the evaluation process.

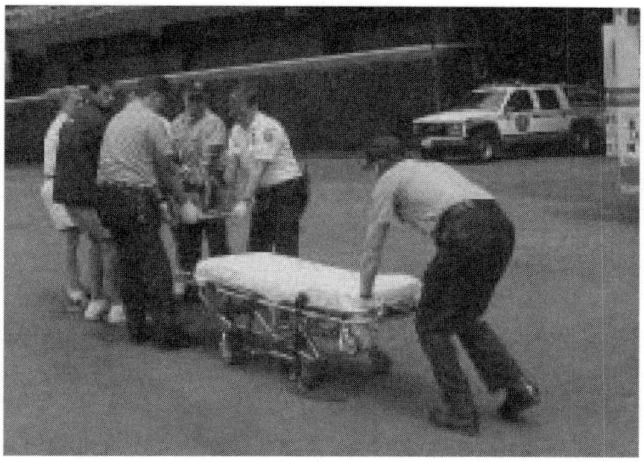

Figure 5: When the player has been stabilized, he may be moved to the sidelines or transported off the field for further evaluation.

Sideline Assessment

When an athlete has not lost consciousness and a thorough onfield evaluation has been completed, he/she may frequently be moved to the sidelines (Figure 5). As with any head trauma, symptoms may not be obvious during the first 3-5 minutes postinjury. While on the sidelines, and once a spinal injury is no longer a concern, an athlete's helmet should be taken off and given to the equipment personnel. In this way, it can be reasonably certain that the athlete cannot be inadvertently returned to the game without clearance from the medical team.

While on the sideline, the athlete should be re-assessed every 5 minutes for neurological trauma. Once a normal neurological and mental status examination is demonstrated, specific functional tests to assess strength, balance, and coordination are carried out prior to return to play. If the athlete is allowed to return, the medical staff should maintain direct contact with that athlete during the remainder of the contest and observe any signs suggesting compensation or loss of function during play.

Following a Traumatic Incident

When a traumatic injury has occurred, each staff member should have a list of individuals who must be contacted. In the high school and college settings, the athlete's parents and coaches should be contacted concerning the athlete's condition and status. In the professional levels, the procedure varies by sport, team personnel, and league as well

TABLE 2
TESTS USED BY ATHLETIC TRAINERS FOR SIDELINE CRANIAL NERVE ASSESSMENT

Nerve	Sensory Test	Motor Test
II Optic	vision screening	
III Oculomotor		medial gaze, eye lid elevation, pupillary constriction
IV Trochlear		downward gaze
V Trigeminal	tongue, chin, and cheek	mastication
VI Abducens		lateral gaze
VII Facial	taste tip of tongue	facial expression
VIII Vestibulocochlear	hearing screening	balance
IX Glossopharyngeal	gag reflex	gag reflex
X Vagus	gag reflex	gag reflex
XI Spinal accessory		shoulder shrug
XII Hypoglossal		tongue protrusion

as the team policy regarding such matters. At no time should any specific information be provided to the public prior to team and family notification.

Planning or assisting the athlete with referral sources for outside needs, such as specialists for evaluation and rehabilitation, is the responsibility of the medical staff. In the high school setting, the injured athlete often becomes distant from the team and the coordination of follow-up services may not occur. Following an injury to an athlete, it is important to allow the athlete and parents to feel that they remain an important part of the team.

In the higher levels of athletics, a rehabilitation staff specialist is responsible for overseeing the specific protocols and medical treatment as outlined by the team physician. In such a setting, an athlete is able to rehabilitate under the direct supervision of a team staff member while maintaining a close relationship with teammates during the rehabilitative phases.

Precontest Preparation
Developing an Emergency Plan

It is in everyone's best interest to allow the personnel with expertise in a given situation to take charge regarding the multitude of needs following a spinal trauma while on the field. Preseason coordination of such skills allows the event to be handled smoothly and professionally, with each member of the medical staff understanding his/her role in the care of the athlete who presents with head or spinal injury. An appreciation for the variety of expertise involved in covering an athletic event will allow for optimal care to be delivered if the time arises.

A variety of items should be included when developing a sound emergency plan for hosting athletic contests.

- A primary concern is sufficient medical staff on the sidelines. Optimally, these include at least one physician, at least one certified athletic trainer and assistant, emergency medical personnel with state-of-the-art transportation available, qualified medical personnel in the emergency room of choice, and an institutional administrator. This is often an athletic director who oversees the legal and support concerns of a team.

- State-of-the-art equipment should include oxygen, emergency instrumentation, transportation devices, facemask removal gadgets, a defibrillator, and a transport vehicle. The EMS staff and team physician provide most of these items. The selection of a quality, well-equipped EMS staff can offset the costs of purchasing individual items by athletic teams. The defibrillator has gained significant acceptance as of late due to its user-friendly application.

- Communication devices are a must when dealing with the variety of medical personnel for a large athletic contest. The use of standard walkie-talkie devices is still the acceptable norm; however, technological advances in multifunction communication products allow full access to persons both on- and offsite from the athletic venue. Such devices are certainly necessary when attempting to host multiple events during the same day or weekend. With the increase in sports programs in the high school and college settings, it is no longer uncommon to host more than three sporting events simultaneously, in different facilities at the same campus.

- Proper facilities should be a requirement when hosting an event. All fields should have access for emergency vehicles. The primary hospital should have air transportation available, if necessary, and be reasonably accessible by ground with regard to traffic and distance from the host venue.

Coordinating For Services and Responsibilities Following an Injury

The potential for a variety of medical professionals to be present at an athletic event creates a need for coordination and communication regarding specific services and responsibilities following a severe injury on the field. Prior to each game, a plan including task descriptions and the chain of medical command must be agreed upon by all involved parties. Since each group offers their own medical expertise, a team approach must be developed for assessment of a potential cervical spine and spinal cord injury.

Establishing protocols as to who performs which task and the variety of responsibilities of each medical team player offers the best chance for expedient care for even the most challenging medical emergency. By using preplanned protocols, each staff member realizes the importance of the task at hand and the consequences therein. The preplanning work by the medical coordinator includes contracting for transport services in emergency situations. The use of ambulance services, carts, stretchers, and spine boards requires immediate communication and knowledge of emergency apparatus (Figure 6).

The athletic training staff usually has the sole responsibility for coordinating medical efforts for home contests. Regardless of the level of play, there are general rules that most athletic training staffs adhere to as a host. There are also specific responsibilities as a guest at a foreign site. However, the first responsibility is the care and prevention of injuries to the athletes on the staff's own team.

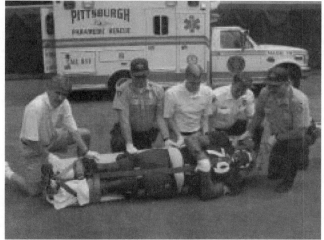

Figure 6: Example of a player properly stabilized on a spine board.

Determining When an Athlete Can Return To Play

Any athlete who has experienced a neurological trauma should be assessed prior to contest participation. A challenge for the medical staff is the determination of when an athlete can return to play. In many instances, the decision is not made until hours prior to an event or game. The determination is often made using a baseline established at the beginning of the season.

Because athletic trainers work on a daily basis with their athletes, they have the opportunity to gain knowledge of personalities of the players prior to injury. Each athlete has a pregame ritual, attitude, and a variety of idiosyncrasies. The athletic trainer interacts with the player on a daily basis in the ritual of taping, padding, and prevention of injuries. This allows the athletic trainer the opportunity to interact with the healthy athlete and increases the trainer's ability to assess an athlete's affective behavior following injury. The medical staff should be skilled to the point where a general affect evaluation could be performed during a nonformal conversation.

A small portion of patients who sustain a neurological injury will sustain further damage secondary to the initial trauma.[8] Educating the athlete regarding the warning signs, or "red flags," of a head or spinal injury allows for better communication between the athlete and medical staff. Avoiding the pitfalls where an athlete may think that a symptom is "normal" will allow the medical staff the opportunity to avoid a potentially debilitating or life-threatening event. In many instances, a second-time trauma can be avoided when a medical professional knows the athlete.

Responsibilities of the Host Medical Staff

The responsibilities of the host athletic training staff include a list of items usually performed prior to the athletic season. Creating a working relationship with the medical community is paramount. Some services require a contractual agreement up to 1 year in advance.

- The host facility should provide the nearest Level I trauma facility with a list of dates, times, and locations of annual contests. Direct communication with the hospital medical staff should be secured prior to beginning the season. Often, the team physician facilitates this process because of familiarity with hospital personnel and policy.

- The host medical staff is responsible for the transportation of an injured athlete, including the use of an onsite ambulance during each event. A relationship with an ambulance service is usually achieved during the off-season, with contractual agreements made with ambulance companies and EMS specialists. These groups provide apparatus such as oxygen and spine boards, as well as highly trained staff who have expertise in moving an injured athlete from the field of play. They also have expertise in life-threatening responses to head or spinal injury, as well as environmental conditions that may arise.

- The host medical staff should contact the visiting staff to address any needs that they may have prior to or during the contest. This allows the visiting team to adjust the amount of equipment and staff needed during travel. In most scenarios, there is a limit as to the equipment the traveling medical staff can bring. In the college and professional levels, this is less a concern than at the high school or club level. In some instances, specifically in international athletic events, it is the visiting medical team's responsibility to bring all components of equipment desired. This is an additional burden a staff must assume due to the variety of technologies that are made available at international venues.

Responsibilities of the Visiting Medical Staff

Upon arrival at the venue, the medical staff from the visiting team should meet with their counterpart from the home team. Athletic trainers, physicians, and various other medical personnel should meet and discuss the emergency plan. Medical team leaders should be introduced to the staff of the opposing team. In many levels of athletics today, leagues and organizations require the host team to provide a list of items qualifying them to be a host for such an event.

It is also recommended that the visiting medical staff take time to familiarize themselves with the facility and its location. In traumatic instances, a member of the medical team will be required to travel with the athlete during transport to a medical facility.

References

1. Anderson C: Neck injuries: backboard, bench, or return to play? **Phys Sportsmed** 21(8):23-24, 1993
2. Bailes JE, Hadley MN, Quigley MR, et al: Management of athletic injuries of the cervical spine and spinal cord. **Neurosurgery** 29: 491-497, 1991
3. Bailes JE, Lovell MR, Maroon JC: **Sports-Related Concussion**. St Louis, Mo: Quality Medical, 1999, p 146
4. DeLorenzo RA, Olson JE, Boska M, et al: Optimal positioning for cervical immobilization. **Ann Emerg Med** 28:301-308, 1996
5. Feuer H: History, examination and acute management of spinal injury, in Nicholas JA, Hershman EB (eds): **The Lower Extremity and Spine in Sports Medicine**. St Louis, Mo: CV Mosby, 1995
6. Johnson DR, Hauswald M, Stockhoff C: Comparison of a vacuum splint device to a rigid backboard for spinal immobilization. **Am J Emerg Med** 14:369-372, 1996
7. Little NE: In case of a broken neck. **Emerg Med** 21(9):22-32, 1989
8. Marks MR, Bell GR, Boumphrey FR: Cervical spine fractures in athletes. **Clin Sports Med** 9:13-29, 1990
9. News from the 24th Annual AOSSM Meeting, The American Orthopedic Society for Sports Medicine Issues: **Football Helmet Removal Guidelines**, July 15, 1997
10. Watkins RG: Neck injuries in football players. **Clin Sports Med** 5: 215-246, 1986

CHAPTER 11

Neuropsychological Assessment of the Amateur Athlete

DONNA K. BROSHEK, PHD, and JEFFREY T. BARTH, PHD

History of Neuropsychological Assessment in Sports

Prior to 1989, mild head injury was not considered to be a significant area of concern within the medical community, nor was it recognized as a public health problem. This lack of concern regarding mild head injury persisted despite the pronouncement by Symonds[88(p4)] in 1962 that "it is questionable whether the effects of concussion, however, slight, are ever completely reversible." By 1968, work by Oppenheimer[64] had identified petechial lesions at autopsy in patients who had sustained concussions, but who had not demonstrated neurological signs or symptoms. It was still believed at that time, however, that most individuals who suffered head trauma with brief or no loss of consciousness made rapid and complete recoveries. Those individuals with persisting symptoms were often diagnosed as depressed, neurotic, hysterical, or malingerers in pursuit of litigation (i.e., "compensation neurosis").

An epidemiological study conducted at the University of Virginia Medical School involving over 1200 head-injured patients was instrumental in changing those perceptions.[72] The University of Virginia study revealed that 55% of their head-trauma sample suffered mild injuries and that these symptoms, including the inability to return to work, persisted for at least 3 months in more than a third of those patients. Subsequent studies at the University of Texas-Galveston, University of Washington, New York University, and the University of California-San Diego also documented neurocognitive impairment in some patients at 1 month postinjury, with most patients significantly improved 2 months later.[24,49,51,77] Persisting symptoms following mild head injury were identified that were typically associated with individual vulnerability (e.g., age or medical history), complications including emotional distress and physical pain, more-severe injury, and neuroimaging evidence of neuropathology.[5,48,76] Postconcussion syndrome symptoms associated with longer recovery periods were identified and included headache, dizziness, memory problems, fatigue, depression, irritability, difficulty in rapid new problem solving and abstract reasoning, sleep disturbance, nausea, tinnitus, and emotional lability.[5] At the same time, primate research by Gennarelli et al[27] demonstrated that mild acceleration-deceleration head injury could result in identifiable axonal injury characterized by shear-strain. The body of research on mild head injury conducted in the 1980s and 1990s provided substantial data in support of the concerns raised earlier by Symonds and Oppenheimer.

In the mid-1980s, the University of Virginia Department of Neurological Surgery undertook a prospective study of acceleration-deceleration concussions involving 2300 football players from 10 universities to further the understanding of mild head injury in the clinical setting.[5,53] This pre- and post-mild head injury neuropsychological outcome study documented that mild neurocognitive deficits were noted 24 hours following mild head injury without loss of consciousness in comparison to players' preseason test scores. Injured players demonstrated gradual cognitive improvement and performed at a level comparable to the non-injured control group at 5 to 10 days postinjury. From a clinical perspective, this research was important in that it documented mild, acute neurocognitive deficits with a potentially rapid recovery curve in a group of young, healthy, and well-motivated individuals with very mild head injury. In addition, the study marked the beginning of modern-day sports concussion neurocognitive research.

The incidence of mild head injury varies widely by sport. A review of the available sports literature determined that "among reported injuries, the chances of any athlete incurring mild head trauma are generally between 2% and 10%, but range as high as 91% (in one study) for equestrian accidents."[74] Head injuries can occur in any sports activity, with the top five estimated ranges of rates of concussion as follows: equestrian 3%-91%, boxing 1%-70%, rugby 2%-25%, soccer 4%-22%, and United States football 2%-20%. In children and adolescents, the greatest incidence of severe head and neck injury is in U.S. football, but serious central nervous system (CNS) trauma is also sustained in equestrian sports, wrestling, baseball, boxing, soccer, and gymnastics.[11] Severe head and neck injury is rare in children under the age of 12 participating in organized sports, but the rate of injury increases significantly in children 15 to 18 years old.

Research on Concussion in Sports

Research has been conducted that specifically looks at the unique aspects of the incidence and prevention of concussion and head injury in many sports activities. Boxing, cheerleading, equestrian sports, ice hockey, rugby, soccer, skiing, tae kwan do, and U.S. football are discussed below.

Boxing

Boxing "stands alone among other contact sports in having as its goal, rendering opponents unconscious and helpless through successive blows to the head."[22] Direct impact and rotational torque on the brain appear to be the primary mechanisms of head injury in boxing. Such forces increase the risk for acute and severe focal and diffuse neurological injury such as intracranial hemorrhage, cerebral edema, and diffuse axonal injury. It has been speculated that boxers who constantly suffer repeated mild head injuries have cumulative and delayed effects, such as early neurodegenerative conditions (e.g., dementia pugilistica) and Parkinson's-like syndromes.[40,41] New evidence indicates that some boxers with the apolipoprotein E e4 allele may have a genetic predisposition for chronic traumatic encephalopathy, which is exacerbated by multiple blows to the head.[42] Neuropathology studies have revealed that chronic traumatic encephalopathy has characteristics similar to those seen in Alzheimer's disease. With the possible exception of amateur competition, boxing clearly represents the most potentially severe end of the head injury spectrum, with cerebral injuries often requiring acute medical management. Between 1918 and 1997, 659 boxing-related fatalities were recorded.[78] Other research, however, has found no significant difference between the neurological signs and symptoms in 33 former amateur champion boxers and a control group of former soccer athletes.[90]

The most common injury documented in a study of amateur boxers in Ireland[65] was concussion and, in contrast to other types of injuries (e.g., hand, wrist, facial, and knees), all of the cerebral injuries were sustained during competition. A study that examined 13 young professional and amateur boxers in the U.S.[50] (mean age 20.5 ± 2.1 years) found a trend toward deficits in reading and verbal learning in the boxers compared to control nonboxing amateur athletes who were matched by age, education, parental socioeconomic status, and race.[50] The results suggested the possibility of subtle deficits in processing verbal information, but may have reflected premorbid verbal learning deficits in those who elected to become boxers. Nine boxers underwent magnetic resonance imaging (MRI) at a 6-month follow-up and studies in all were normal.

In a review of the literature, Mendez[60] stated that most studies of amateur boxers revealed only mild neuropsychological impairment. When amateur boxers are compared with athletes participating in other sports, including soccer, track and field, water polo, and rugby, there are no significant group differences in neuropsychological performance. In contrast, Mendez noted that professional boxers have demonstrated deficits in memory, complex attention, executive functions, information processing speed, finger tapping, and sequencing abilities. Similarly, Mendez reported that while amateur boxers have no apparent changes on computed tomography (CT) or MRI, professional boxers revealed evidence of chronic subdural hematomas, contusions, porencephalic cysts, and previous perivascular hemorrhage.

Mild electroencephalographic (EEG) abnormalities, however, have been found in amateur boxers compared to control groups of soccer players or track and field athletes.[33,34] In a retrospective study of 50 former amateur Swedish boxers, Haglund and Eriksson[33] found no significant differences between boxers and control groups in platelet MAO activity, CT and MRI findings, and neuropsychological performance, with the exception of bilateral upper-extremity fine motor function.

A review of the international literature on 289 neuropsychological assessments of amateur boxers concluded that there are no consistent findings of neurocognitive deficits, with the exception of a slight reduction in fine motor functioning of the nondominant hand.[12] The slight impairment of the nondominant hand was still within normal limits and was hypothesized to be indicative of mild peripheral nerve injury secondary to leading with the nondominant hand in boxing.

The most impressive study of its kind examined neuropsychological and neurological functioning in 484 amateur boxers in the U.S., ranging in age from 13 to 21 years, at baseline and 2-year follow-up.[86] All data were collected between 1986 and 1990. Although there were no significant associations related to the number of bouts between the baseline and follow-up evaluations, the number of bouts prior to the baseline was associated with deficits in memory, perceptual/motor functions, and visuoconstructional abilities. Notably, sparring was not significantly associated with deficits in any test domain. Possible explanations cited by the authors to explain the lack of relationship between competition during the 2-year follow-up period and neuropsychological deficits include that the critical factor in the expression of neurocognitive dysfunction may be the time duration since the first exposure or the increased safety measures instituted between 1984 and 1986 for amateur boxers. These new safety measures include mandatory headgear, matching boxers by skill level, rules that halt competition when a boxer is at risk for head injury, and required suspension for apparent head injuries.[86]

The Association Internationale de Boxe Amateur, the regulatory body that governs amateur boxing, has added rules to increase the safety of its athletes.[78] Additional safety controls include increased medical supervision and intervention for concussed boxers, more thorough preseason medical evaluations by experienced physicians, restrictions on the number of rounds, and increased power accorded to the referee to halt a contest between mismatched competitors. Sadly, there is no universal regulatory system for professional boxing, and state commissions are often motivated by financial interests rather than the welfare of the boxers.[78]

Cheerleading

Although the incidence of head injury has not been well researched in cheerleading, the potential for injury exists due to the increased incorporation of tumbling, partner stunts, and pyramid formations in cheerleading routines.[39] The risk of injury appears to be low (0.17 injuries per 1000 athletic exposures), but 7% of the injuries in high school and college cheerleaders occurred to the head and neck. Notably, a comparison of 23 sports revealed that cheerleaders lost more days (mean 28.8 days) per injury than athletes in other sports.[4] Further research is needed to determine the incidence and severity of head injury in cheerleading and any persisting neurocognitive deficits.

Equestrian Sports

A prospective study of all patients with equestrian-related CNS trauma admitted to the University of Kentucky Medical Center between 1992 and 1996 found that, of 59 such injuries, 47% required neurosurgical intervention.[47] Twenty-four patients sustained head injuries, six underwent craniotomy, and five died. Severe head injury with subsequent herniation was the cause of all fatalities. In 63%, the injured riders were recreational equestrians and the remainder were professionals. Of the seven children injured, three were bystanders who were kicked or crushed by a horse, suggesting that safety precautions are paramount when children are in the vicinity of horses. Notably, 80% of those injured were not wearing helmets at the time of injury, including the patients who required craniotomy or ventriculostomy and all of the fatalities. According to the authors, "no one wearing a helmet suffered serious head injury or death."

A 20-year follow-up study of equestrian injuries in the Oxford, England catchment area revealed that, compared to the initial prospective survey in 1971-1972, the incidence of head injury decreased from an average of 51 to 11 per year.[19] The significant decline in head injury was associated with the increased use of helmets and improvements in helmet design. The initial survey noted seven skull fractures annually and one fatality, but no such injuries were recorded in the 20-year follow-up.

A retrospective examination of 156 equestrian-related injuries in southern Alberta, Canada revealed that 91.7% were head injuries.[35] Of these, 121 were considered minor (Glasgow Coma Scale score $\geq$13), four were moderate (score 9-12), and 18 were severe (score $\leq$8). Eleven patients in the severe head-injury group were fatalities, and three had persisting moderate to severe disability.

In a 2-year study of pediatric equestrian injuries conducted at the University of Virginia, 32 children under the age of 15 were identified.[8] Eight patients had loss of consciousness and two had a concussion. One fatality secondary to intracranial hemorrhage was noted, and one child had a fatal basilar skull fracture. Neither of the latter patients was wearing a helmet at the time of injury, and wearing a helmet was associated with a reduced risk of head injury and decreased severity of head injury.

Equestrians also appear to be at risk for multiple injuries, raising concern that they might be susceptible to the cumulative effects of multiple head injuries.[26] Research indicates that the most frequently injured group is young, female amateur equestrians.[19,26,47] Despite the high incidence of head injuries, there are no known studies of neuropsychological functioning in concussed equestrians.

Ice Hockey

The incidence of concussion among elite semiprofessional Swedish hockey players was examined by Tegner and Lorentzon.[89] In a retrospective survey, they found that 22% of the 227 participating players reported a total of 87 concussions during their hockey careers. Of this group, 38 players sustained one concussion and 11 had between two and five concussions. One player reported six concussions and another sustained nine. In the prospective portion of the study, which covered four seasons of competition, a total of 805 injuries and 52 concussions were reported. Three players sustained three concussions, and three had two concussions. Most of the concussions were due to body checking or boarding, while concussions due to contact with the puck or stick accounted for only 10%. Of note is that Tegner and Lorentzon reported that two players stopped playing ice hockey due to multiple concussions. One player sustained 12 concussions during his career and developed irritability and deficits in memory and concentration. Although CT and EEG were normal in this player, neuropsychological testing revealed evidence of cerebral dysfunction. Residual symptoms were noted after 3 years of abstaining from play, and neuropsychological reevaluation revealed continued neurocognitive impairment. The second player sustained four concussions in two seasons and was advised to stop playing. Three years later, he demonstrated no symptoms of brain injury, EEG and CT were normal, and he returned to play. Also of importance is that this study documented only those injuries diagnosed by a physician, and the authors noted that this may have resulted in an underreporting of minor concussions without loss of consciousness.

The prevalence of injuries to the face, head, and neck in recreational hockey athletes in Ontario was examined by gathering data on the individuals who presented to the emergency room of a tertiary care medical center.[68] Of 226 total injuries, 85% were to the face, 13% to the head, and 6% to the neck. The most common source of injury in these recreational players was being struck in the face with the stick or puck. Minor head injuries accounted for 20 of the injuries, and one adolescent had a severe spinal cord injury resulting in quadriplegia. No cerebral contusions or intracranial bleeds were identified, and only 1% of the athletes required further assessment or treatment by a neurosurgeon.

Rugby

In a review of CNS trauma in children and adolescents who participated in Rugby, Bruce et al[11] indicated that severe head injury was rare and that the prevalence of concussion was not well documented. Others have noted, however, the high incidence of concussion in amateur and professional Rugby.[2,28,81]

Professional Rugby players (n=54) who sustained a mild head injury without loss of consciousness during league play demonstrated deficits in information processing speed when assessed 24-48 hours after injury compared to their non-injured teammates.[36] The average number of previous concussions in the head-injured group was 2.6 and in the control group was 2.8, suggesting that neuropsychological assessment is sensitive to the acute effects of mild head injury in previously concussed patients. These authors noted that baseline assessments were useful in determining impaired performance on tests administered after mild head injury.

Skiing

Increased attention to the risk of head injury in skiing has occurred since the recent deaths of Michael Kennedy and Sonny Bono,[66] and some physicians have been advocating the use of helmets for skiing and snowboarding in order to reduce the incidence of concussion and more severe head trauma.[10] A survey obtained over 15 seasons at Sugarbush Ski Resort in Vermont identified 309 head injuries.[66] Of these, three were fatal, 10 were skull fractures, eight were severe head trauma, and 288 were concussions.

Examination of records at the University of Calgary revealed that 145 downhill skiers sustained CNS trauma over a 5-year period.[62] Five of these patients died and 88 sustained a head injury. Another survey at Blackcomb Mountain in British Columbia identified 2092 injuries during one season.[54] The majority of the injured were male, and the highest rate of injury was to adolescents and children. In 39%, the injuries occurred to the face or neck, and 22% of these injuries resulted in clinical evidence of concussion or loss of consciousness. Despite the significant incidence of head injury, there is no known literature on the neuropsychological assessment of skiers who sustained head injuries.

Soccer

Soccer is by far the most popular international sport, and it has become increasingly popular in the U.S. As reported by Nafpliotis,[63(p270)] "soccer is a combative sport, and, as a result, the chances of colliding with other players and sustaining an injury in the process are rather large." Potential head injuries for most soccer players will occur through kicks to the head, head-to-head contact, head-to-ground impact, head to goalpost, and heading the ball.

In soccer, severe or fatal head and neck injuries include skull fracture, subdural hematoma, cerebral hemorrhage, epidural hematoma, and spinal cord transection.[83] Head injuries are not evenly distributed in soccer, and limited data suggest that the goalie appears to be at about three times the risk for significant head injury (kicks to the head, head to goalpost, and head to ground) than other position players, and that defensive players (fullbacks and halfbacks) head the ball more often than do forwards.[38]

Although severe head trauma, as well as mild concussions, can occur via multiple mechanisms, "heading" the ball is a high-frequency aspect of the game that has significant potential for neurocognitive disruption and that has only recently gained scientific scrutiny. In addition to other mechanisms of head trauma, it is estimated[4] that professional soccer players head the soccer ball 350 times per year in games, producing an average game career of 5250 headings.[84] The latter findings do not include heading drills performed in practice. Smodlaka[84] estimated that the 14-16 ounce ball can travel at speeds up to 120 kilometers per hour, and that heading the ball can be traumatic to the brain and cervical spine. Although it has often been suggested that proper heading technique will prevent neurocognitive dysfunction, a 10-15 minute demonstration of proper heading by 10 professional players resulted in half developing headaches.[57]

As reported by Boden et al,[7] 18 people, primarily children, died after impact with a goalpost while participating in soccer over a period of 13 years in the U.S.[92] Surprisingly, a study of amateur boxers that used soccer players as a control group found that neither group showed neurological or neuropsychological impairment, but that the soccer players reported more head injuries and 70% reported persistent memory and concentration deficits.[90] A study of injuries conducted by the Norwegian Football Association between 1970 and 1974 found that 22% of the 480 adolescent and 70 adult soccer players sustained head and neck injuries.[73]

Mild EEG disturbances and complaints of chronic postconcussion syndrome were found in a sample of Norwegian professional soccer players.[91] Follow-up studies of 69 active and 37 retired professional players revealed postconcussion symptoms in 30% of the retired players and unexpected cerebral atrophy on CT in 33%.[91] Neurocognitive deficits were demonstrated in 81% of the players compared to 40% of the age-matched controls. This research has been criticized, however, for failing to assess for alcohol or drug use and previous head injuries.[7]

A neuropsychological study of 31 college soccer players and a control group of tennis players revealed that an increased number of games played was significantly correlated with a decrement in rapid, complex mental processing in the soccer group.[1] These players also had a significantly greater incidence of blurred vision, dizziness, headache, and loss of consciousness. A study based on the research of Abreau et al[1] involved a brief neuropsychological assessment of 20 high school, 20 college, and 20 professional soccer players, as well as 12 age-equivalent nonsoccer athletes.[98] The results revealed that increased heading of the soccer ball and years of experience were associated with decreased neuropsychological functioning, including impaired attention, concentration, mental flexibility, and general intellectual ability.

Research with New Zealand winter soccer players suggested that 33% of the soccer injuries were attributable to heading the ball.[59] Among 20 members of the U.S. National Team, seven soccer players reported a history of head injury sustained during participation and five of these involved loss of consciousness.[43] Self-reported symptoms of head and neck injury were significantly correlated with acute head injury, but not with age, years of play, or estimated exposure to heading the ball. None of these variables was associated with positive findings on MRI. These data were interpreted to indicate that self-reported symptoms of head injury are associated with previous acute head injury and are not secondary to heading.

A recent study of 53 Dutch professional soccer players found that they demonstrated neuropsychological impairment in memory, planning, and visuoperceptual tasks compared to a group of elite athletes participating in noncontact sports.[56] These deficits were positively associated with an increased number of concussions and heading frequency; the forward and defensive players demonstrated greater impairment relative to midfield players and goalkeepers.

A prospective examination of the incidence of concussion in elite amateur college soccer players from Atlantic Coast Conference teams during the 1995 (162 males and 188 females) and 1996 (163 males and 188 females) seasons found that 59% of the men and 41% of the women sustained concussions.[7] Three players sustained a concussion in both seasons. The concussions occurred primarily during games (69%), with the remainder sustained during practices. In 28% the concussion was due to head-to-head collision, and in 24% they were due to contact with the soccer ball (i.e., when a player was hit in the head by a ball kicked full force and the injured player did not have sufficient time to react or failed to see the ball coming). None of the injuries due to head-to-ball contact involved routine or prepared heading. One player lost consciousness for 5 minutes, and 28% had a loss of consciousness of less than 2 minutes. In 76%, the players were disoriented or confused ranging from seconds to 30 minutes after injury, and 93% reported headaches that lasted up to 4 days. Other reported symptoms included concentration deficits (62%), vomiting or nausea (52%), posttraumatic amnesia (17%), temporary personality change (14%), and retrograde amnesia (10%). Findings by Boden et al[7] revealed a surprisingly high level of concussion in competitive amateur soccer. They suggest that evidence of chronic traumatic encephalopathy found in soccer players is more likely due to multiple concussions rather than to routine heading of the ball.

Taekwondo

Taekwondo is a full-contact sport and, although punching to the head is not allowed, kicks to the head and face earn points in tournaments and are legal.[25] Tournament competitors typically wear protective equipment covering the head, chest and abdomen, groin, shins, and forearms.

Feehan and Waller[25] conducted a retrospective study of competitors at a full-contact tae kwon do tournament in New Zealand to assess the incidence of injuries in the prior year. The sample consisted of 39 males and eight females, with the incidence of injury in males (69%) and females (67%) roughly equivalent. Nine participants reported head and neck injuries and, of these, four were described as closed-head injuries. Although this is a limited sample, the occurrence of four closed-head injuries in 1 year out of a total of 48 participants suggests that taekwondo carries a significant risk of head injury. It should also be noted that this study asked participants to report only those injuries that required medical intervention or interfered with training, suggesting that the incidence of concussion may be significantly greater.

U.S. Football

U.S. football has the potential for serious and catastrophic head injury. A fatality from either head or cervical spine injury sustained in football has occurred every year between 1945 and 1994 with the exception of 1990.[61] A total of 684 fatalities due to football participation occurred during that time period, with 68% of the fatalities secondary to head trauma. The overwhelming majority of fatal head traumas were linked to subdural hematoma. Approximately 74% of the injuries were in high school football players, and the majority were sustained during games. Most of these players were injured while executing a tackle or being tackled.

As previously noted, the University of Virginia study[5,53] of 2300 football players focused attention on the presence of mild cognitive dysfunction with rapid recovery in amateur athletes who sustained a mild head injury without loss of consciousness. This prospective study assessed all players at preseason with a brief neuropsychological battery, a history questionnaire, and a symptom checklist. After sustaining an injury, players were assessed at 24 hours, 5 days, 10 days, and postseason. A matched control group was also assessed at the same intervals. This study focused on the sequelae of single injuries, with the 12 players sustaining multiple injuries excluded from analysis. Although the injured players showed little decrement in performance relative to their preseason performance, their failure to demonstrate improved performance on the neuropsychological tests as shown by the control group (i.e., practice effects) revealed the presence of impaired sustained attention and visuomotor speed. The neuropsychological impairment generally resolved by Day 5 postinjury. Players also reported significant increases in headache, dizziness, and memory deficits after injury, which generally decreased to baseline levels by Day 10. The results documented that mild head injury resulted in very real, but generally brief, neurocognitive dysfunction. The University of Virginia study also demonstrated the importance of baseline assessment in detecting mild cognitive change after a concussion.[53]

A neuropsychological test battery designed for preseason assessment of the Pittsburgh Steelers football team was also administered to a Division 1A college football team.[52] Of the 63 participating athletes who underwent baseline testing, four sustained documented concussions. Exclusive of the concussed players, 40 returned for postseason assessment. Although those who underwent postseason testing demonstrated statistically significant improvement on a measure of simple processing speed and a decline on verbal fluency, these differences were not deemed clinically significant. The former was attributed to practice effects and the latter was considered to reflect the effects of alternate forms, fatigue, or continued mild postconcussion symptoms. Neuropsychological assessment of the four injured players within 24 hours postinjury revealed that they performed below their baseline on a majority of the 10 tests in the battery. The most sensitive measures were those that assess verbal fluency and information processing speed.

Protection of the Athlete

Mild head injury and concussion occur quite frequently in sports, yet are often over-looked since they seldom produce loss of consciousness or medical symptoms that are reported by the players. A problematic issue is that athletes typically minimize symptoms in order to remain in the game and/or return to play. As in the clinical literature, sports mild head injury may be referred to as the "silent epidemic" that can have catastrophic, cumulative, and long-term effects.

Neuropsychological assessment is especially useful as a sensitive measure of neurocognitive functioning in concussed athletes, particularly when neurological and radiological evaluations are normal. Preseason neuropsychological assessment of athletes is important in providing a baseline for comparison of performance after injury for several reasons.[52] Because of the variability in cognitive performance among athletes, it is useful to compare each injured player's performance to his/her own preseason performance in determining the presence of cognitive dysfunction. Second, some players may have attention deficit/hyperactivity disorder, learning disabilities, or emotional factors (e.g., anxiety) that may impair their performance on more complex tasks and mimic concussion symptoms. The presence of a baseline enables an examination of change in performance to identify postconcussion neurocognitive dysfunction. Preseason neuropsychological assessment is also helpful in determining whether impaired neuropsychological performance is due to a current concussion or past concussions in multiply injured athletes.

Optimal protection of the athlete involves a brief neuropsychological evaluation administered to every player as part of the preseason physical. Testing a large group of individuals in a short period of time requires a 20-30 minute baseline evaluation.[52] Such brief assessments are a radical departure from the 4- to 6-hour evaluations typically administered by neuropsychologists in outpatient clinical settings. The use of a brief screening sacrifices sensitivity and comprehensiveness in favor of establishing baseline data on a large number of players in the domains most typically affected by concussion. A more comprehensive neuropsychological evaluation is recommended for injured players and should occur within 24 hours after trauma.

Careful consideration of return to play is essential after an athlete has sustained a concussion (see below). The second-impact syndrome, described by Schneider[80] in 1973 and Saunders and Harbaugh[79] in 1984, occurs when an athlete returns to play after a mild head injury before he/she is fully recovered and then sustains a second mild head injury with devastating consequences.[16-18] A second blow to the head may stun the athlete, but not typically cause loss of consciousness, and the athlete may even complete the play or walk off the field. "What happens in the next 15 seconds to several minutes sets this syndrome apart from a concussion or even a subdural hematoma. Usually within seconds to minutes of the second impact, the athlete—conscious yet stunned—quite precipitously collapses to the ground, semicomatose with rapidly dilating pupils, loss of eye movement, and evidence of respiratory failure."[16(p38)]

A loss of autoregulation of the brain's vascular supply is believed to be the underlying mechanism of second-impact syndrome.[16] As a result, craniovascular engorgement occurs with a subsequent increase in intracranial pressure, followed by herniation of the

"Return to Play" Practice Options

The AAN Quality Standards Subcommittee[3] established return-to-play practice options based upon a review of the literature and consensus of experts in the field. The suggestions below are based on the AAN concussion severity classification system.[63]

Grade 1

- Remove from contest.
- Examine immediately and at 5-minute intervals for the development of mental status abnormalities or postconcussion symptoms at rest and with exertion.
- May return to contest if mental status abnormalities or postconcussion symptoms clear within 15 minutes.
- A second Grade 1 concussion in the same contest eliminates the player from competition that day, with the player returning only if asymptomatic for 1 week at rest and with exercise.

Grade 2

- Remove from contest and disallow return that day.
- Examine onsite frequently for signs of evolving intracranial pathology.
- A trained person should re-examine the athlete the following day.
- A physician should perform a neurological examination to clear the athlete for return to play after 1 full asymptomatic week at rest and with exertion.
- CT or MRI is recommended in all instances where headache or other associated symptoms worsen or persist longer than 1 week.
- Following a second Grade 2 concussion, return to play should be deferred until the athlete has had at least 2 weeks symptom-free at rest and with exertion.
- Terminating the season for that player is mandated by any abnormality on CT or MRI consistent with brain swelling, contusion, or other intracranial pathology.

uncus of the temporal lobe or lobes below the tentorium or herniation of the cerebellar tonsils through the foramen magnum. Careful assessment of an athlete's concussion and adherence to recommended return-to-play guidelines are of paramount importance in protecting athletes and preventing the tragedy of second-impact syndrome.

Protection of athletes is also based on proper conditioning and technique. For football players, proper strengthening of head and neck muscles is essential to minimizing head and neck injury.[55] Proper head-up tackling and blocking techniques are also critical in reducing football-related head and neck injury.[37,55] Changes in rules that emphasize safety, such as the 1976 rule that outlawed tackling or blocking by making initial contact with the head (spearing), have made a significant impact on reducing head and neck injuries in football.[61] The use of helmets certified by the National Operating Committee on Standards for Athletic Equipment is now mandatory for all high school and college football players. The presence of physicians or a certified athletic trainer at all games and practices is also crucial to the quick identification of head injury and treatment and/or referral for further medical and neuropsychological assessment and intervention.[61]

Measurement of Severity of Concussion

One of the primary difficulties in determining the incidence and severity of concussion is that there is no agreed upon definition of concussion.[13] According to Cantu,[13] a generally accepted working definition of concussion was proposed by the Committee on Head Injury Nomenclature of the Congress of Neurological Surgeons[20] that states, "a clinical syndrome characterized by immediate and transient post-traumatic impairment of neural function, such as alteration of consciousness, disturbance of vision, equilibrium, etc., due to brainstem involvement." The practice parameter established by the Quality Standards Committee of the American Academy of Neurology (AAN)[3] defines concussion as a "trauma-induced alteration in mental status that may or may not involve loss of consciousness. Confusion and amnesia are hallmarks of concussion." The AAN practice parameter also describes typical features of concussion, including vacant stare, slow verbal and motor responses, confusion and deficits in focused attention, disorientation, altered or incomprehensible speech, gross incoordination, emotional lability or overreactivity, memory impairment, and any loss of consciousness. The practice parameter identified the following symptoms that occur within minutes or hours of the concussion: headache, dizziness or vertigo, nausea or vomiting, and lack of awareness of surroundings. Problematic symptoms for days or weeks after concussion (postconcussion syndrome symptoms) include persisting headache, lightheadedness, attention and concentration deficits, memory impairment, fatigue, low frustration tolerance and irritability, sensitivity to bright light or loud noise, difficulty focusing vision, anxiety or depression, and sleep disturbance.

Cantu[14] created a system for classifying the severity of concussion that is based upon both loss of consciousness and length of posttraumatic amnesia. No loss of consciousness and less than 30 minutes of amnesia characterize a Grade 1 concussion (mild). A Grade 2 concussion (moderate) is associated with a loss of consciousness of less than 5 minutes or amnesia ranging from 30 minutes to 24 hours. A Grade 3 concussion (severe) refers to those injuries in which loss of consciousness is greater than 5 minutes and amnesia lasts 24 hours or more.

An alternative concussion classification system has been proposed as part of the practice parameter established by the AAN[3] and was based upon a review of all existing scales including the 1991 guidelines developed by the Colorado Medical Society. In the AAN system, a Grade 1 concussion is marked by transient confusion, no loss of consciousness, and resolution of mental status abnormalities or symptoms of concussion within 15 minutes. A Grade 2 concussion is also marked by transient confusion and no loss of consciousness, but mental status abnormalities or concussion symptoms do *not* resolve within 15 minutes; if symptoms persist for more than 1 hour, medical observation is warranted. A Grade 3 concussion refers to any loss of consciousness from seconds to minutes. Cantu[13] has expressed some concern about the AAN system, noting that it classifies a concussion with brief loss of consciousness as more serious than one without loss of consciousness, but with posttraumatic amnesia of greater than 24 hours. Cantu believed that the latter concussion, with a profound amnesia, represents a greater cerebral insult than the former.

A variety of neuropsychological tests may be administered during preseason assessment or during the more comprehensive neuropsychological evaluation of athletes who have sustained a head injury. Although the specific tests chosen by various neuropsychologists may vary, the neuropsychological evaluation of a head-injured athlete will typically include assessment of information processing speed, memory, and attention/concentration. The following tests have been identified as particularly helpful in the assessment of sports-related head injury:[52]

- *California Verbal Learning Test:*[23] A multitrial verbal list learning task that also assesses the ability to improve memory performance with conceptual organization.

- *Computerized Neuropsychological Tests:* In addition to the traditional neuropsychological measures, a number of computerized neuropsychological assessments have been used with some success,[52] including: the Continuous Performance Test,[21] MicroCog,[67] CogScreen,[44] Automated Neuropsychological Assessment Metrics,[69] and Vigil.[93]

- *Controlled Oral Word Association Test:*[85] Assesses rapid verbal fluency.

- *Digit Span Subtest of the Wechsler Adult Intelligence Scale (WAIS-R)-Revised or WAIS-III:*[94,95] Assesses auditory attention and working memory.

- *Grooved Pegboard Test:*[45,46] A timed test of manual dexterity, fine motor control, and eye-hand coordination.

- *Hopkins Verbal Learning Test:*[9] A multitrial verbal list learning task with semantic categories that is used to assess noncontextual verbal memory.

- *Letter and Number Sequencing Subtest from the Wechsler Memory Scale-III:*[96] Assesses auditory attention, working memory, and sequencing.

- *Paced Auditory Serial Addition Task:*[31,32] A measure of rapid new problem solving on an auditory test of serial addition.

- *Rey Auditory Verbal Learning Test:*[71] Assesses immediate and delayed noncontextual verbal memory using a multitrial verbal list learning task.

- *Ruff's 2s and 7s:*[75] A measure of selective visual attention.

- *Standardized Assessment of Concussion:*[58] A brief assessment of orientation, concentration, memory, and neurological screening designed for sideline administration and screening.

- *Stroop Color and Word Test:*[29,30,87] Measures sustained attention and the ability to inhibit typical response patterns.

- *Symbol Digit Modalities Test:*[82] Measures rapid figural encoding and visual scanning with a motor component.

- *Trail Making Test Parts A and B:*[70] Assesses simple and complex cognitive processing speed.

Practice Options continued—

Grade 3

- Transport the athlete from the field to the nearest emergency department by ambulance if still unconscious or if worrisome signs are detected (with cervical spine immobilization, if indicated).

- A thorough neurological evaluation should be performed emergently, including appropriate neuroimaging procedures when indicated.

- Hospital admission is indicated if any signs of pathology are detected or if the mental status of the athlete remains abnormal.

- If findings are normal at the time of the initial medical evaluation, the athlete may be sent home. Explicit written instructions will help the family or responsible party observe the athlete over a period of time.

- Neurological status should be assessed daily thereafter until all symptoms have stabilized or resolved.

- Prolonged unconsciousness, persistent mental status alterations, worsening postconcussion symptoms, or abnormalities on neurological examination require urgent neurosurgical evaluation or transfer to a trauma center.

- After a brief (seconds) Grade 3 concussion, the athlete should be withheld from play until asymptomatic for 1 week at rest and with exertion.

- After a prolonged (minutes) Grade 3 concussion, the athlete should be withheld from play for 2 weeks at rest and with exertion.

- Following a second Grade 3 concussion, the athlete should be withheld from play for a minimum of 1 asymptomatic month. The evaluating physician may elect to extend that period beyond 1 month, depending on clinical evaluation and other circumstances.

- CT or MRI is recommended for athletes whose headache or other associated symptoms worsen or persist longer than 1 week.

- Any abnormality on CT or MRI consistent with brain swelling, contusion, or other intracranial pathology should result in termination of the season for that athlete and return to play in the future should be seriously discouraged in discussions with the athlete.

TABLE 1
GUIDELINES FOR RETURN TO PLAY AFTER CONCUSSION

	First Concussion	Second Concussion	Third Concussion
Grade 1 (mild)	May return to play if asymptomatic* for 1 week	Return to play in 2 weeks if asymptomatic at that time for 1 week	Terminate season; may return to play next season if asymptomatic
Grade 2 (moderate)	Return to play after asymptomatic for 1 week	Minimum of 1 month; may return to play then if asymptomatic for 1 week; consider terminating season	Terminate season; may return to play next season if asymptomatic
Grade 3 (severe)	Minimum of 1 month; may then return to play if asymptomatic for 1 week	Terminate season; may return to play next season if asymptomatic	

*No headache, dizziness, or impaired orientation, concentration, or memory during rest or exertion. (Reprinted from Cantu RC with permission)

Return-to-play Criteria

Neuropsychological testing can be important in determining when an athlete can return to play.[52,97] Neuropsychological assessment "represents the most sensitive method of detecting post concussion symptoms and involves the application of neuropsychological test instruments that are sensitive even to subtle changes in attention/concentration, memory, information processing, and motor speed or coordination."[52(p10)] In contrast to neurodiagnostic procedures that provide information on brain structure, such as CT and MRI, neuropsychological procedures assess cognitive abilities and related brain functioning. According to Lovell and Collins,[52] players should not return to play if they demonstrate impaired performance on any neuropsychological measure relative to their baseline performance.

Neuropsychological data can also be helpful in more accurate classification of concussion. In a study by Lovell and Collins,[52] impairment on a neuropsychological evaluation postinjury suggested that four injured athletes initially diagnosed as having Grade 1 concussions may have been more accurately diagnosed with Grade 2 concussions due to lingering cognitive deficits with subsequent implications for return to play. MRI is clearly more sensitive than CT in detecting mild cerebral dysfunction, and it is recommended that MRI studies be obtained in those injured athletes with persisting neuropsychological impairment or postconcussion symptoms.[97]

Return-to-play guidelines based upon the Cantu criteria and suggestions for medical interventions are described in Cantu,[15] and are found in Table 1.

Future Directions

A panel of neurologists and neuropsychologists with an interest in sports-related concussion began meeting in 1995 to address issues in the field.[52] Recommendations for future directions were proposed after a meeting in February 1997, and a summary of those are presented here. Concern was raised with the current limited use of neuropsychological assessment in evaluating younger amateur athletes, including those in junior and senior high school, to determine the short- and long-term effects of mild head injury sustained in sports. The few studies collected on this population failed to utilize adequate control groups or had other methodological problems. Research to date has focused primarily on football and male athletes, with less attention to other sports and female athletes. Future research needs to focus on other sports with potential for mild head injury, such as lacrosse, Rugby, soccer, and wrestling, and to examine the neuropsychological sequelae in concussed female athletes.

Many professional athletic teams, including teams in the National Football League and National Hockey League, have begun baseline neuropsychological testing of their athletes. These data will provide valuable information in the treatment and recovery of injured individuals, but will also shed light on the sequelae of head injury by the creation of sports neuropsychology databases. Additional areas for future research include consideration of language and cultural issues in the neuropsychological assessment of non-English-speaking athletes and a focus on research into treatment for concussion. Further development of computerized, complex reaction-time measures for identification of subtle neuropsychological deficits related to concussion has also been proposed based on research that suggests reaction-time dysfunction after concussion.[6] Finally, equestrian sports have the highest risk of head injury, but little research has been conducted into the neurocognitive sequelae of these head injuries. Particularly since equestrians appear to be at risk for multiple head injuries, research on the short- and long-term neuropsychological effects of repeated head trauma is needed.

References

1. Abreau F, Templer DI, Schuyler BA, et al: Neuropsychological assessment of soccer players. **Neuropsychology** 4:175-181, 1990
2. Adams ID: Rugby football injuries. **Br J Sports Med** 11:4-6, 1977
3. American Academy of Neurology: Practice parameter. The management of concussion in sports (summary statement). **Neurology** 48: 581-585, 1997
4. Axe MJ, Newcomb WA, Warner D: Sports injuries and adolescent athletes. **Del Med J** 63:359-363, 1991
5. Barth JT, Diamond R, Errico A: Mild head injury and postconcussion syndrome: does anyone really suffer? **Clin Electroencephalogr** 27: 183-186, 1996
6. Bleiberg J, Halpern EL, Reeves D, et al: Future directions for the neuropsychological assessment of sports concussion. **J Head Trauma Rehabil** 13:36-44, 1998
7. Boden BP, Kirdendall DT, Garrett W: Concussion incidence in elite college soccer players. **Am J Sports Med** 26:238-241, 1998
8. Bond GR, Christoph RA, Rodgers BM: Pediatric equestrian injuries: assessing the impact of helmet use. **Pediatrics** 95:487-489, 1995
9. Brandt J: The Hopkins Verbal Learning Test: development of a new memory test with six equivalent forms. **Clin Neuropsychologist** 5: 124-142, 1991
10. Brown JM, Ramsey LC, Weiss AL: Ski helmets: an idea whose time has come. **Contemp Pediatr** 14:115-125, 1997
11. Bruce DA, Schut L, Sutton LN: Brain and cervical spine injuries occurring during organized sports activities in children and adolescents. **Primary Care** 11:175-194, 1984
12. Butler RJ: Neuropsychological investigation of amateur boxers. **Br J Sports Med** 28:187-190, 1994
13. Cantu RC: Athletic head injuries. **Clin Sports Med** 16:531-542, 1997
14. Cantu RC: Guidelines for return to contact sports after a cerebral concussion. **Phys Sportsmed** 14(10):75-83, 1986
15. Cantu RC: Return to play guidelines after a head injury. **Clin Sports Med** 17:45-60, 1998
16. Cantu RC: Second-impact syndrome. **Clin Sports Med** 17:37-44, 1998
17. Cantu RC: Second impact syndrome: immediate management. **Phys Sportsmed** 20:55-66, 1992
18. Cantu RC, Voy R: Second impact syndrome: a risk in any contact sport. **Phys Sportsmed** 23(6):172-177, 1995
19. Chitnavis JP, Gibbons CLM, Hirigoyen M, et al: Accidents with horses: what has changed in 20 years? **Injury** 27:103-105, 1996
20. Committee on Head Injury Nomenclature of the Congress of Neurological Surgeons: Glossary of head injury including some definitions of injury to the cervical spine. **Clin Neurosurg** 12:386-394, 1966
21. Conners J: **Conners' Continuous Performance Test.** North Tonowanda, NY: Multi-Health System, 1967
22. Council for Scientific Affairs, American Medical Association: Head injury in boxing. **JAMA** 249:254-257, 1983
23. Delis DC, Kramer JH, Kaplan E, et al: **California Verbal Learning Test: Adult Version.** San Antonio, Tx: Psychological Corp, 1987
24. Dikmen S, McLean A, Temkin N: Neuropsychological and psychological consequences of minor head injury. **Neurosurgery** 48:1227-1232, 1986
25. Feehan M, Waller AE: Precompetition injury and subsequent tournament performance in full-contact tae kwon do. **Br J Sports Med** 29: 258-262, 1995
26. Frankel HL, Haskell R, Digiacomo C, et al: Recidivism in equestrian trauma. **Am Surg** 64:151-154, 1998
27. Gennarelli TA, Adams JH, Graham DI: Acceleration induced head injury in the monkey: I. The model, its mechanical and physiological correlates. **Acta Neuropathol Suppl** 1:23-25, 1981
28. Gibbs N: Common rugby league injuries. Recommendations for treatment and preventive measures. **Sports Med** 18:438-450, 1994
29. Golden JC: Identification of brain disorders by the Stroop color and word test. **J Clin Psychiatr** 32:654-658, 1976
30. Golden JC: **Stroop Color and Word Test.** Chicago, Ill: Stoelting, 1978
31. Gronwall DMA: Paced Auditory Serial Addition Task: a measure of recovery from concussion. **Percept Motor Skills** 44:367-373, 1977
32. Gronwall DMA, Sampson H: **The Psychological Effects of Concussion.** Auckland, NZ: Auckland University Press, 1974
33. Haglund Y, Eriksson E: Does amateur boxing lead to chronic brain damage? A review of some recent investigations. **Am J Sports Med** 21: 97-109, 1993
34. Haglund Y, Persson HE: Does Swedish amateur boxing lead to chronic brain damage: 3. A retrospective clinical neurophysiological study. **Acta Neurol Scand** 82:353-360, 1990
35. Hamilton MG, Tranmer BI: Nervous system injuries in horseback-riding accidents. **J Trauma** 34:227-232, 1993
36. Hinton-Bayre AD, Geffen G, McFarland K: Mild head injury and speed of information processing: a prospective study of professional rugby league players. **J Clin Exp Neuropsychol** 19:275-289, 1997
37. Hodgson VR, Thomas LM: Play head-up football. **Natl Fed News** 2: 24-27, 1985
38. Hunt M, Fulford S: Amateur soccer: injuries in relation to field position. **Br J Sports Med** 23:265, 1990
39. Hutchinson MR: Cheerleading injuries: patterns, prevention, case reports. **Phys Sportsmed** 25:83-96, 1997
40. Jordan BD: Chronic neurological injuries in boxing, in Jordan BD (ed): **Medical Aspects of Boxing.** Boca Raton, Fla: CRC Press, 1993, pp 177-185

41. Jordan BD: Neurological aspects of boxing. **Arch Neurol 44:**453-459, 1987

42. Jordan BD, Relkin NR, Ravdin LD, et al: Apolipoprotein E ε4 associated with chronic traumatic brain injury in boxing. **JAMA 278:** 136-140, 1997

43. Jordan SE, Green GA, Galanty HL, et al: Acute and chronic brain injury in United States National Team soccer players. **Am J Sports Med 24:**205-210, 1996

44. Kay G: **CogScreen.** Odessa, Fla: Psychological Assessment Resources, 1995

45. Klove H: Clinical neuropsychology, in Forster FM (ed): **The Medical Clinics of North America.** New York, NY: WB Saunders, 1963

46. Klove H, Matthews CG: Neuropsychological studies of patients with epilepsy, in Reitan RM, Davidson LM (eds): **Clinical Neuropsychology.** Washington, DC: Hemisphere, 1974

47. Kriss TC, Kriss VM: Equine-related neurosurgical trauma: a prospective series of 30 patients. **J Trauma 43:**97-99, 1997

48. Leininger BE, Gramling SE, Ferrel AD, et al: Neuropsychological deficits in symptomatic minor head injury patients after concussion and mild concussion. **J Neurol Neurosurg Psychiatry 53:**293-296, 1990

49. Levin HS, Eisenberg HM, Benton AL: **Mild Head Injury.** New York, NY: Oxford University Press, 1989

50. Levin HS, Lippold SC, Goldman A, et al: Neurobehavioral functioning and magnetic resonance imaging findings in young boxers. **J Neurosurg 67:**657-667, 1987

51. Levin HS, Mattis S, Ruff RM, et al: Neurobehavioral outcome following minor head injury: a three-center study. **J Neurosurg 66:**234-243, 1987

52. Lovell MR, Collins MW: Neuropsychological assessment of the college football player. **J Head Trauma Rehabil 13:**9-26, 1998

53. Macciocchi S, Barth JT, Alves W, et al: Neuropsychological functioning and recovery after mild head injury in collegiate athletes. **Neurosurgery 39:**510-514, 1996

54. Macnab AJ, Cadman R: Demographics of alpine skiing and snowboarding injury: lessons for prevention programs. **Injury Prevent 2:** 286-289, 1996

55. Maroon JC, Steele PB, Berlin R: Football head and neck injuries—an update. **Clin Neurosurg 27:**414-429, 1980

56. Matser JT, Kessels AGH, Jordan BD, et al: Chronic traumatic brain injury in professional soccer players. **Neurology 51:**791-796, 1998

57. Matthews WB: Footballer's migraine. **Br Med J 2:**326-327, 1972

58. McCrea M, Kelly J, Randolph C: **The Standardized Assessment of Concussion: Manual for Administration, Scoring, and Interpretation.** Alexandria, Va: Brain Injury Association, 1997

59. McKenna S, Borman B, Findlay J, et al: Sports injuries in New Zealand. **NZ Med J 99:**899-901, 1986

60. Mendez MF: The neuropsychiatric aspects of boxing. **Int J Psychiatry Med 25:**249-262, 1995

61. Mueller FO: Fatalities from head and cervical spine injuries occurring in tackle football: 50 years' experience. **Clin Sports Med 17:**169-182, 1998

62. Myles ST, Mohtadi NG, Schnittker J: Injuries to the nervous system and spine in downhill skiing. **Can J Surg 35:**643-648, 1992

63. Nafpliotis H: Neurologic injuries in soccer, in Jordan BD, Tsairis P, Warren RF (eds): **Sports Neurology.** Rockville, Md: Aspen Press, 1989, pp 269-278

64. Oppenheimer RD: Microscopic lesions in the brain following head injury. **J Neurol Neurosurg Psychiatry 31:**229-306, 1968

65. Porter M, O'Brien M: Incidence and severity of injuries resulting from amateur boxing in Ireland. **Clin J Sports Med 6:**97-101, 1996

66. Potero C: Celebrity ski deaths inspire helmet debate. **Phys Sportsmed 26:**21-22, 1998

67. Powell D, Kaplan E, Whitla D, et al: **Manual for MicroCog: Assessment of Cognitive Functioning.** San Antonio, Tx: Psychological Corp, 1993

68. Rampton J, Leach T, Therrien SA, et al: Head, neck, and facial injuries in ice hockey: the effect of protective equipment. **Clin J Sports Med 7:** 162-167, 1997

69. Reeves D, Kane R, Winter K, et al: **Automated Neuropsychological Assessment Metrics (ANAM): Test Administration Manual (Version 3.11).** St Louis, Mo: Missouri Institute of Mental Health, 1995

70. Reitan R: Validity of the Trail Making Test as an indicator of organic brain damage. **Percept Motor Skills 8:**271-276, 1958

71. Rey A: **L'Examen Clinique en Psychologie.** Paris: Press Universitaire de France, 1964

72. Rimel RW, Giordana MA, Barth JT, et al: Disability caused by minor head injury. **Neurosurgery 9:**221-228, 1981

73. Roaas A, Nilsson S: Major injuries in Norwegian football. **Br J Sports Med 13:**3-5, 1979

74. Ruchinskas R, Francis J, Barth JT: Mild head injury in sports. **Appl Neuropsychiatr 4:**43-49, 1997

75. Ruff RM, Allen CC: **Ruff 2 & 7 Selective Attention Test.** Odessa, Fla: Psychological Assessment Resources, 1996

76. Ruff RM, Crouch JA, Troster AI, et al: Selected cases of poor outcome following minor brain trauma: comparing neuropsychological and positron emission tomography assessment. **Brain Inj 8:**297-308, 1994

77. Ruff RM, Levin HS, Mattis S, et al: Recovery of memory after mild head injury: a three center study, in Levin HM, Eisenberg HM, Benton AL (eds): **Mild Head Injury.** New York, NY: Oxford University Press, 1989, pp 176-188

78. Ryan AJ: Intracranial injuries resulting from boxing. **Clin Sports Med 17:**155-168, 1998

79. Saunders RL, Harbaugh RE: The second impact in catastrophic contact-sports head trauma. **JAMA 252:**538-539, 1984

80. Schneider RC: **Head and Neck Injuries in Football.** Baltimore, Md: Williams & Wilkins, 1973

81. Seward H, Orchard J, Hazard H, et al: Football players in Australia at the elite level. **Med J Aust 159:**298-301, 1993

82. Smith A: **Symbol Digit Modalities Test.** Los Angeles, Calif: Western Psychological Services, 1991

83. Smodlaka VM: Death on the soccer field and its prevention. **Phys Sportsmed 9:**101-107, 1981

84. Smodlaka VM: Medical aspects of heading the ball in soccer. **Phys Sportsmed 12:**127-131, 1984

85. Spreen O, Benton AL: **Neurosensory Center Comprehensive Examination for Aphasia (NCCEA) (Revised Edition).** Victoria: University of Victoria, Neuropsychology Laboratory, 1977

86. Stewart WF, Gordon B, Seines O, et al: Prospective study of central nervous system function in amateur boxers in the United States. **Am J Epidemiol 139:**573-588, 1994

87. Stroop JR: Studies of inference in serial verbal reaction. **J Exp Psychol 18:**643-662, 1935

88. Symonds C: Concussion and its sequelae. **Lancet 1:**1-5, 1962

89. Tegner Y, Lorentzon R: Concussion among Swedish elite ice hockey players. **Br J Sports Med 30:**251-255, 1996

90. Thomassen A, Juul-Jensen P, de Fine OB, et al: Neurological, electroencephalographic and neuropsychological examination of 53 former amateur boxers. **Acta Neurol Scand 60:**352-362, 1979

91. Tysvaer AT, Storli OV, Bachen NI: Soccer injuries to the brain. A neurological and electroencephalographic study of former players. **Acta Neurol Scand 80:**151-156, 1980

92. United States Consumer Product Safety Commission summary reports. **National Electronic Injury Surveillance-System: 1990-1992.** Washington, DC: US Consumer Product Safety Commission, 1993

93. Vigil. San Antonio, Tx: Psychological Corp, 1997

94. Wechsler D: **Wechsler Adult Intelligence Scale—Revised.** San Antonio, Tx: Psychological Corp, 1981

95. Wechsler D: **Wechsler Adult Intelligence Scale—Third Edition.** San Antonio, Tx: Psychological Corp, 1997

96. Wechsler D: **Wechsler Memory Scale—Third Edition.** San Antonio, Tx: Psychological Corp, 1997

97. Wilberger JE: Minor head injuries in American football: prevention of long term sequelae. **Sports Med 15:**338-343, 1993

98. Witol A: Neuropsychological deficits associated with differing exposure to heading and experience in soccer. **Arch Clin Neuropsychol** (In press)

CHAPTER 12

Neuropsychological Assessment of the Head-Injured Professional Athlete

MARK R. LOVELL, PhD, AND MICHAEL W. COLLINS, PhD

All contact and collision sports carry the risk of mild traumatic brain injury (MTBI) or concussion. Although all professional athletes assume some risk when they take to the field or ice, there has been increasing interest in protecting and improving the health of the professional athlete. Not only is this important on humanitarian grounds, but efforts to protect the health of the professional athlete also make economic sense. Professional sports franchises invest millions of dollars in purchasing the services of their athletes and naturally desire to protect their investment.

The majority of professional athletes who experience an MTBI recover quickly and have no apparent neurological sequelae. However, some athletes experience persistent cognitive and/or neurobehavioral difficulties. Preliminary research has indicated that the risk of permanent neurological injury appears to be particularly great if the athlete has experienced multiple MTBIs.[9] Efforts to protect athletes from career-ending and potentially disabling neurological injuries have led to increased efforts in professional sports to more effectively evaluate the injured athlete. Specifically, large-scale neuropsychological evaluation programs have recently been created within both the National Football League (NFL) and the National Hockey League (NHL).[16]

This chapter reviews the use of neuropsychological testing in professional athletes. The current neuropsychological testing programs within professional football and hockey are reviewed and the use of this approach to assist in making return-to-play decisions is discussed. Neuropsychological research in other professional sports, such as boxing, soccer, and Australian Rules football, is also reviewed.

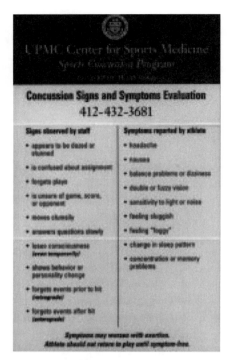

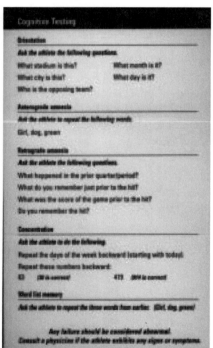

Figure 1: Field mental status examination.

Timeline for the Evaluation of the Professional Athlete

The initial evaluation of the concussed athlete begins on the playing field, with the first assessment of the athlete's status usually completed by the team physician or athletic trainer. The player should be evaluated for both signs and symptoms of concussion. To facilitate the identification of concussion on the field, the authors have developed a pocket-sized card that lists the frequently observed signs and symptoms of concussion (Figure 1).

This evaluation should involve an assessment of the player's orientation to place, game, and details of the contest. The athlete's recall of events preceding the collision (retrograde amnesia) should be evaluated. The ability to learn and retain new information (anterograde amnesia) should be tested via a brief sideline memory test. The player should be asked to repeat three to five words until they can do so consistently. They should be checked for recall of this list within 5 minutes. Brief tests of attentional capacity, such as the recitation of digits in backward order or the backward recitation of months of the year, are also useful. Finally, the player should be observed for emerging postconcussion symptoms such as headache, nausea, imbalance, or onfield confusion.[13] A second onfield assessment approach has recently been standardized to allow for the more systematic evaluation of MTBI in athletes.[24] However, it should be emphasized that this type of brief sideline evaluation is not a substitute for more formal neuropsychological testing and should not serve as the primary basis for making decisions regarding return to the field, court, or ice.

The neuropsychological evaluation of the athlete should take place within 24 to 48 hours of the suspected MTBI, whenever possible. Although many athletes may appear to be symptom-free, the authors suggest a neuropsychological evaluation to assess more subtle aspects of cognitive functioning such as information processing speed and memory. If the athlete displays any cognitive deficits on testing or continues to exhibit postconcussion symptoms, a follow-up neuropsychological evaluation is recommended within 5 to 7 days after injury, prior to return to competition. This time interval represents a useful and practical time span and also appears to be consistent with animal brain metabolism studies which have demonstrated metabolic changes in the brain that persist for several days following injury.[10]

The Historical Roots of Neuropsychological Testing in Professional Sports

The systematic study of MTBI in athletics has been a recent phenomenon. Although neuropsychological testing was first undertaken in professional boxing, the original clinical introduction occurred in the sport of football. The first large-scale study of concussion in athletes (football players) was carried out at the college level and involved the cooperative efforts of the University of Virginia, the Ivy League schools, and the University of Pittsburgh. This study was directed by Dr. Jeffrey Barth at the University of Virginia in the early 1980s and involved more than 2300 athletes.[1,18] These athletes were given a "baseline" evaluation prior to the beginning of the season and repeat testing was completed if the player suffered an MTBI during the season. Follow-up testing was conducted at 24 hours after an MTBI, and again at 5 days, 10 days, and postseason. This study revealed subtle and rapidly resolving diffi-

TABLE 1

NFL NEUROPSYCHOLOGICAL TEST BATTERY

Test	Ability Evaluated
Brief Visuospatial Memory Test-Revised (BVMT-R)[2] Delayed recall from BVMT-R	Visual memory Delayed recall for designs
Controlled Oral Word Association Test[3]	Word fluency, word retrieval
Hopkins Verbal Learning Test (HVLT)[4] Delayed recall from HVLT	Memory for words (verbal memory) Delayed recall for words
Orientation Questions	Retrograde and anterograde amnesia, orientation to place and time
Postconcussion Symptom Inventory[16]	MTBI symptoms
Trail Making Test[28]	Visual scanning, mental flexibility
WAIS-III Digit Span[34]	Attention span
WAIS-III Digit Symbol[34]	Visual scanning, information processing
WAIS-III Symbol Search[34]	Visual scanning, visual search

culties in cognitive functioning on tests sensitive to information processing speed, as compared to a control group.

Based on the need for more sensitive MTBI evaluation procedures in professional football players, a neuropsychological evaluation program was instituted with the Pittsburgh Steelers in 1993 by Drs. Joseph Maroon and Mark Lovell and with the active participation of John Norwig, ATC, and Dr. Julian Bailes.[16] This represented the first clinically oriented project structured to assist team medical personnel in making return-to-play decisions following a suspected MTBI. This approach involved the formal evaluation of each player prior to the beginning of the season to provide the basis for comparison, in the event of an MTBI during the season. Testing was then repeated within 24 hours after a suspected MTBI and again prior to the return of the athlete to contact (approximately 5 days postinjury).

The preseason baseline evaluation of the athlete is important for several reasons. Individual players vary with regard to their level of performance on tests of memory, attention/concentration, mental processing speed, and motor speed. Some players perform poorly on the more demanding tests because of pre-injury learning disabilities, attention deficit disorder, or other factors such as test-taking anxiety.

Table 1 provides a list of the neuropsychological tests originally used with the Pittsburgh Steelers; this list has now been adopted by a number of other NFL teams. This test battery has recently been revised with the addition of the several tests from the Wechsler Adult Intelligence Scale-III (WAIS-III; Digit Span, Digit Symbol, and Symbol Search).[34]

The Hopkins Verbal Learning Test (HVLT)[4] consists of a 12-word list that is presented to the athlete on three consecutive trials. The athlete is assessed for recall after each presentation and again following a 20-minute delay period. The Brief Visuospatial Memory Test-Revised (BVMT-R)[2] evaluates visual memory and involves the presentation of six abstract spatial designs on three consecutive trials. Similar to the HVLT, the athlete's recall following each trial and his/her delayed recall is evaluated. Both tests have multiple equivalent forms that minimize practice effects and make them ideal for use with athletes who are likely to undergo evaluation on multiple occasions throughout the course of their careers.

The Trail Making Test[28] consists of two parts and requires the athlete to utilize spatial scanning and mental flexibility skills. The Controlled Oral Word Association Test[3] requires the athlete to recall as many words as possible that begin with a given letter of the alphabet, within a 60-second time period. This is completed for three separate letters and provides a measure of verbal fluency. In addition to the neuropsychological tests mentioned above, it is important to monitor the athlete's symptoms. The Postconcussion Symptom Inventory[16] has recently been developed and is currently being utilized by a number of teams within the NFL and NHL.

As can be seen in Table 1, the NFL test battery was constructed to evaluate multiple aspects of cognitive functioning. It is heavily oriented toward the evaluation of attention processes, visual scanning, and information processing, although the test battery also evaluates verbal memory, coordination, and speech fluency. The tests that made up the battery were administered using standardized instructions to avoid variation in results across testing sessions and across teams.

Neuropsychological Testing in Ice Hockey

Similar to the sport of football, ice hockey is a collision sport that can and does result in MTBIs. The recent interest in conducting neuropsychological testing in professional hockey players developed as a result of several converging forces. First, heightened media exposure led to a general awareness of the potential danger of MTBI by both the players and the team medical staff. Second, the large-scale neuropsychological testing projects underway in professional football and at a number of universities have demonstrated the feasibility and utility of conducting neuropsychological testing in large groups of athletes.[6,17] This section reviews some of the unique aspects of ice hockey with regard to MTBI and details some of the work that is currently underway in this sport.

Although athletes who participate in the sports of football and hockey share many characteristics, there are differences between hockey and other sports (such as football) that are worth mentioning. For example, the high speed at which professional athletes typically skate as well as the rules of the game result in a continuation of high-speed play, with minimal stoppage of play for substitutions. This results in players being at near-peak physical performance during their shift and throughout the game. The high speed of the game increases the potential for high-velocity collisions on the ice. In addition, maneuverability on skates is poorer in certain situations, which may result in difficulty in avoiding high-speed collisions on the ice. Finally, the sideboards in hockey represent a potential source of injury that does not exist in football or other sports that are played in the open field.

A Model for the Use of Neuropsychological Assessment Procedures in Ice Hockey

A number of factors need to be considered prior to the implementation of a neuropsychological evaluation program for professional-level hockey players. In particular, the benefit of baseline testing and the need for brief but sensitive test procedures are as important in working with hockey players as they are with football athletes. The need to perform a baseline evaluation of more than 20 athletes, often during a 1-day period, creates a challenge to the neuropsychologist.

While the time pressures in working with large groups of athletes are similar in both football and hockey, several factors make the evaluation of the hockey athlete particularly challenging. First, multiple languages are spoken within the professional hockey ranks (e.g., French, English, Russian, Czechoslovakian, Swedish, Finnish, and German). While examination of each athlete in his native language may appear to be the most effective way of evaluating the athlete both at baseline and following an MTBI, this is highly impractical and would require the availability of multilingual neuropsychologists in all cities within a given league. For this reason, it is far more practical to utilize test procedures that are not heavily language-dependent. The assessment of players in their native tongue would also impede league- or sport-wide efforts to study performance on standardized tests due to limitations in directly translating languages. Another, more realistic alternative is for the neuropsychologist to rely on measures that are not heavily language-based. Such an approach should focus on information processing speed or psychomotor functioning, which are known to be affected by MTBI.

In addition, a typical hockey schedule differs significantly from football. In professional football, most games are played on weekends and the teams return home, often immediately after the game. This allows for the neuropsychological assessment of injured athletes in the home city within 24 to 48 hours of injury. However, in the professional hockey ranks, teams often embark on lengthy road trips (2-3 weeks) and typically receive medical treatment outside of their home city. Therefore, any league-wide program aimed at the systematic evaluation of MTBI needs to be structured so that all athletes have access to neuropsychological testing, regardless of where the game is being played. This requires cooperation at the conference or league level.

Selection of a Neuropsychological Test Battery for Ice Hockey

As noted earlier, the application of neuropsychological assessment strategies to ice hockey provides specific challenges. As is the case with professional football, the need for brevity must be balanced against the need for sampling of functioning across multiple cognitive domains. The test battery should be constructed to evaluate the athlete's functioning in the areas of attentional processes, information processing speed, fluency, and memory. Although there are numerous tests that can provide information regarding the athlete's ability to function in these domains, procedures should also be selected that have equivalent multiple forms or that have been thoroughly researched with regard to the expected "practice effects." Although much more research needs to be completed that investigates the use of specific neuropsychological tests with athletes, a test battery has been developed for use with hockey players, which has been supported by the NHL/NHL Players Association (NHLPA) Neuropsychological Advisory Board members. This group is composed of Dr. Mark Lovell, Dr. Ruben Echemendia (program co-directors), Dr. William Barr, Dr. Elizabeth Parker, and Dr. W. Gary Snow (NHLPA representative). The test battery can be administered in approximately 30 minutes and samples from multiple cognitive domains. In keeping with the authors' previous experience with amateur and professional athletics, preseason baseline testing, follow-up testing within 24 to 48 hours of a suspected MTBI and a 5-day follow-up evaluation are recommended. The authors' suggested test battery is seen in Table 2.

The Hopkins Verbal Learning Test[4] has been discussed previously in the section on the assessment of football athletes. The Ruff Figural Fluency Test[29] is a relatively new test that requires the athlete to rapidly draw a series of unique designs while under a time pressure. Although the use of this test has yet to be formally evaluated with athletes, its nonverbal nature may be ideal for use with athletes for whom English is a second language.

The Color Trail Making Test[8] was developed to provide a culture-fair alternative to the widely used Trail Making Test.[28] This test requires the athlete to utilize visual scanning and sequencing skills while under a time pressure. The Symbol Digit Modalities Test[31] mea-

TABLE 2
NHL NEUROPSYCHOLOGICAL TEST BATTERY

Test	Ability Evaluated
Color Trail Making Test[8]	Visual scanning, mental flexibility
Controlled Oral Word Association Test[3]*	Word fluency, word retrieval
Hopkins Verbal Learning Test (HVLT)[4]* Delayed recall from HVLT	Word learning Delayed recall for words
Orientation Questions	Retrograde and anterograde amnesia, orientation to place and time
Penn State Symbol Cancellation Test	Visual scanning, attention
Postconcussion Symptom Inventory[16]	Postconcussion symptoms
Ruff Figural Fluency Test[29]	Design fluency
Symbol Digit Modalities Test[31]	Visual scanning, immediate memory

*Suggested for English-speaking athletes only.

sures mental processing speed. The Penn State Symbol Cancellation Test (R. Echemendia, personal communication) is a test that measures visual scanning and attentional processes and requires the athlete to cross-out symbols that are imbedded within an array of other symbols.

In addition to the neuropsychological tests listed above, the neuropsychologist should be careful to evaluate noncognitive symptoms of MTBI. The Postconcussion Symptom Inventory[16] scale has been found to be useful in this regard. This scale is presented in Figure 2. Finally, the athlete should be checked for orientation to year, month, date of the month, and day of the week, and should also be questioned regarding their last memory prior to the hit (retrograde amnesia) and first memory following the hit (anterograde amnesia).

Neuropsychological Testing in Other Sports

Virtually all sports and recreational activities carry a risk of sustaining head injury. Clearly, sports such as basketball, soccer, and rugby have a risk of injury due to the high velocity of the game and the potential for the head to strike the opponent, turf, or a goalpost. Even recreational activities such as roller-blading, hang-gliding, or diving carry a certain risk of injury for obvious reasons. The authors have attempted, thus far, to introduce two comprehensive neuropsychological programs in the NFL and NHL that have been organized to evaluate both the short- and long-term effects of MTBI. Although much less systematic, other circumscribed neuropsychological projects have been implemented in high-risk sports, especially in boxing, soccer, and Australian Rules football. A review follows of these projects and a critical analysis of associated findings. It should be mentioned that all of the works presented, without exception, have been implemented for the purpose of research, rather than for clinical decision-making (i.e., return to play following injury).

Patient/Athlete:_____   Team: _____

SYMPTOM	RATING			BASELINE Date:	TESTING 2 Date:	TESTING 3 Date:
	None Mod. Severe					
Headache	0 1 2 3 4 5 6					
Nausea	0 1 2 3 4 5 6					
Vomiting	0 1 2 3 4 5 6					
Balance problems	0 1 2 3 4 5 6					
Dizziness	0 1 2 3 4 5 6					
Fatigue	0 1 2 3 4 5 6					
Trouble falling asleep	0 1 2 3 4 5 6					
Sleeping more than usual	0 1 2 3 4 5 6					
Sleeping less than usual	0 1 2 3 4 5 6					
Drowsiness	0 1 2 3 4 5 6					
Sensitivity to light	0 1 2 3 4 5 6					
Sensitivity to noise	0 1 2 3 4 5 6					
Irritability	0 1 2 3 4 5 6					
Sadness	0 1 2 3 4 5 6					
Nervousness	0 1 2 3 4 5 6					
Feeling more emotional	0 1 2 3 4 5 6					
Numbness or tingling	0 1 2 3 4 5 6					
Feeling slowed down	0 1 2 3 4 5 6					
Feeling mentally "foggy"	0 1 2 3 4 5 6					
Difficulty concentrating	0 1 2 3 4 5 6					
Difficulty remembering	0 1 2 3 4 5 6					
TOTAL SCORE						

Figure 2: Postconcussion scale-revised. (Reproduced from Lovell[16] with permission)

Professional Boxing

The goal of boxing is to render the opponent unconscious, with the knockout set as the standard by which champions are judged. As such, the major health concern in the sport of boxing is the cumulative effects of sustaining blows to the head. In terms of neuropathology, four basic mechanisms may account for injury. These include rotational/acceleration forces (e.g., left or right hook), linear or translational acceleration (e.g., a direct blow to nose/mouth), carotid injury (e.g., a blow to neck resulting in brief ischemia), and impact deceleration (e.g., a dazed boxer hitting canvas). Martland[21] delineated the earliest description regarding the cumulative effects of boxing-related head injury. In an article entitled "punch drunk," the outlined constellation of symptoms included initial confusion and unsteady gait, followed by increased speech and motor latencies (i.e., bradyphrenia or bradykinesia), upper-extremity and head tremors, general cognitive decline (e.g., memory, attention, and intellectual functioning), and parkinsonian-like motor deficits. Similar symptom profiles have more recently been labeled chronic boxer's encephalopathy,[23] traumatic boxer's encephalopathy,[30] and dementia pugilistica.[14] Recent research has indicated that genetic factors, such as apolipoprotein E polymorphism, may be associated with the manifestation of dementia pugilistica.[12]

Although less systematic and comprehensive than the previously outlined NFL and NHL programs, a number of neuropsychological studies have been conducted with professional boxers. Importantly, however, a paucity of well-designed studies exists. Most studies compared data to normative, rather than baseline, values and many have not incorporated appropriate control groups. Variables such as education, age, vocational history, and prior drug/alcohol history are critical to examine when determining whether deficits are secondary to boxing, rather than being more representative of pre-morbid abilities. Obtaining baseline (pre-injury) data and using the athlete as his/her own control eliminate the impact of extraneous factors.

One widely cited study in the area of boxing was conducted by Casson et al.[5] For this study, boxers underwent a neurological examination, computed tomography (CT), electroencephalography (EEG), and neuropsychological testing. Baseline testing was not conducted and athletes were not chosen at random. Nonetheless, findings suggested that 87% of all boxers exhibited abnormal findings on at least two of the four examinations. In terms of neuropsychological data, each boxer performed in the impaired range on more than one measure, including the Trail Making Test (attention/concentration), the Symbol Digit Modalities Test (concentration, visual memory), the Wechsler Memory Scale (story learning), and the Bender Visual-Motor Test (visual-spatial functioning). Casson et al found that the percentage of impaired neuropsychological test scores correlated significantly with age, number of professional fights, and abnormalities on CT. They deduced that a direct relationship existed between the length of a professional boxing career and the presence of cumulative brain damage.

A study with professional boxers was also conducted by McLatchie and colleagues.[26] Twenty active Scottish boxers (four to 200 fights), aged 18-49 years, were evaluated cross-sectionally with neuropsychological tests, EEG, and CT scanning. When compared to controls (outpatients with limb fractures or university students), boxers performed significantly worse on several neuropsychological measures, including the Digit Span Test (attention), the Wechsler Logical Memory Test (story learning), reaction-time measures, and the Paced Auditory Serial Addition Task (complex attention). Although CT and EEG were compared to normative values, one boxer had an abnormal CT and eight demonstrated abnormal EEG findings. These researchers concluded that neuropsychological testing was the most sensitive indicator of neurological dysfunction in this population.

Levin and colleagues[15] compared baseline and follow-up (6 months) neuropsychological performance in 13 boxers and 13 recreational athletes. Although there was no mention of bouts fought in the interim, they found no significant differences between the groups across any measure comprising a comprehensive neuropsychological test battery. These researchers warned that a low frequency of fights during the study period and/or a delayed onset of symptoms may have contributed to the lack of findings.

Murelius and Haglund[27] conducted a cross-sectional case control study assessing neuropsychological performance in 50 former Swedish amateur boxers versus 25 soccer and track and field athletes. Results suggested a significant correlation between the nondominant finger-tapping speed, the length of boxing or soccer career, and the total number of bouts. All athletes displayed normal neurological examination and unremarkable magnetic resonance imaging (MRI) and CT examinations. In a more recent study, Jordan[11] conducted cross-sectional analyses of 42 professional boxers using a comprehensive neuropsychological battery and CT scanning. Abnormal findings on CT were revealed in two boxers, 17 had borderline findings, and normal findings were present in 23 boxers. Conversely, robust relationships were found between poorer performance on select neuropsychological measures and variables such as frequency of sparring, number of rounds fought per week, and sparring intensity. Jordan concluded that increased sparring exposure resulted in neuropsychological deficit, especially in the domains of attention, concentration, and memory.

Professional Soccer

Although less severe than boxing, professional soccer players may also experience cumulative blows to the head. First, a soccer player may experience mild head trauma secondary to deceleration forces, such as striking a stationary object (e.g., the opponent's head) or hitting the ground after a fall. Second, although subtle, soccer players experience cumulative rotational effects placed on the brain secondary to "heading" the ball. As outlined by Tysvaer,[32] there are two main techniques in heading the ball; a standing jump and running jump. If the head is fixated, via strong neck muscles, the force of the blow is distributed throughout the rest of the body and the rotational effects on the brain are attenuated. However, the timing of this becomes difficult in the case of a running jump. Often, the athlete's neck is less rigid, resulting in greater acceleration of the cranium (and the brain lagging behind in a rotational fashion). Further, greater velocities and resultant forces are involved since the athlete accelerates into a jump. Thus, individuals who head the ball with greater frequency (i.e., forwards and defensive players) would appear to be at greater risk for morbidity. Two studies have utilized neuropsychological testing in professional soccer players.

Tsyvaer and Løchen[33] examined 37 former Norwegian professional players, cross-sectionally, 4 to 35 years after completion of their careers (mean 14 years). A group of non-head-injured hospitalized patients matched for age and education served as the comparison. Across a comprehensive neuropsychological battery, soccer players revealed lower scores on the Trail Making Test (attention/concentration), the Digit Span Test (attention/concentration), and the Benton Visual Retention Test (visual memory). In this study, 73% of former players showed impairment on at least one measure (3% severe, 38% moderate, and 32% mild). There was no significant difference between those athletes deemed "typical headers" versus the "nonheaders," although a trend did exist (20% of "headers" were impaired compared to 8% of "nonheaders").

Matser and colleagues[22] recently performed a cross-sectional study. They administered a comprehensive battery of neuropsychological measures in 53 active, rather than retired, professional players from the Netherlands. These athletes were compared with a control group of 27 elite noncontact sport athletes (swimming and track athletes). Age, education, occupational history, and drug and alcohol history were used as covariates. Professional soccer players, relative to controls, exhibited impaired performances across tests of visual and verbal memory (Logical Memory Test and Visual Reproduction Test), executive functioning (Wisconsin Card Sorting Test), and visuoperceptual processing (Rey Complex Figure Test). Further, performance on testing was related to position, as forwards and defensive players exhibited more impairment. Matser et al concluded that neurocognitive impairment might be associated with professional soccer players. Based on their findings, these authors recommended that a thorough medical evaluation be conducted following all concussions. Specifically, they recommended that all athletes receive a baseline neuropsychological evaluation so that following injury, objective measures could delineate potential impairment and help determine when the player can safely return to play.

Australian Rules Football and Rugby

It can be argued that the extent of injury and neuropathological features associated with mild brain injury during Australian Rules football or rugby are similar, and potentially more severe, to that seen in football in the United States. A major dissociating feature is that the Australian Rules athletes do not wear protective headgear, likely resulting in greater rotational/linear forces associated with trauma and an increase in injuries, such as skull fracture or hematoma, that tend to be more severe.

Several neuropsychological studies have been conducted in the area of Australian Rules football, and to a lesser extent, rugby. Cremona-Meteyard and Geffen[7] utilized reaction times to assess postconcussion functioning in nine Australian Rules athletes. All athletes were assessed 2 weeks following concussion, and six players were retested after 1 year. Twelve athletes from various contact and noncontact sports were used as controls. Age, gender, IQ, and education were included as covariates. Diminished response times were seen in concussed athletes versus controls at both 2 weeks and 1 year. The study authors concluded that concussion may pose further risk for an athlete since he/she is unable to take action as quickly as before a concussive injury. Notably, however, a lack of baseline data makes it difficult to ascertain whether poor reaction time pre-existed injury in the relatively few studies.

Maddocks and Saling[20] conducted baseline testing on 130 Australian Rules football players using the Paced Auditory Serial Addition Task (complex attention), the Digit Symbol Test (visual memory, concentration), and a cued reaction-time test. Concussions were identified in 10 players, and repeat testing was conducted at 5 days post-injury. Controls were umpires matched for age and education. A symptom questionnaire was also used. The Digit Symbol Test and reaction-time measure were selectively affected (when compared to controls) at 5 days. Further, no significant differences were found on the self-report measure. In a previous study, Maddocks et al[19] evaluated 28 Australian Rules football players in the acute phase of recovery following concussion. Using a battery of questions designed to evaluate orientation and memory, they assessed athletes at 10 minutes after injury. Results were compared to control athletes with injuries other than concussion. Results suggested that questions assessing recently acquired information (e.g., word list) were more sensitive to concussion than orientation questions (e.g., day of the week or opposing team characteristics). It was recommended that anterograde amnesia be thoroughly assessed on the sidelines following concussion.

Lastly, McCrory et al[25] evaluated 17 Australian Rules football players and two rugby players who had sustained postconcussion convulsions (all had resolved within 150 seconds). These athletes were assessed at 60 minutes and 5 days postinjury using a cued reaction-time task and Digit Symbol Substitution Test (concentration and visual memory). Baseline testing was not conducted and controls were not used. There was no exclusionary criteria. Results suggested that both tests were abnormal at 60 minutes, but resolved by 5 days. MRI and CT findings were unremarkable. EEG abnormalities were seen in one athlete.

Summary

This chapter reviewed the potential uses of neuropsychological testing with professional athletes and described current research taking place in the area. The large-scale programs currently being conducted with the NFL and NHL are reviewed. Although this area of research is in its initial stages, these neuropsychological assessment programs should yield important new information in the months and years to come.

From the studies reviewed in boxing, soccer, and Australian Rules football and rugby, it is evident that neuropsychological testing represents the most sensitive method available for delineating neurobehavioral sequelae following mild brain injury. Although CT and MRI are invaluable in discerning more serious intracranial pathology (e.g., a hemorrhagic lesion), it appears that neuropsychological assessment is the better tool to quantify and outline recovery or loss of function. Research methodology, however, is crucial to this endeavor. The need for baseline testing (at an early age) and longitudinal studies (of longer duration) is clearly indicated. Further, a comprehensive neuropsychological battery, measuring different aspects of brain functioning, seems indicated given the variable nature of pathology. From this review, it is clear that there is a paucity of such studies. Further, most studies have only included male-oriented team sports. The authors are hopeful that additional studies/clinical projects using female athletes across a range of sports will take place. A more systematic and comprehensive approach of study, such as seen in the league-wide NFL or NHL programs, are warranted if we are to understand more clearly the specific effects of injury. Such work would possess great research merit and, from a clinical standpoint, would provide athletes, their families, and physicians a more informed and quantitative basis from which to make return-to-play decisions.

References

1. Barth JT, Alves WM, Ryan TV, et al: Mild head injury in sports: neuropsychological sequelae and recovery of function, in Levin H, Eisenberg H, Benton A (eds): **Mild Head Injury.** New York, NY: Oxford University Press, 1989, pp 257-275

2. Benedict RHB: **Brief Visuospatial Memory Test-Revised.** Odessa, Fla: Psychological Assessment Resources, 1997

3. Benton A, Hamsher K: **Multilingual Aphasia Examination.** Iowa City, Ia: University of Iowa Press, 1978

4. Brandt J: The Hopkins Verbal Learning Test: development of a new memory test with six equivalent forms. **Clin Neuropsychologist 5:** 125-142, 1991

5. Casson IR, Siegal O, Sham R, et al: Brain damage in modern boxers. **JAMA 251:**2663-2667, 1984

6. Collins MW, Grindel SH, McKeag D: Neuropsychological testing in college football: a multi-center analysis of sports-related concussion. Presented at the American Medical Society for Sports Medicine/World Congress of Sports Medicine, Orlando, FL, June, 1998

7. Cremona-Meteyard SL, Geffen GM: Persistent visuospatial attention deficits following mild head injury in Australian Rules football players. **Neuropsychologia 32:**649-662, 1994

8. D'Elia L, Satz P: **The Color Trail Making Test.** Odessa, Fla: Psychological Assessment Resources, 1989

9. Gronwall DMA: Cumulative and persisting effects of concussion on attention and cognition, in Levin H, Eisenberg H, Benton A (eds): **Mild Head Injury.** New York, NY: Oxford University Press, 1989

10. Hovda DA, Prins M, Becker DP, et al: Neurobiology of concussion, in Bailes JE, Lovell MR, Maroon JC (eds): **Sports-Related Concussion.** St Louis, Mo: Quality Medical, 1998

11. Jordan BD: Sparring and cognitive function in professional boxers. **Phys Sportsmed 24:**87-98, 1996

12. Jordan BD, Relkin NR, Ravdin LD, et al: Apolipoprotein E e4 associated with chronic traumatic brain injury in boxing. **JAMA 278:** 136-140, 1997

13. Kelly JP, Rosenberg JH: Diagnosis and management of concussion in sports. **Neurology 48:**575-580, 1997

14. Lampert PW, Hardman JM: Morphological changes in brains of boxers. **JAMA 251:**2676-2679, 1984

15. Levin HS, Lippold SC, Goldman A, et al: Neurobehavioral functioning and magnetic resonance imaging findings in young boxers. **J Neurosurg 67:**657-667, 1987

16. Lovell MR: Evaluation of the professional athlete, in Bailes JE, Lovell MR, Maroon JC (eds): **Sports-Related Concussion.** St Louis, Mo: Quality Medical, 1998

17. Lovell MR, Collins MW: Neuropsychological assessment of the college football player. **J Head Trauma Rehabil 13:**9-26, 1998

18. Macciocchi S, Barth JT, Alves W, et al: Neuropsychological functioning and recovery after mild head injury in collegiate athletes. **Neurosurgery 39:**510-514, 1996

19. Maddocks DL, Dicker GD, Saling MM: The assessment of orientation following concussion in athletes. **Clin J Sport Med 5:**32-35, 1995

20. Maddocks DL, Saling MM: Is cerebral concussion a transient phenomenon? **Med J Aust 162:**167, 1995 (Letter)

21. Martland HAS: Punch drunk. **JAMA 19:**1103-1107, 1928

22. Matser EJT, Kessels AGH, Jordan BD, et al: Chronic traumatic brain injury in professional soccer players. **Neurology 51:**791-796, 1998

23. Maudsley C, Ferguson FR: Neurological disease in boxers. **Lancet 19:** 795-801, 1963

24. McCrea M, Kelly JP, Kluge J, et al: Standardized assessment of concussion in football players. **Neurology 48:**586-588, 1997

25. McCrory PR, Bladin PF, Berkovic SF: Retrospective study of concussive convulsions in elite Australian Rules and rugby league footballers: phenomenology, aetiology, and outcome. **Br Med J 314:**171-174, 1997

26. McLatchie G, Brooks N, Galbraith S, et al: Clinical neurological examination, neuropsychology, electroencephalography and computed tomographic head scanning in active amateur boxers. **J Neurol Neurosurg Psychiatry 50:**96-99, 1987

27. Murelius O, Haglund Y: Does Swedish amateur boxing lead to chronic brain damage? A retrospective neuropsychological study. **Acta Neurol Scand 83:**9-13, 1991

28. Reitan R: Validity of the Trail Making Test as an indicator of organic brain damage. **Percept Motor Skills 8:**271-276, 1958

29. Ruff R: **Ruff Figural Fluency Test.** Odessa, Fla: Psychological Assessment Resources, 1988

30. Serel M, Jaros O: The mechanisms of cerebral concussion in boxing and their consequences. **World Neurol 3:**351-358, 1962

31. Smith A: **Symbol Digit Modalities Test Manual.** Los Angeles, Calif: Western Psychological Services, 1982

32. Tysvaer AT: Head and neck injuries in soccer. Impact of minor trauma. **Sports Med 14:**200-213, 1992

33. Tysvaer AT, Løchen EA: Soccer injuries to the brain: a neuropsychologic study of former soccer players. **Am J Sports Med 9:**56-60, 1991

34. Wechsler D: **Wechsler Adult Intelligence Scale-III.** San Antonio, Tx: Psychological Corp, 1997

CHAPTER 13

Head, Spine, and Peripheral Nerve Injuries in Sports and Dance: An Encyclopedic Reference

VINCENT J. MIELE, BS, RPH, and JULIAN E. BAILES, MD

American football, ice hockey, and boxing are commonly referred to when discussing sports-related neurological injury, probably because they involve frequent and obvious violent contact. While they do represent activities with inherent risks, debilitating injuries to the nervous system have been commonly observed in activities considered less violent. The United States Consumer Product Safety Commission (USCPSC) reported in 1990 that of the top five sports that cause head injury requiring hospitalization, only football is a traditional "collision" sport; the others are basketball, bicycling, baseball, and playground activities.[483] The catastrophic sports injury registry considers gymnastics and wrestling to be among those sports with the greatest chance of causing catastrophic head injury.[78] Other sports with a significant risk of head injury include automobile racing, equestrian sports, martial arts, Rugby, and skiing. This chapter reviews each of these sports as well as others; the frequency and type of reported injuries associated with them are also discussed.

Archery/Bow Hunting: History

Artifacts of archery date back 25,000 years. The sport first appeared in the Olympic Games in Paris in 1900. Because of a lack of uniform international rules, archery events in these games varied widely, and it was dropped from the program in the early 1900s. The Federation Internationale de Tir a l'Arc, the international governing body of the sport, was founded in 1931 and implemented standardized rules for competition. The first World Championship was held that same year, and it led to the reinstatement of archery at the 1972 Munich Games.

Hunting with bow and arrow has become popular also; in many regions, seasons have been established for taking game in this manner.

Archery/Bow Hunting

Epidemiology

The most common cause of neurological injury in archery is accidental falls out of hunting tree stands. These falls have long been associated with injuries, most commonly to the back. They result in significant long-term disability, expensive and lengthy hospitalization, and even death. The hazards related to the tree stands are not widely appreciated. A study by Crites and Moorman[107] examined the types and sequelae of spinal injuries resulting from these falls. Significant neurological deficits occurred in 44% of the injured. In the patients studied, burst fractures occurred in 17, wedge compression fractures in eight, fractures involving the posterior elements in four, and coronal fracture of the sacral body in one. One third of the injuries required open reduction, internal fixation, or spine fusion. One patient was treated with a halo jacket and the remaining patients were treated with braces alone. A report using spinal cord injury (SCI) surveillance data by the Oklahoma State Department of Health examined the incidence and circumstances surrounding hunting-related injuries.[364] In that study, all of the injuries resulted from falls from trees or tree stands. The rate of injury was fewer than one per 100,000 licensed hunters. One half of the injuries resulted in neurological damage significant enough to cause permanent paralysis or death. Urquhart et al[482] analyzed 19 patients admitted to the Medical College of Georgia Hospital and Clinics for injuries related to falls from deer stands. One death occurred, and six of the 18 survivors remain paralyzed. Fracture of the spine and long bones accounted for the majority of the injuries, with seven of the survivors hospitalized for more than 4 weeks and eight remaining permanently disabled.

When falls are excluded, the archer is most at risk for nerve injuries in the upper extremities. In some cases, archers have lacerated the digital nerve and artery with the razor-sharp broad head used for hunting. Compression neuropathies of digital nerves in the fingers that pull back the bowstring have also been reported. Chronic injuries include bilateral medial epicondylitis, median nerve compression at the wrist, de Quervain's tenosynovitis, and median nerve compression at the elbow.[369] Naraen et al[331] reported an overuse injury of the coracoid process in an 11-year-old archer. Shimizu et al[420] reported a case of isolated long thoracic nerve palsy resulting from recurrent injury to the nerve in a 20-year-old archer. The patient presented with classic winging of the left scapula secondary to weakness and atrophy of the left serratus anterior muscle. The injury was believed to be secondary to repeated overstretching and compression of the long thoracic nerve while practicing. A case of suprascapular nerve palsy presenting as selective atrophy of the infraspinatus muscle in an archer was reported by Hashimoto et al.[185]

Bow Hunter's Stroke

Bow hunter's stroke is a condition resulting from vertebrobasilar insufficiency caused by mechanical occlusion or stenosis of the vertebral artery at the C1-2 level during head rotation. It may also be caused by atlantoaxial anomalies. It commonly occurs on head rotation of 90° or more to the left, as does an archer when aiming.

An interesting risk of archery is vertebral artery spasm and injury secondary to the repeated cervical rotations associated with the sport. There have been numerous reports of infarction of the brain and spinal cord associated with head movement. In fact, the Stroke Council of the American Heart Association has 360 registered cases,[380] and at least 38 cases have been reported in the literature.[113,254] Chiropractic manipulation of the neck is another etiology, as are various sports requiring extreme head turning. This occurrence is rare, suggesting that the victim may have predisposing factors such as vertebral artery anomalies, tortuosity, or atherosclerosis. The duration and force of the head rotation also appear to be factors in these injuries.[28,206,458] One case report of this condition involved a 39-year-old archer. A right dorsolateral medullary syndrome that was believed to be the result of right vertebral artery spasm with an aneurysm distal to the spasm evolved over a period of minutes.[431]

Australian Rules Football and Rugby Union/Rugby League

Several studies have described the incidence and circumstances of injury experienced by Rugby Union, Rugby League, and Australian Rules players. While differences exist in the types and frequency of injury between the various forms of Rugby and Australian Rules football, some trends are common in all three. While the lower limbs are the most frequently injured body part, injuries to the head and neck also occur. Competitions result in more injuries per exposure, while practice accounts for a greater percent of the total number of injuries. The majority of injuries occur during tackles; the forwards, who have greater physical involvement in the game both in attack and in defense, appear to be at the highest risk. Foul play accounts for a significant percentage of injuries.

Epidemiology

A prospective study by Davies and Gibson[117] followed a cohort of 356 male and female Rugby Union players throughout the 1993 competitive club season. Detailed information was collected for 4403 player-games and 8653 player-practices. A total of 569 Rugby-related injury events were reported. The injury rate for games was much higher than that for practices, and the lower limb was the region most often injured. Per 100 player-games, the injury rate for males was 10.9 and that for females was 6.1. In a prospective study of 185 participants in Rugby clubs, 151 injuries were found among 98 players during a single season. Forwards were found to be at significantly more risk than backs. The skill level of the Rugby team, the player's body weight, the degree of fitness, and the presence of joint hypermobility did not appear to affect a player's risk of injury. Injuries to the head and neck were significantly more common when play was static and on wet pitches. Almost half of the injuries occurred during the last quarter of the game, and foul play might have been the cause in as many as one third of the reported injuries. Adams[3] reviewed 1000 injuries secondary to Rugby Football and found a 14% incidence of head injuries. The majority of these were mild, but four players required immediate hospital admission for the injury. Injury rates varied by position, with male locks and female inside backs having the highest rate in their respective genders. In games, the tackle was the phase of play in which the most injuries occurred (40%), followed by rucks (17%) and mauls (12%).[36] Sparks[434] reported an incidence of 197.7 injuries per 10,000 player-hours.

Stephenson et al[438] investigated the incidence of injury in an English professional Rugby League over a period of four playing seasons. The overall injury rate was found to be 114 per 1000 playing hours, with muscular injuries being the most common injuries and the head and neck region being the most frequently injured site. Players received the largest percentage of injuries when being tackled, and forwards had a higher injury rate than backs. Injury rates in the elite football competitions in Australia over the 1992 season were examined by Seward et al.[416] Some 2398 injuries were recorded from 26 clubs in competitions, which included the Australian Football League (AFL), the New South

Australian Rules Football and Rugby: History and Rules

The origins of Rugby date back to 1823. Legend has it that the game started at Rugby School in England, when one of the students, William Webb Ellis, picked up the ball during a game of soccer in 1823 and ran with it. In the following years, the sport was adopted in private schools and universities throughout the United Kingdom, and in 1871 the first Rugby Union was founded in London. Rugby Union remains the most popular amateur form of the game. Also known as rugger, the game is played with 15 men to a side. The players do not usually wear any protective equipment. The game does not allow time-outs or substitutions (except for injury) and consists of two 40-minute halves.

Rugby became a professional sport in 1895 when 22 Rugby clubs in northern England called for compensation of lost wages for their players of Saturday matches. This action led to the formation of a Rugby League, which introduced adapted rules for professionals. Rugby League uses 13 players to a team and allows substitutions during the game.

Australian Rules football began in Melbourne, Australia in 1858 and is played with teams of 18 players, with three substitutes allowed to replace players at any time during the game. The game is divided into 25-minute quarters. Sixteen national teams compete with each other throughout the season to play in the grand final, which is held in Melbourne.

Wales Rugby League, and the New South Wales Rugby Union. In the Rugby codes, minor injuries to the head and neck were more common, particularly in forwards. In Rugby League and Union, head and facial lacerations were the most common injuries, followed by concussion. While Rugby League players tended to suffer the most injuries, AFL injuries were on average more severe.

Head Injury

Head injuries occur with some frequency in Rugby and Australian Rules football. A few such injuries, especially diffuse cerebral swelling, second-impact syndrome, and subdural hematomas, can result in death. The more minor cerebral injuries, mostly concussions, have unknown but potential long-term consequences.

The effects of Rugby-related concussions could be long lasting. Hinton-Bayre et al[193] found that 16 of 20 concussed professional Rugby League players had impaired information processing 1-3 days following injury. The study also demonstrated that seven players still displayed cognitive deficits at 1-2 weeks, and did not return to preseason levels of cognitive function until 3-5 weeks had passed. Maddocks and Saling[281] studied subjects with mild concussive injuries received while playing Australian Rules football in an attempt to determine whether neuropsychological sequelae are detectable. Analyses of covariance showed poorer performances on several neuropsychological performance measures. Their results suggested that neuropsychological deficits persist after neurological symptoms resolve in the early stages following mild concussive injury in this sport.

Players who have had at least one previous traumatic brain injury (TBI) have an increased risk for a second similar episode. Delaney et al[122] found that a history of loss of consciousness or a diagnosed concussion were both associated with increased odds of experiencing a concussion. They also reported that 70% of all concussed players experienced repeated concussions. The odds of experiencing a concussion increased 13% with each game played. This increase in risk of subsequent head injuries could be the result of a decreased ability to take action quickly in response to expected events. This idea was studied in two groups of Australian Rules football players who had sustained mild head injuries during competition. Their reaction times were compared to a control group of 12 non-injured sportsmen. Nine footballers tested within 2 weeks of sustaining their injury showed decreased reaction times to targets in expected locations compared to controls. Their reaction time to objects in unexpected locations did not appear to be affected. This pattern has been previously observed in moderate to severely injured patients.[93] When the nine subjects were retested a year later, their pattern of performance had not altered but their overall reaction time had improved. These findings were replicated in another eight players tested at least 1 year after sustaining mild head injuries.[105]

McCrory et al[301] retrospectively studied Australian football-related fatalities from 1990 through 1999 to determine the frequency and nature of fatal brain injuries. The authors identified 25 deaths associated with Australian football. Of these, nine were secondary to brain injury. The most common findings in deaths due to brain injury were intracranial hemorrhages, including one subarachnoid hemorrhage from a vertebral artery injury. Intracranial hemorrhages were found in eight patients, and an infarct in the territory of the middle cerebral artery in one. In three of four cases of subarachnoid hemorrhage, vertebral artery trauma was noted. In all but one case, the fatal injury occurred as an accidental part of play.

Death secondary to diffuse axonal injury has been reported in a Rugby player following a fall.[367] The player died 15 hours after being tackled. Sections of a player's cerebrum, cerebellum, and brainstem underwent staining using an immunoperoxidase technique to detect beta-amyloid protein. Sections of the pons revealed axonal spheroids in the base, and those of the cerebellum showed axonal spheroids in deep white matter, which are findings consistent with diffuse axonal injury.

Spinal Cord Injury

According to the U.S. National Spinal Cord Injury Data Research Center (NSCIDRC), the mean age of Rugby-related SCI in 1980 and 1981 was 21 years (range 20-22). All injuries occurred in men, were in individuals considered adept at the sport, and resulted in quadriplegia (K. Clarke, personal communication, 1983). There has been a decline over the last decade in Rugby-associated SCIs in England, Australia, and New Zealand.[67,422,467]

Injuries in South African Rugby players have remained constant. The average number of players per year admitted to the Spinal Cord Injury Center in Cape Town has risen.[406] For every serious Rugby-associated SCI, 10 severe neck injuries occur that do not involve the cord.[238]

Kew et al[238] performed a retrospective study of SCIs in Rugby from 1960 through 1989. They identified 117 catastrophic neck injuries and reviewed the risk factors for such injuries. Match play, as opposed to practice, was overwhelmingly associated with the highest risk. This is despite the fact that the majority of playing time is spent in practice, and is probably secondary to the much higher intensity of competitive play. Age was also determined to be a significant risk factor, with 69% of all injuries occurring in adults. The risk to adults could be as high as 10-12 times the risk in youths. This is contrary to an earlier study by Torg et al[467] suggesting that players of student age had a higher risk of SCI. The lower risk for school-aged participants was welcome news, since the vast majority of Rugby players are in this population. In the Cape Province area, the ratio of youth to adult participants is as high as 10 to 1.[406] Higher levels of play are associated with greater risk and incurred 69% of injuries. This population of players is relatively small when compared to the entire population of Rugby participants. Once again, the higher rate of injury is likely associated with the more competitive attitudes of the participants.

The playing position of the Rugby player also influences the risk. Studies by authors in the U.S., Australia, and New Zealand found the hooker to be the highest risk position.[7,68,238,460] Centers and flyhalves were found to have the greatest risk for backline players in a study by Kew et al.[238] There are national differences in position risk. For example, in South Africa the least frequently injured player on the team is the prop, while in Australia the prop is the second most commonly injured player on the team. Props and hookers are most often injured during scrums, and up to 85% of injuries to backline players occurred during tackling. Forwards are most vulnerable during loose play.[422,460] Risks of serious neck injury during particular phases of the game also appear to be dependent on location. In South Africa and New Zealand, more than half of the injuries occur during tackling and fewer than 25% during scrums.[67] In Australia, Canada, Eire, and Northern Ireland, the majority of injuries occur during scrums.[299,343,433,460] Crashing the scrum is a problem in the U.S., Australia, and to a lesser extent, England. In the U.S., more than 30% of all injuries occur during this phase. The various phases of game play are described below.

The beginning of the season and the period following the midseason break carry higher risks for all Rugby injuries. These periods are traditionally considered high risk in most sports, probably secondary to athletic deconditioning and disuse of skills[299,332,467,515] (Figure 1).

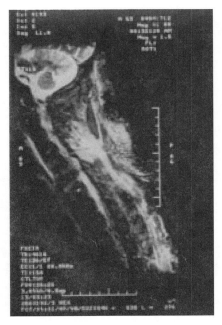

Figure 1: Sagittal MRI illustrating posterior cervical ligamentous injury with no evidence of vertebral column damage in a Rugby player.

Mechanisms of Spinal Injury

Three specific activities during the game of Rugby result in the majority of injuries to the cervical spine. They are the tackle, tight scrum, and loose play (ruck and maul).[405]

Tackling Injury

In a study by Kew et al,[238] 21% of SCIs occurred while tackling and 30% occurred while being tackled. Injury during the tackle can occur to both the perpetrator and the recipient of the tackle. The perpetrator's greatest cause of injury is poor technique. The tackled player can be injured by the force of the collision with the opponent or the ground. Scher[402,403] analyzed tackling injuries and discovered three common mechanisms of injury. These are injury of the tackler secondary to head impact, injury to the recipient from a high tackle, and injury from a double tackle. Injury from impact to the tackler's head occurs when the head suddenly stops forward progress from contact with the ground or the body of the opponent (usually the thigh). This can result in compression fractures of the vertebral bodies from axial forces transmitted down the spine. These forces are increased significantly if the player's neck is flexed, as if diving, which eliminates the normal lordosis of the cervical spine. As in American football, if a tackler's first point of contact with an opponent is the vertex of his/her head, there is a substantial risk of injury.[469] Injuries secondary to high tackles can be from behind or to the side of the recipient. If the tackle is from behind, hyperextension injuries are likely secondary to the head being pulled back and down. If the tackle is from the side, a hyperflexion injury often results. Rotational forces are also a factor in these injuries, especially if the tackle is performed with only one arm. Double tackles, often referred to as sandwich or high-low tackles, can be quite dramatic and occur both intentionally and by chance. They are more common near the goal, with a concentration of defenders merging on the ball carrier. This tackle can cause injury to both the offensive and defensive player. If the defensive players miss their target, they may collide into each other with considerable force at unexpected angles. If the tackle is successful, the offensive player's body is forced in two directions. This inhibits the player from moving with either force completely, increasing rotational and shearing stresses to the spine.

Scrum Injury

The force on the back of a player's neck in the middle of a scrum has been calculated to be as high as 1.5 tons.[406] Kew et al[238] determined that 21% of cervical spine injuries occurred during tight scrum. The most common serious neck injury during the scrum is caused by hyperflexion trauma, resulting in anterior dislocation of the cervical spine. The majority of these injuries involve bilateral locking of the facets, which is much less common in non-Rugby cervical spine injuries.[55] In this type of injury, the upper vertebral laminar arch at the level of injury compresses the dorsal aspect of the spinal cord against the posterosuperior surface of the inferior vertebrae, and usually results in permanent quadriplegia or death. A smaller subset incurs unilateral locking of the facets, which is due to rotational force during the injury.[406]

The scrum collapse is a common time for this type of hyperflexion injury. It is a consequence of the front row of players collapsing and being unable to free themselves and the remainder of the players continuing to push. Crashing the scrum also has the potential for neck injury. The front-row players distance themselves from the opponent and then rush toward them, creating considerable force on contact. Although this is against the rules of the sport, it occurs commonly and can cause hyperflexion injuries.

Loose Play Injury

Rucks and mauls are similar and are referred to as loose scrums or loose play. A ruck occurs when the ball is on the ground and one or more players from each team are on their feet in physical contact, closing around the ball between them. A maul is formed by one or more players from each team on their feet and in close contact closing around a ball carrier (South African Rugby Board, 1981). Kew et al[238] determined that 18% of cervical spine injuries occur during this phase of the game. These activities account for a substantial number of general Rugby injuries, often caused by kicks and trampling. They also spawn a substantial portion of illegal play. Spinal injury from loose play results from forced flexion of the ball carrier's neck, forced neck flexion of the player at the bottom of the ruck, and head and neck injury from charging into a group of players.[406]

In addition to catastrophic injuries to the spinal cord, participants are at risk for long-term degenerative changes in the structure of their spines. Scher[404] reported an increased incidence of cervical spine osteoarthritis in Rugby players. That study compared cervical spine radiographs of 150 Rugby players with 150 controls. Premature degenerative disease was found in the Rugby population compared to the control group. Individuals playing the tight-forward position had the most dramatic changes. Importantly, players with these degenerative changes are at greater risk for future cervical spine injury from hyperextension.

Scher[407] reported cases of transient paralysis in Rugby players believed to be the result of spinal cord concussion, which is defined as a transient disturbance of spinal cord function resulting from trauma, usually resolving in 48 hours. This can be associated with osteogenic changes of the vertebral canal, congenital fusion of the vertebrae, or bony narrowing of the spinal canal.

Ashworth[17] described migraine attacks provoked by facial impact during a Rugby tackle. Some only have attacks in this particular circumstance, but the majority have spontaneous episodes at other times. Similar to other forms of migraine, the presentation is usually in childhood or early adult life. The condition appears to be benign but may cause the patient to give up playing football. Migraine symptoms precipitated by head trauma have also been reported. Bennett et al[31] found that the head trauma is usually minor and not associated with amnesia. Following a symptom-free interval usually lasting several minutes, visual, motor, sensory, or brainstem signs and symptoms begin. These symptoms last for 15 to 30 minutes, are followed by a headache, and are frequently accompanied by nausea and vomiting. It is not known whether this apparently "benign" condition can cause long-term sequelae, especially in athletes with repeated episodes.

Automobile Racing

In the U.S., automobile racing boasts the second largest attendance of all sports. It can be categorized by whether the vehicle is open- or closed-wheeled. Open-wheel vehicles are considered the fastest closed-course vehicles. They range from the Go-kart, to Formula 1 cars that can attain speeds in excess of 240 mph, to the dragster that is capable of speeds in excess of 300 mph.

Closed-wheel vehicles are exemplified by those used in NASCAR today. This is the most popular form of racing in the U.S. and takes advantage of the "stock car," a highly modified version of everyday passenger vehicles. Stock car drivers at short asphalt tracks often sustain minor injuries. The neck and the knee are the most commonly injured areas.[69] Chapman and Oni[83] conducted a 1-year study in 1991 of motorcycle and automobile racing accidents and reported that 70 of 33,184 competitors required hospital treatment. The authors concluded that the number of participants requiring admission

Automobile Racing: History

The first automobile "competition" dates back to 1894 in Paris, France. It was a 79-mile race to Rouen, and the purpose was actually to test the reliability of the vehicles. This was followed in 1895 by a 732-mile endurance race, which included a roundtrip from Paris to Bordeaux, France. In the U.S., the first oval track race was held in 1896 in Cranston, Rhode Island. The U.S. gained prestige in the sport of auto racing when Carl Fisher opened the 2.5-mile brick-surfaced Indianapolis Motor Speedway in Indianapolis, Indiana. As were the first races in France, the "brickyard's" main purpose was as a proving ground for automobiles. The first 500-mile race at this track was held in 1911 and resulted in 11 fatalities (nine spectators and two drivers). Gradually, the inception of specially built tracks for racing decreased the risk to spectators. They did not do the same for the driver.

In the early 20th century, drivers were usually killed instantly from massive head injuries or burns when accidents occurred. Primitive helmets were worn but offered little protection. They were often constructed of cloth or leather. Helmet material changed to metal in 1953 and to fiberglass in the 1960s. Current helmets are made of a carbon fiber, often have built-in radios, and weigh more than three pounds. All major organizations today require the use of helmets while racing. The 1950s brought the seatbelt, which was originally treated with disdain by many drivers who felt that they would be safer in an accident if thrown clear of the vehicle. Acceptance grew as it became apparent that this was not the case, and by the end of the decade, full-restraint systems were in place.

to the hospital is broadly similar for car and bike races (less than 0.1%). As expected, this injury rate was higher than on the public highway.

More than 90% of the neurological injuries suffered in the sport are to the head, and are usually mild closed head injuries. These injuries would be much more severe if not for the use of helmets, safety restraints, and well-constructed safety cells in which the driver is positioned. Because of these safety devices, 85% of head injuries in auto racing are mild versus 60%-80% of those incurred in the general public. Also, because of the use of effective head protection in the sport, epidural and subdural hematomas occur much more frequently in the general population than in the auto racing population. Since 1981, 29% of all racing injuries have been to the head, according to statistics provided by the professional racing organization CART.[475] The group reported four fatalities in this period, all of them secondary to severe head injury.

Head Injury

The mechanisms of head injury are usually acceleration, deceleration, or rotational forces transmitted to the brain. Diffuse axonal injury can result from high-energy impacts that transfer significant shearing forces to the brain. Passengers involved in motor-vehicle accidents often suffer from this type of injury, which is caused by shearing of multiple axons secondary to rotational forces. Severe cases of this type of injury exhibit several characteristic features. Focal lesions of the corpus callosum and associated intraventricular hemorrhages occur; focal lesions can also be present on the dorsolateral aspect of the rostral brainstem. Finally, the brain's white matter exhibits diffuse axonal injury.[498] This accounts for 16% of all severely head-injured patients in the general population and for 51% of the occurrences.[156] In auto racing, diffuse axonal injury accounts for just 5% of all head injuries secondary to the protective equipment utilized by the driver. Race car drivers who sustain this injury also appear to fare better than the general public. However, when this injury is combined with other open- or closed-head injuries, the prognosis becomes dismal. Of the four fatalities in CART racing since 1981, all have involved this type of combined head injury.

Spinal Injury

Data collected by CART reveals that 20% of injuries sustained since 1981 have been to the axial skeleton.[474] Between 1981 and 1991, 50 Indy car drivers incurred competition-related injuries. Nine of these involved the axial skeleton and three the cervical spine.[474] In 1997 and 1998, 25 SCIs related to race car driving were reported.[512] Left-sided sprains and strains are the most common injury of the cervical spine in CART drivers, and are secondary to the lateral forces endured on oval tracks, which can exceed 5.5 G. The drivers frequently report transient brachial plexus injury secondary to straps looped around their arms and then connected to their helmets to combat these forces. These injuries present as left upper-extremity paresthesias. Cervical spine fractures are rare. The most commonly reported vertebral fractures are spinous process avulsions or compression fractures of the cervical vertebral bodies.[156] Rear impacts can cause whiplash and result in flexion-extension injuries. The rollover accident carries the greatest risk of cervical spine injury. A burst fracture of C5 has been reported from a rollover accident following a collision with a retaining wall. The fracture was not the result of the driver's head contacting the ground, but flexion-distraction secondary to momentum. A hangman's fracture of C2 has been reported secondary to a side impact that propelled the driver's head against a shoulder strap.

Thoracolumbar injuries are uncommon in this sport, mainly due to the driver being so well attached in the cockpit. Unlike cervical spine injuries, thoracolumbar injuries are associated with direct frontal impacts. Injury results when the vehicle strikes an object with enough force to cause the back wheels to lift off the ground. When the back of the car comes down, significant axial loads can be transmitted to the driver's spine. Studies performed by General Motors Research have found that the more reclined a driver is, the more neck load he/she receives during a crash.[346] There is a give-and-take of injury risk between open- and closed-wheel vehicles based on this. In the open-wheel vehicle, the driver sits in a more reclined position. This results in greater force transferred to the neck during an accident. On the other hand, because the seat is lower, the driver is at less risk of being hit in the head by debris or other object. It appears that drivers of closed-wheel vehicles are particularly immune to these injuries secondary to their being seated nearly upright. In the past 25 years of NASCAR racing, there have been three cervical spine fractures and no thoracolumbar fractures reported.[474]

Peripheral Nerve Injury

Peripheral nerve injuries are fairly common in this sport. As mentioned above, transient brachial plexus injuries occur secondary to compression by straps used to combat the lateral forces on the driver's head. The strap usually attaches to the left side of the helmet, loops around the axilla, and returns to the helmet. The injuries present as paresthesias and usually affect the left arm. Ulnar, peroneal, and sciatic nerve injuries can result from constant pressure against the seat or objects in the driver's cockpit.

Other Areas of Injury

Carbon monoxide exposure may potentially modify a neurological presentation. Professional racing drivers are confined in a small cockpit for a significant period of time during a race and toxicity can be a problem. Holley et al[198] studied the effects of carbon monoxide on race car drivers. Closed-vehicle professional racing drivers were questioned after competition regarding symptoms consistent with poisoning and underwent expired carbon monoxide monitoring before and after a race. All of the tested drivers were found to have elevated carboxyhemoglobin concentrations after competition. Although drivers who were cigarette smokers had higher baseline levels than nonsmokers, they did not experience symptoms at a greater rate than nonsmokers. The majority of drivers had post-race symptoms such as fatigue, nausea, headache, and weakness. No correlation was found, however, between post-race carbon monoxide levels and symptoms.

Obviously, automobile racing should be avoided in epileptics with uncontrolled seizures. The Netherlands requires a 2-year seizure-free period and an annual check-up for an epileptic to participate in this sport.[486]

The Use of Helmets and Other Safety Measures

The use of helmets, six-point restraints, and uniforms have significantly decreased the risk of serious injury to the automobile racer. A HANS device that decreases neck loading during accidents by keeping the head and neck locked together as one unit has been developed at Michigan State University. It has already been used successfully in both stock car and sports car racing events. The system is bulky and consists of a shoulder yoke attached to the driver's torso and the helmet. Some drivers feel that the device limits their peripheral vision. Aside from these shortcomings, which can be easily overcome, the system may have the potential to reduce injuries. To avoid acute and chronic injuries, the driver's cockpit should be properly padded with energy-absorbing materi-

Early car design also contributed to driver fatalities. Cars were not constructed to dissipate energy and usually transmitted the forces directly to the driver. In contrast to today's vehicles that literally disintegrate in a collision, older vehicles sustained little damage and could often be driven after the driver was killed. The idea of the car absorbing much of the energy of a collision developed in the 1950s with the introduction in Europe of the rear-engine car. These cars came apart in a collision, and every piece that came off dissipated some of the lethal force of the accident. The 1970s were notoriously dangerous years in the sport. Severe head injury was still the main cause of fatalities. Automobile racing was second only to the piloting of self-built aircraft in sports fatalities.[346] Over the last two decades, however, advances in safety technology have been catching up to the technology that allows cars to travel in excess of 300 mph. While speeds have increased more than 20% in the last 15 years, both the injury and fatality rates have declined.[475]

als. Brachial plexus injuries from head-restraining straps are being reduced by replacing the straps with head supports. Injuries to the ulnar, peroneal, and sciatic nerves can be prevented by a proper fit in the seat and the elimination or repositioning of objects in the cockpit that apply constant pressure to the driver's upper or lower extremities. Proper physical conditioning and strength are necessary for a long race to combat the G forces endured and to avoid accidents precipitated by exhaustion. The evolution in recent years of technologically advanced vehicles capable of speeds exceeding 300 mph mandates commensurate sophistication in new safety equipment development. It is hoped that with this effort, the sport will continue to become safer.

Ballet and Dance: History

The origin of ballet dates back to performances in the courts of Renaissance Italy. Modern dance began in the 1920s on the eastern and western coasts of the U.S. as a revolt against the classical ballet, which was considered by some to be too European and snobbish. Modern dance was inspired by the more popular sorts of dance in the U.S., such as tap and jazz, as well as the dances of other cultures. It became accepted as an art form in the 1930s and flourishes today.

Modern dance differs from classical ballet in many aspects. The modern dancer does not wear shoes, uses different techniques, and the style is more a "fall and recover" than formal steps. These differences produce different types of injuries than those seen in the classical ballet dancer.

Ballet and Dance

Whether as participants or spectators, dance is enjoyed by more people today than ever before. Its extraordinary range extends from classical ballet and modern dance to new forms such as breakdancing. Classical ballet is a popular but physically taxing activity. Although not thought of as a "rough" sport, professional dancers practice extreme and repetitive movements daily and present with all of the problems of a more traditional athlete. As with other athletes, the dancer is often highly motivated to suppress pain and ignore injuries, and participants often do not present until the injury is affecting their performance. This hesitance may be due to fear of losing performance opportunities or status, or to financial concerns. Participants may be underinsured and must absorb the costs of treatment. The financial outcome of ballet dancers' injuries was studied over three seasons for a large professional ballet company. In this time, 104 dancers sustained 309 injuries that resulted in medical costs of $398,396. The average cost per injury was $1289, and in 4% of the injuries medical costs exceeded $5000. Nine injuries resulted in medical costs in excess of $10,000 each.[153]

There is a distinct difference between ballet injuries and sports injuries in general. While acute, severe injuries are rare in dancers, the chronic microtraumas endured lead to a variety of overuse syndromes. The practice of dancing on the toes, turning the feet out in an exaggerated fashion, and the extreme flexibility of the dancer's hips and spine all lead to unusual injuries. Most of the problems occurring in dancers develop subtly over a period of time rather than through a single traumatic episode. Dance movements can be stressful to the body, and the required extreme positions may place physiological structures at risk for acute, subacute, or chronic injury.

Ballet dancers are vulnerable to various stress-related injuries, and muscle strains represent more than a third of all injuries in dancers. Neurological injuries predominantly affect the lumbar spine and peripheral nerves and, to a much lesser extent, the cervical spine. The National Organization of Dance and Mime surveyed 141 dancers from seven professional ballet and modern dance companies regarding chronic and recent injuries.[53] Of the participants, 67 (48%) had experienced a chronic injury and 59 (42%) had received an injury in the previous 6 months that had affected their performance. Garrick and Requa[153] reported 2.97 injuries per injured dancer in a large professional ballet company. The foot (74 injuries), lumbar spine (71), and ankle (41) were the most frequently injured body parts.

Spondylolysis

Back problems are fairly prevalent in ballet and dance, with 10%-17% of injuries occurring in the vertebral column.[318] Spinal conditions often result from hyperextension and hyperlordosis of the lumbar spine. Spondylolysis is a form of overuse injury secondary to chronic microtrauma to the spine. It is usually caused by damage to the posterior elements of the lumbar spine. Although the facets, pedicles, lamina, and spinous processes can be affected, the pars interarticularis is most commonly injured. This area of the spine is particularly vulnerable to the stress of hyperextension. The condition often presents with occasional pain during dancing and can progress to continuous pain with activity or at rest. It is important to diagnose the injury quickly to avoid spondylolisthesis or a frank fracture. The unusually high incidence of spondylolysis in ballet dancers is partially the result of strength imbalances between agonists and antagonists muscle groups. Koutedakis et al[249] investigated the relationship between knee flexion-to-extension peak torque ratios and low back injuries. The authors found that the lower the knee flexion-to-extension peak torque ratio, the greater the degree of low back injury and that hamstring strength training can decrease the risk of low-back injury. They also concluded that isokinetic assessment of the quadriceps and hamstring muscles obtained at lower velocities compared to higher angular velocities is more prognostic of low-back injury. The frequency of spondylolysis in dancers is similar to that of gymnasts. Steiner and Micheli[437] found an association of this condition and spina bifida occulta in 20% of young athletes.

Fractures

Microfractures of the anterior vertebral bodies from repetitive trauma is another cause of back pain in the dancer. Repetitive flexion results in injury to the anterior portions of the vertebrae. This can result in wedging and Schmorl's nodes at the thoracolumbar junction. This condition is known as atypical Scheuermann's disease, and is also commonly seen in young gymnasts. The definition of classical Scheuermann's disease is the wedging of at least three consecutive thoracic vertebrae with Schmorl's nodes and a structurally round back.[191,432] This condition can also be the result of lumbar extension contracture with excessive flexion demands transferred to the thoracic spine, with resultant anterior vertebral plate fractures and secondary bony deformation of the vertebrae.[49,313] The risk of atypical Scheuermann's disease is high in dancers with a tight lumbosacral fascia. This causes forward flexion in the dorsal spine versus the lower lumbar spine. Also at risk are dancers with a sagittal flat-back alignment with lumbar hypolordosis and thoracic hypokyphosis. This posture is frequently seen in mature ballerinas. The most commonly fractured area of the vertebral body is the pars interarticularis. Shear forces are concentrated here, and this area is structurally weaker than other areas. Fractures of the pars usually begin in the posteromedial region, which is the thinnest area of bone.[174,313] Injuries to the pedicles can also occur. The inferior margin of the pedicle is the most vulnerable for spondylitic defects secondary to the high concentration of stress at this point. Ireland and Micheli[211] reported a stress fracture of both second lumbar pedicles in an 18-year-old ballet dancer.

Lumbar Spondylosis/Premature Arthrosis

Premature arthrosis and lumbar spondylosis can result in low back pain in the dancer. Arthritic degeneration secondary to chronic microtraumas usually occurs to the facet joints. This is referred to as facet syndrome and is an overuse injury resulting from repetitive microtrauma and hyperextension.[197] The risk for this injury increases in the older dancer due to erosion of the joint's cartilage and osteophyte formation. Teitz and Kilcoyne[461] attempted to determine whether arthrosis begins at an unusually early age in professional dancers by studying 14 retired dancers who had performed professionally for a minimum of 10 years. The authors found the prevalence of arthrosis in dancers to be higher than that of nondancers in the same age group. Van Dijk et al[484] also reported a relationship between long-term ballet dancing and arthrosis in 19 former professional female dancers. In this condition, pain commonly radiates into the legs from nerve root compression and irritation at the facet. Rest and anti-lordotic bracing may be helpful in these athletes.

Discogenic Back Pain

While discogenic pain is rare in children, its incidence increases in proportion to athletic participation.[123] This is especially true with activities that involve axial compression, such as dancing. Some athletes may be genetically predisposed to the development of this condition. Steiner and Micheli[437] reported that some young dancers have a clover-shaped spinal canal with short pedicles, which increases the chances of discogenic back injury. DeOrio and Bianco[123] determined that athletes with this might have a higher incidence of continued back complaints through adulthood. Sciatic pain occurs in dancers for a variety of reasons. It is often present with disc injury and can also be associated with spondylolysis secondary to nerve root compression at L4 or L5. Dancers also have less adipose tissue on their buttocks and might be at higher risk of traumatic sciatic nerve injury.[394] Sammarco[394] reported sciatic neuritis resulting from repetitive extreme lower-back and hamstring stretching and poor landing techniques with jumps. The nerve courses through the piriformis muscle and can become entrapped if the muscle becomes hypertrophic or spasms. The secondary pain can mimic symptoms of discogenic disease. The condition often presents with pain in the deep gluteal area that radiates down the leg in the distribution of the sciatic nerve.

Mechanical Back Pain

Acute or chronic musculotendinous and ligamentous injuries of the spine can lead to mechanical back pain. This type of injury presents as a backache that worsens with prolonged standing or sitting. Radiographic workups are usually negative. This problem is believed to be the result of tight extensor structures or weak abdominal musculature. It can also be secondary to postural lordosis and poor technique. The condition can be improved by avoiding a hyperlordotic posture. Hyperlordosis is a problem in many dancers. Dancers are frequently required to perform movements involving hyperflexion of the spine, such as an arabesque, that emphasize hyperlordosis.

Mechanical back pain appears to be especially prevalent in the younger population. Muscular strength imbalance plays a major role in its acquisition, with the strong back muscles overpowering the weaker abdominal muscles. It can occasionally be the result of genetic disorders such as chondroplasia or cleidocranial dystosis. Mechanical back pain may also be secondary to more rapid growth of the bony elements of the spine in comparison to the tendons and ligaments during the second growth spurt. This condition is more common in males and results in posterior decompensation of the torso over the pelvis. A rounded-back posture is often adopted when the dancer attempts to correct this decompensation, which can result in vertebral body wedging. The majority of these conditions can be improved by correcting strength imbalances with abdominal exercise. Anti-lordotic braces are also available for refractory cases.

Male ballet dancers are often required to lift partners. Lifting with a swayed back, especially in a dancer with a lordotic back, increases the risk of injury. This tendency is often the result of inadequate strength and can be improved with the reinforcement of proper technique and weight training. One other source of lower back pain in dancers is the presence of an abnormal transitional vertebra in the lumbosacral junction. This can lead to sacroiliac pseudoarthritis, especially when the dancer has enlarged transverse processes or a laterally fused mass. These can elicit painful symptoms from rubbing against the iliac wing or sacrum and occasionally requires resection of the bony protrusion.[400]

Scoliosis/Osteopenia

The young ballet dancer is at risk for osteopenia and scoliosis secondary to endocrine abnormalities, low body weight, and inadequate nutrition. Idiopathic scoliosis occurs in approximately 10% of the general population, and the incidence is significantly higher in young dancers.[499] Warren reported a 24% prevalence of scoliosis in a survey of 75 professional ballet dancers with a mean age of 24 years. The dancer's risk for this rises substantially with delayed menarche or secondary amenorrhea, which are both common in this population. Delayed menarche and prolonged intervals of amenorrhea can increase the risk of stress fractures in ballet dancers.

Steps that require rapid sequential spinning on one foot, such as the pirouette and fouette in classical ballet, have been shown to lead to cervical radiculopathy. This can be the result of "spotting," which is done to prevent vertigo. The participant fixes their eyes on a distant object as their body spins until their head cannot rotate further on its axis. At that point, it is quickly rotated 360° following the body to again rest the eyes on the same object. Cervical spine injury secondary to spotting presents with neuralgias resulting in paresthesias and hyperesthesias from the neck to the fingers. Lifting of partners has also been reported to cause this condition.

Peripheral Nerve Injury

Nerve entrapment, neuropathy, and nerve dysfunction in the legs, ankles, and feet of athletes are common and due mainly to overuse syndromes. Femoral nerve injuries occur in both modern and ballet dancers.[319,397] Both Sammarco and Stephens[394,397] and Miller and Benedict[319] have reported femoral nerve neuritis in this population. Femoral neuropathy is often secondary to the repeated stretching of the femoral nerve that occurs over months in an established dance routine. Steps involving simultaneous knee flexion and hip extension, such as the "Horton hinge" modern dance step, amplify this effect. Sammarco and Stephens reported a case of acute-onset neurapraxia of the femoral nerve in a pure modern dancer that presented as left hip and sacroiliac joint pain followed by a significant loss of strength in her thighs.

Peripheral nerve injuries distal to the nerve root are most common in the dancer's foot. The cutaneous branch of the deep peroneal nerve is vulnerable to injury where it runs over the tarsus, and external trauma can cause neuritis presenting as forefoot paresthesia between the first and second phalanges and tenderness over the nerve.[396] The external pressure of the ribbons or elastic used to secure toe shoes to the foot can also cause this condition. Injury to the subcutaneous sural nerve can result from foot and ankle traumas. These injuries cause pain in the lateral forefoot and a positive Tinel's sign. This type of injury is especially prevalent in the modern dancer because of the increased vulnerability of bare feet.[396] Dorsal cutaneous neuritis has also been reported in modern dancers. This results from the dancers sitting on their feet, which puts pressure on the dorsum of the foot. As with peroneal neuritis, dorsal cutaneous neuritis presents with pain and paresthesias between the first and second phalanges.[393] Bony injury to the tibial sesamoid under the head of the first metatarsal can lead to interdigital neuroma or digital neuritis.[395,396] While interdigital neuromas have not been shown to be more prevalent in dancers, their occurrence in this population causes more difficulties since the dancer must place continuous pressure on the metatarsal heads. The third and fourth metatarsal heads are most commonly affected. Conservative treatment that decreases the pressure on the neuroma is often effective; however, recalcitrant cases may require excision.[395]

Different patterns of injury exist between age groups in dancers. Mechanical back injury is more common in the older population. Injury often involves anterior disc elements made vulnerable secondary to the spinal degeneration associated with age. This can result in discogenic pain with sciatica ensuing. As an athlete ages, spinal canal stenosis and nerve encroachment may also develop secondary to bony overgrowth at the facets. This increases the risk of nerve injury due to minor traumas. Injuries to children and adolescents tend to be more severe and are often related to spondylolysis. Pain is more often associated with posterior element dysfunction resulting from stress fractures of the pars interarticularis and other vertebral regions.[315]

Other Forms of Dance

Participants in less formal styles of recreational dance are not devoid of risk for neurological injury. McNeil et al reported a young breakdancer with multiple subdural hematomas. This form of dance includes spinning on various parts of the body, including the head, dorsal spine, and hands. Head spins are the likely etiology for the reported dancer's injury. "Head banging" is another current trend in dancing to heavy metal music, which involves extreme flexion, extension, and rotation of the head and cervical spine. The motions can be performed so violently as to cause whiplash injury to the cervical spine. Kassirer and Manon[233] studied a group of 37 eighth graders participating in a dance marathon during which head banging occurred. Of the children participating in the activity, 82% of the girls and 17% of the boys had resultant cervical spine pain that lasted 1-3 days. Belly dancers are not immune to neurological injury. Axial lateropulsion cervical dystonia is informally referred to as "belly dancer's head."[215]

Baseball: History

While it is difficult to determine the exact origin of baseball, experts agree that it is highly unlikely that Abner Doubleday developed the game as it is played today. It is believed that the sport most likely evolved from cricket and the medieval English game of "rounders." The modern game likely began in 1842 when a group of men from Manhattan got together to play different varieties of Base Ball. By the fall of 1842, at the insistence of member Alexander Cartwright, this group formally organized and became known as the New York Knickerbockers Base Ball Club. Cartwright and the Knickerbockers president, Daniel Lucius Adams, devised a formal set of rules for the game. These rules included: a diamond-shaped infield, defined foul lines, and that the ball could no longer be thrown at the runner for an out. On June 19, 1846, the first official game using the rules developed by Cartwright and Adams was played. After being a demonstration sport in 1984 and 1988, baseball in the Olympic Games is now recognized as a full medal sport.

Baseball/Softball

Baseball was the first organized sport for children in the U.S. Today, an estimated 16 million youths play the game. Of these, 4.5 million participate in official leagues (F. Mueller, 1995). Approximately half of these belong to teams sponsored by Little League of America, Inc.[129] There are currently 500,000 baseball players in high schools and 20,000 in colleges (F. Mueller and R. Cantu, 1996). Minor injuries are fairly common and catastrophic injuries do occur. In fact, more documented deaths occur in youth baseball than in any other youth team sport (N. Rytina, 1995). The USCPSC (1994) estimated that approximately half of baseball injuries are secondary to being struck by the ball. This makes sense when one considers that players as young as 12 years are able to throw the hard ball at 70 miles per hour. Injuries appear to occur more frequently in younger players, likely because of their lower skill level, slower reaction time, and a wider variation in abilities (C. Morehouse, 1983).

In organized softball in the U.S., it is estimated that 23 million games are played each year. It has been reported that this sport causes more injuries leading to emergency room visits than any other. Between 1983 and 1989, more than 2.6 million emergency room visits were documented throughout the U.S.[218] The most common softball injuries are those that occur while sliding into a base. Janda et al[219] determined that base sliding was responsible for 71% of recreational softball injuries. Injuries also occur from collisions or falls.

General Injury Statistics

Injuries resulting from playing recreational softball and baseball are among the most frequent causes of sports-related emergency room visits in the U.S., accounting for an estimated 321,000 injuries in 1989.[427] The reported incidence of injury varies significantly between sources. This is most likely due to variations in the definition of injury. Some only report an event that leads to missed participation, while others consider any scrape or contusion an injury. Major organizations such as the USCPSC, the American Academy of Pediatrics, and Little League Baseball, Inc., have reported injury rates of between 2% and 8% per season (G. Rutherford et al, 1984). The majority of these are minor soft-tissue traumas. An internal Little League study reported an injury rate of 2% a season.[184] A study of baseball participants in an Oklahoma high school claimed a comparable injury rate of 1%. However, in a similar study of Seattle participants, a rate of 18% was found.

Pasternack et al[351] studied patterns of injury in 2861 Little League baseball players aged 7 to 18 and reported 81 total injuries, with 66 acute injuries and 15 due to overuse. Of the acute injuries, 11 were considered severe. The calculated overall injury rate was found to be 0.057 injuries per 100 player-hours. As in other studies, the most frequent cause of all injuries was being struck by the ball (62%). The severe-injury rate was 0.008 per 100 player-hours. Of the serious injuries, five were secondary to being hit by the ball and three were the result of collisions between players. No catastrophic injuries were reported. Of note, 68% of the ball-related injuries occurred while the player was on defense. This emphasizes the point that protection is not needed only while at bat. Over the season, 2% of participants incurred an acute injury, including 18 injuries to the head (16 secondary to impact of the ball and two severe). Again, the vast majority of these injuries (16) occurred while the player was on defense. Most injuries to defensive players occur in the more crowded infield. A substantial number also occur while the players are warming up. The USCPSC described 164,800 baseball-related injuries to children during 1993, with 46% of the injuries being to the head. Being struck by the ball accounts for more than 50% of the acute injuries in the game. As in other studies, most occurred while the player was on defense.

McFarland and Wasik[302] recorded injury epidemiology for National Collegiate Athletic Association (NCAA) Division 1 baseball players over a 3-year period and found a rate of 5.83 injuries per 1000 exposures. The injuries occurred in practice in 46% and in games in 54%. The most common injuries were strains, sprains, and contusions. Injuries were to the upper extremity in 58%, to the trunk/back in 15%, and to a lower extremity in 27%. Upper-extremity injuries accounted for 75% of the total time lost from the sport. When divided by position, the shoulder injuries occurred most frequently in pitchers and rotator cuff tendinitis was the most frequent complaint and resulted in the most time lost from the sport.

Catastrophic Injury

In baseball players aged 5 to 14 years, 88 fatalities were reported by the USCPSC between 1973 and 1995. Of these, 14 occurred in 1994 and 1995. The majority of these deaths (77%) resulted from being hit with the ball on either the head or the chest; 30 deaths were caused by the ball impacting the head or neck and 38 were secondary to impact with the chest. The other deaths were due to being struck with a bat or other mechanisms (P. Adler, 1995). Catastrophic injury is far less common in the older athlete. Three deaths were reported in high school baseball players between 1982 and 1993. During this same period, two college players died from injuries (F. Mueller and R. Cantu, 1996). The greatest risk appears to be to the pitcher or batter.

Softball: History

Softball was created around the beginning of the 20th century by American professional baseball players who wanted to keep in practice during the off-season. The first national amateur softball tournament took place in Chicago, Illinois, in 1933 in connection with the World's Fair. Also in 1933, the Amateur Softball Association was founded to standardize the rules and govern the sport, and the first world softball championship was played in 1966. Softball has become a popular sport among women, particularly at the youth and college levels. More than 600 NCAA member institutions sponsor women's softball teams, and national championship tournaments for women are held for three collegiate divisions. Women's fast-pitch softball was selected to be an event at the Olympic Games in 1996.

The USCPSC produced a detailed hazard analysis of baseball-related injuries in children (G. Rutherford et al, 1984). The study examined 51 baseball-related deaths between 1973 and 1983 in children aged 5 to 14 years. The most common cause of fatality was secondary to chest impact from the ball. The arrhythmias that result from chest trauma varied from sinus tachycardia to ventricular fibrillation. The majority of the fatalities involved the catcher or batter; pitching machines accounted for two deaths. This occurrence is termed "commotio cordis."[288,489] The mechanism involved in deaths secondary to balls striking the chest is unclear. In the majority of cases, the baseball is traveling at less than 40 mph and internal tissue damage to the heart or surrounding structures is rarely found. The patient usually has no prior medical problems. An experimental model of low-energy chest-wall impact suggested that commotio cordis events are due largely to the exquisite timing of blows during a narrow window within the repolarization phase of the cardiac cycle, 15 to 30 msec prior to the peak of the T wave.[287] Link et al[268] developed a swine model of commotio cordis in which a low-energy impact to the chest wall was produced by a wooden object the size and weight of a regulation baseball. The authors also found that the likelihood of ventricular fibrillation was proportional to the hardness of the ball, with the softest balls associated with the lowest risk. The American Academy of Pediatrics Committee on Sports Medicine and Fitness suggested that both batters and pitchers use chest protectors and that softer low-impact baseballs be used if they are proven to be safer.[374]

Head Injury

The USCPSC reported in 1990 that for every 100,000 head injuries in baseball, 174 athletes required hospitalization.[483] Between 1982 and 1995, 0.21 annual head injuries per 100,000 high school baseball players and 0.74 annual head injuries per 100,000 college baseball players were reported. Five fatalities related to head trauma were recorded in both high school and college baseball (F. Mueller and R. Cantu, 1996). Recently, mild TBI has been found to have potential serious consequences to the athlete in general. Powell and Barber-Foss[360] studied its occurrence in high school varsity athletes over a 3-year period (see Chapter 7). Of 23,566 reported injuries, 1219 (5.5%) were mild TBIs. Of the mild TBIs, baseball accounted for 15 (1.2%) and softball for 25 (2.1%). The injury rates per 100 player-seasons were 0.23 for baseball and 0.46 for softball. Head injuries are much more common in the younger baseball player. Caveness[80] found that in the 5- to 14-year-old group, 40% of injuries are in this location versus 19% in players age 15 years and older (Figure 2).

Sliding

Approximately 71% of softball-related injuries are caused by sliding.[473] Hosey and Puffer[201] studied the incidence of sliding-related injuries in seven softball and three baseball NCAA Division 1 teams. The authors reported 37 injuries in 3889 slides over 637 games and 7596 athlete-game exposures. The overall incidence of sliding injuries was 9.51 per 1000 slides and 4.87 per 1000 game exposures. The majority of injuries were minor, with four (11%) causing the athlete to miss more than 7 days of participation. Softball players were found to have a significantly higher incidence of sliding injuries than did baseball players (12.13 vs. 6.01 per 1000 slides). The injury rate was higher in baseball for feet-first slides than for head-first slides or divebacks. Conversely, softball participants had a higher rate of injury for head-first slides than for feet-first slides or divebacks.

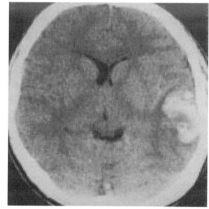

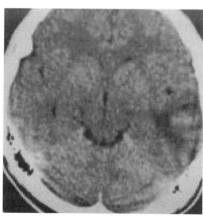

Figure 2: *Top:* CT scan demonstrating a large left temporal hematoma in a 36-year-old recreational softball pitcher who was hit by a line drive. *Bottom:* Following 4 weeks of conservative management, the hematoma spontaneously resolved as well as this patient's aphasia.

Slides can be categorized as either feet- or head-first on the basis of the leading part of the body during the slide. The head-first slide into a base appears to cause the most risk of catastrophic SCI for a baseball player. If the hands separate, the top of the runner's head can collide with the leg of the defensive player, creating a great deal of axial-load transmission to the vertebral column. While the use of breakaway bases substantially decreases the risk for occurrence of sliding-related injuries, serious injuries can still occur. The use of low-profile bases and the outlawing of sliding have also been suggested.[329] According to the NSCIDRC, baseball accounted for 1% of all sports-related SCIs between 1973 and 1981 (J. Young et al, 1982).

Injury Risk of Various Positions

The pitcher's arm must withstand more repetitive stress throughout a season than any other body part on the team. Considering this, it is not a surprise that Long et al[273] reported that every major league baseball pitcher, most minor league pitchers, and several amateur pitchers studied had reduced sensory nerve action potentials in their throwing arm. This is probably secondary to an overuse syndrome affecting the brachial plexus. Acute fractures of the humerus and ulna have also been reported in pitchers' arms. Ogawa and Yoshida[344] studied 90 recreational baseball players with humeral shaft fractures. All of the injuries were external rotation spiral fractures, which resulted in radial nerve palsy in 14 patients (16%). Tanabe et al[455] reported three cases of fatigue fracture of the ulna in male fast-pitch softball pitchers. The authors observed that these ulnar fractures are torsionally induced and tend to occur at the middle one third of the bone.

Softball pitching is commonly performed underhand. While a perception exists that, compared with overhead pitching, the underhand motion creates less stress on the arm and results in fewer injuries, fast-pitch softball pitchers withstand maximum compressive forces at the elbow and shoulder equal to 70%-98% of their body weight.[27] These stresses predispose the pitcher to both overuse and peripheral nerve injuries. Radial neuropathy resulting from "windmill pitching" in competitive softball has been reported by Sinson et al.[426]

The throwing arm of the baseball player can also develop neurovascular deficits. Circulatory disturbances in the throwing arms of baseball pitchers have been described by several authors. Itoh et al[212] reported three detailed cases that they had observed. In two, the injuries were believed to be caused by hypertrophy of the lumbrical muscles or thickening of the palmar aponeurosis. This resulted in compression within the lumbrical canal of the vascular supply to the index and middle finger. In the third, the injury was caused by neurovascular bundles of the long finger being entrapped by the proximal edges of Cleland's ligaments. Surgical releases were successful in all cases.

In the complex movement that makes up the baseball pitch, the shoulder appears to be the weakest link and by far the most commonly injured site. Chronic shoulder injury and pain are frequent complaints of pitchers. This can be secondary to extreme subluxation and shearing forces to the rotator cuff or suprascapular neuropathy.[151,349] The latter condition results in shoulder pain and weakness of abduction and external rotation. Ringel et al[373] reported this condition in two professional baseball pitchers who experienced shoulder pain when cocking for the pitch. Both athletes were treated surgically by resection of the superior transverse scapular ligament, which released the nerve at the suprascapular notch. This nerve originates from the superior trunk of the brachial plexus and extends laterally through the posterior triangle of the neck, innervating the supraspinatus and infraspinatus muscles of the rotator cuff. The bulk of the nerve passes underneath the suprascapular ligament. Through cadaveric studies, the authors identified five areas of potential nerve trauma:[373]

1. the passage of the spinal roots at C5-6 and upper trunk of the brachial plexus between the fascial encasements of the anterior and middle scalene muscles;
2. the course of the suprascapular nerve and its accompanying artery in the fascia of the subclavius and omohyoid muscles;
3. the suprascapular notch where the nerve passes inferior to the transverse scapular ligament to enter the supraspinous fossa;
4. the fascial compartment between the supraspinatus muscle and the base of the coracoid process; and
5. the spinoglenoid notch where the suprascapular nerve and artery enter the infraspinous fossa to innervate the infraspinatus muscle.

The authors also found that, as the season progressed, suprascapular nerve conduction decreased in many healthy pitchers and was accompanied by minimal asymmetrical hypertrophy of the muscles in the throwing arm and decreased deep tendon reflexes.

Long thoracic nerve injury and the resulting "winged scapula" can occur in baseball. This nerve arises from branches of the anterior division of C5-7, courses down the outer surface of the serratus anterior posterior to the midaxillary line, and gives off branches to each digitation of the muscle as it progresses. Injury has been shown to occur with chronic vigorous activity.[147,170] Mechanisms of injury are theorized to be secondary to traction forces. Schultz and Leonard[413] reported a case of long thoracic neuropathy with secondary serratus anterior weakness in a 26-year-old professional baseball player. The only precipitating factor was a recent change in batting stance, with the right arm abducted and forward flexed and the elbow flexed at 90°. Electromyography (EMG) of the associated right serratus anterior demonstrated complete absence of voluntary motor activity. The injury was treated with range of motion and strengthening exercises. Six months after the therapy was started, repeat EMG demonstrated reinnervation. Traction injuries to this nerve generally have a good prognosis, with an average recovery time of 9 months. However, if no EMG evidence of reinnervation occurs within 2 years, the chances of spontaneous recovery are slim.[170]

Sugawara et al[442] studied digital ischemia in eight baseball players. Three shortstops, two first basemen, one second baseman, one third baseman, and one outfielder developed digital ischemia on their catching hands, presenting as cyanosis, paleness, and numbness. Four were found to have occluded index digital arteries. Importantly, the authors discovered that the sequelae of ball catching on the circulation of the hand is related to the number of years played, the frequency of practice, and the position played. This conclusion was the result of additional studies of baseball players from junior high school to college. The authors found no instance of digital ischemia in junior high school players; ischemia was present in 22% of the high school players and in 40% of the college players. The condition occurred most frequently in catchers and first basemen.

Baseball catchers receive up to 200 pitches a game, many of which exceed 90 mph. Their catching hand is consequently vulnerable to neurovascular injury. Twenty professional and one college catcher were studied by Lowrey et al,[279] who found that fewer than half of the players had normal circulation in their catching hands. All of the athletes with normal circulation used thick golf or handball gloves under their catcher's mitt. This method is not foolproof, however, considering that more than 50% of the catchers with impaired circulation also used similar protection.

Injury Prevention

Because the majority of catastrophic injuries are the result of being hit by the ball, the ball has been scrutinized in an attempt to make it safer. In 1994, the National Youth

Sports Foundation for the Prevention of Athletic Injuries theorized that the introduction of softer balls into the game should decrease the frequency and severity of injuries.[317] At that time, softer balls were being used in Japan and both injury incidence and severity were reported to be decreasing. The Foundation recommended that a reduced-injury factor (RIF) ball be used in youth baseball leagues. RIF balls have cores that compress over a larger area for a longer period, which decreases the severity of impact. Experimental animal studies also suggest that the use of safety baseballs, as compared with regulation balls, may reduce the risk of commotio cordis.[268] Softer balls are currently available commercially, but are only used sporadically.

Traditionally, baseball players have worn little or no protective equipment. In 1957, Little League Baseball recognized the need for head protection and developed the batter's helmet.[269] Injection-molded polycarbonate facemasks became available in 1977.[80] In 1980, the General Assembly of the American Society for Testing and Materials' Committee on Sports Equipment and Facilities was presented with a need for face protection in baseball. The standard for baseball faceguards, published in 1985, considered the product a failure if any contact occurred between a ball traveling at a minimum speed of approximately 67 mph and the head/face. Currently, organized youth leagues require certain protective equipment, including the use of approved batting helmets, facemasks, and chest and neck protectors for catchers. While readily available, most leagues do not require chest protection for the batter and only catchers consistently use one. This is likely due to conflicting reports concerning their effectiveness. A study by Janda et al[217] reported that this equipment could actually increase the chances of injury.

Pasternack et al[351] concluded that 14% of injuries could be prevented if the players wore helmets with facemasks on both offense and defense. In their study, the use of facemasks only during batting would not have prevented 86% of the injuries from the ball. They concluded that facemasks on batters could reduce or eliminate facial injuries to players on offense, but only slightly reduce the overall occurrence of ball-related facial injuries because the majority are sustained while on defense. Concerns over the use of facemasks include restricted visibility and a theoretical risk of cervical neck injury secondary to rotational forces on the neck if the mask is grabbed or caught (G. Rutherford et al, 1984; USCPSC, 1994).

Basketball

While not considered to be a true collision sport, the injury rate of basketball rivals such games in many studies. An Injury Surveillance System in the District of Columbia found that 17% of all injuries occurred while participating in one of six sports: baseball/softball, basketball, biking, football, skating, and soccer. The most common mechanisms of injury were falls and being struck by or against objects. Basketball injury etiology included striking against the basketball pole or rim or being struck by a falling pole or backboard.[88] Prebble et al[363] conducted a study of basketball injuries occurring in a rural setting. Of more than 6000 patients with sports-related injuries presenting between 1988 and 1994, 1189 (19%) were injured playing basketball. Approximately two thirds of those injured were males; four fifths of injuries occurred in persons between the ages of 10 and 19 years. Most injuries (53%) occurred during school-related activities. Gomez et al[166] studied the incidence of injury in high school girls' varsity basketball in 1993 and 1994. Of 890 athletes, 436 injuries were reported, for a rate of 0.49 per athlete per season. Although game time accounted for only 12.5% of exposure time, it represented one half of the total injuries. Actual neurological injury accounts for 1%-3% of all injuries. The timing of injury differs between amateur and professional players. Most injuries in the high school and college player occur during practice, while the professional is most often injured during competition.[190,368]

Basketball: History

Dr. James Naismith, at the International YMCA Training School in Springfield, Massachusetts, invented basketball in the winter of 1891. Within a few years, high schools and colleges started basketball teams and, by 1905, it was a recognized winter sport. The popularity of basketball continues to grow and spread. Today, the sport enjoys millions of spectators and hundreds of thousands of fans.

Gender

Participation of women in basketball at all levels has increased dramatically in recent years. Some reports have noted a higher susceptibility to various injuries in female athletes compared with their male counterparts.[82,322,526] A cohort observational study tested this hypothesis in high school sports. The study reported that the knee injury rates per 100 players for girls' basketball was higher than for their male counterparts. Major injuries also occurred more often in girls' basketball, and there were a higher number of surgeries required for female basketball participants.[359] A similar study of Texas high school basketball players found that the risk of injury per hour of exposure was not significantly different between the two groups, although female athletes did have a significantly higher rate of knee injuries.[310]

Hickey et al[192] analyzed injuries retrospectively among elite female basketball players at the Australian Institute of Sport from 1990 to 1995. They found a total of 223 injuries, of which 139 were acute and 84 were chronic. The regions most frequently injured were the knee (19%), ankle (17%), lumbar spine (12%), and lower legs (11%). Mechanical low back pain was diagnosed in 4% of the patients. In a comparison of mens' and women's professional basketball injuries, injuries occurred in women 1.6 times more frequently than in men. The female players sustained significantly more knee and thigh injuries as well as sprains, strains, and contusions, while males had significantly more muscle spasms.[526]

Head Injury

Head injuries in basketball can be caused by the sudden deceleration of the head when an athlete's head strikes an immobile object, such as the floor, or the sudden acceleration of the head following being struck by an opponent. These forces can cause tearing of the bridging veins of the sagittal sinus, resulting in subdural hematoma. They can also cause damage to the middle meningeal artery and associated epidural hematoma. Finally, direct contusion of the brain may occur. Between 1982 and 1995, 0.17 annual head injuries per 100,000 high school basketball players were reported. No fatalities were recorded related to head trauma (F. Mueller and R. Cantu, 1996). The USCPSC reported in 1990 that for every 100,000 head injuries in basketball, 258 required hospitalization.[483] In a study by Powell and Barber-Foss et al,[360] girls' and boys' basketball accounted for 63 (5%) and 51 (4%), respectively, of the 1219 mild TBIs reported during the 1995-1997 academic years.

Several reports of acute subdural and epidural hematoma related to playing basketball are in the literature. Datti et al[115] reported an acute left temporal epidural hematoma in a 35-year-old basketball player that required surgical drainage. An acute subdural hematoma was reported by Tudor[478] following a blow from a basketball. Keller and Holland[236] reported a rare basketball-related chronic subdural hematoma. Toro-Gonzalez et al[470] evaluated the death of a previously healthy 17-year-old female basketball player after a fall during a game. An acute cerebral fibrocartilaginous embolism from the nucleus pulposus had caused complete occlusion of the right middle cerebral artery. Fibrocartilaginous embolisms from the nucleus pulposus have been previously reported as a rare cause of spinal cord ischemia.

Back Injury

The most common neurological risk in basketball is to the player's spine. According to the NSCIDRC, basketball accounted for 1% of all sports-related SCIs between 1973 and 1981 (J. Young et al, 1982). Because the sport involves rapid changes in direction and explosive movements, repeated stress on the vertebrae of the spine can result in spondylolysis. Secondary to the athletes' rapid growth, adolescent players with these defects in the pars interarticularis are at a higher risk of vertebral slippage and spondylolisthesis;[517] early detection in the adolescent is critical to reverse this degenerative process. If the injury is not corrected early, spinal stenosis and narrowing of the foramen can result in radiculopathy. Acute back injuries associated with basketball include lumbosacral sprains, contusions, facet joint and pars interarticularis injuries, spinal stenosis, and lumbar disc injuries or fractures.[213,214,314,333,428,448]

A herniated disc frequently has a sciatic nerve distribution, and pain usually extends below the knee. Often, this injury is accompanied by dermatomal dysfunction and an increase in symptoms when coughing or bearing down. The herniation is usually posterior or posterolateral. While discogenic disease is rare in the non-active young population, its incidence increases with involvement in sporting activity. Clark[94] reported the case of a 12-year-old athlete incurring a lumbar disc herniation with apophyseal fracture that occurred during an athletic activity. Disc herniation in athletes is a consequence of numerous microtraumas of the intervertebral disc, which are further compounded by the syndrome of chronic overstraining. Basketball is a leading cause of sports-related disc disease and was the second most common cause of disc herniation among a series of 55 athletes reported by Kovac et al.[250] Other injuries can resemble disc disease. Garth and Van Patten[155] reported a fracture of the lumbar lamina with epidural hematoma simulating herniation of a disc.

Facet syndrome can cause lower back pain in the basketball player. This pain radiates into the posterior buttocks and thigh and rarely descends below the knees. The pain is often increased with hyperextension and decreased with ambulation.[195,213,321] These patients may be treated with rest, facet injection, or rhizotomy. Spinal stenosis can cause chronic lower back pain and radiculopathy. It is often associated with disc disease or injury as well as recurrent pain while playing the game.

Pars interarticularis defects can cause areas of spinal instability and low back pain in the player.[135,195,213,214,314] Pain from this source is greatest with hyperextension or twisting of the spine and may be unilateral. Patients with spondylolysis or spondylolisthesis with less than 50% slippage can be treated with rest. More severe injuries require bracing of the lumbosacral spine or surgical fusion.[213,312,314]

Fractures of the lumbar spine are rare occurrences in basketball.[333] If a fracture occurs, timely diagnosis and treatment are essential. Compression and burst fractures are treated in a similar fashion as in other trauma patients.[11,135] Fractures of the spinous or transverse processes can be treated symptomatically. These may occur secondary to trauma or from strong muscular contraction.[135,213] They more frequently affect the lumbosacral area than the cervical spine.

Cervical cord neurapraxia has been reported in basketball players.[468] It is a transient neurological phenomenon not often associated with any permanent injury. No permanent morbidity has occurred in patients who returned to contact activities. Once a player experiences neurapraxia, however, there is a greater than 50% chance of recurrence. This risk is strongly and inversely correlated with the athlete's sagittal canal diameter.

The basketball player with lower back pain or radicular pain needs careful evaluation. This includes a careful history of any previous injuries or symptoms and a specific history of the new injury. Low back pain in the basketball player usually responds well to rest and conservative therapy.[92] In recalcitrant cases of chronic lower back pain, a functional restoration program consisting of isolated lumbar extensor progressive resistance exercise has been reported to be effective.[125] Anti-inflammatory medications, steroid injections, and surgical intervention can be used in a stepwise fashion for players who do not respond to conservative treatment.[104,118]

Peripheral Nerve Injury

Peripheral nerves are susceptible to injury in the basketball player because of the excessive stresses made to both the neurological structures and the soft tissues that protect them. Because many injuries remain subclinical, they are not recognized before neurological damage is permanent. A high index of suspicion for this type of injury in the basketball player would increase the opportunity for a good outcome.

Although primarily a football injury, "burners" have been reported in basketball as a result of acute head, neck, and/or shoulder trauma. They are usually self-limiting, but they occasionally produce permanent neurological deficits.[143] Peripheral nerve injuries are more common in the upper extremities. The suprascapular, musculocutaneous, ulnar, and median nerves are susceptible to entrapment. Tsur and Shahin[477] reported a basketball player with acute suprascapular neuropathy without any history of shoulder girdle trauma. The injury was the result of chronic microtraumas secondary to nerve traction over the coracoid notch while "'dunking'" the basketball. The patient presented unable to abduct his arm, had some difficulty in external rotation, and developed atrophy of both the supra- and the infraspinatus muscles. The injury responded well to conservative treatment, and after 3 weeks of inactivity, recovery was nearly complete. A case of median nerve entrapment resulting in carpal tunnel syndrome was reported in a patient following intensive basketball training.[110] The athlete's symptoms improved upon terminating participation in the sport. The wrist is a complex joint, with injury incidence in sports participants at approximately 25%. This figure is higher in sports such as basketball that use the hand and wrist extensively. Nerve injuries in this area are most commonly compressive neuropathies.[202] Hand injuries also occur fairly commonly in basketball players.

Stress on the anterior joint structures of the shoulder (i.e., the capsule, ligaments, and subscapularis tendon) with resultant anterior instability often occurs due to the substantial amount of overhead action in basketball. These stresses can cause anterior subluxation, impingement syndromes, or even dislocation. If shoulder dislocation occurs, the axillary nerve is commonly injured. Lo et al[272] conducted a study of shoulder impingement among different athletic groups that demanded vigorous upper arm activities. Of 372 athletes, 163 (44%) indicated that they had shoulder problems, with basketball believed to be the source of the problem in 10 patients.

The sciatic and common peroneal nerves can be injured by trauma. Peroneal palsy is the most common lower-extremity nerve injury and has a poor prognosis after traction injury. Because of the frequent incidence of knee injuries in basketball, the player has a high risk of injury to this nerve.

Bowling

The sport of bowling can be both physically and psychologically demanding. Strong muscular forces are impelled throughout a bowler's stance, approach, pivot step, forward arm swing, release, follow through, and finish position. While the annual incidence of injury is relatively low (0.5 per 1000 participants), the sport can cause a variety of hand and upper-extremity injuries due to either acute or repetitive forces. Bowling involves repetitive stress to the upper extremity (e.g., the fingers, wrist, and elbow) while delivering the ball. Overuse syndromes caused by repetitive microtrauma often occur.

Injuries to the fingers and digital nerves can occur in this sport. Mauch and Bauer[290] presented the case of a 55-year old male bowler who suffered a traumatic dislocation of the four long fingers. Participants can develop what is referred to as a "bowler's thumb," which is actually a neuroma of the digital nerve. Cases of thumb neuroma have been

---

Bowling: History

The sport of bowling can be traced back to Egypt more than 7000 years ago where the implements for such a game have been found in an Egyptian tomb. The modern sport likely grew from a German religious ceremony. In the 3rd century AD, German peasants carried a club called a kegel for protection. It became a customary test of faith in many churches for the parishioner to set up his kegel as a target representing a heathen and then rolling a stone in an attempt to knock it down. Dutch settlers brought bowling to North America during the 1620s in the form of a game called ninepins. Because the game involved gambling, it was outlawed in many areas. It is believed that participants added a tenth pin to circumvent these laws, thus creating modern tenpin bowling.

Today, automatic scoring machines, which calculate scores using computers, and faster pin-setting machines are increasing the popularity of bowling. Variations on the game, such as cosmic bowling where participants use glow-in-the-dark balls and pins, have also attracted new participants. Approximately 60 million people in the U.S. "go" bowling at least once a year, and 7 million compete in league play. The sport was an exhibition game at the 1988 Olympic Games in South Korea.

reported by various authors, including Kitagawa et al.[242] Dobyns et al[127] reported 17 cases of this ailment. The condition presents with a positive Tinel's sign and skin atrophy or callusing over the neuroma. While no true neuroma is usually observed pathologically, the nerve becomes atrophied and there is a proliferation of fibrous tissue at the site.

The sport of bowling can also result in lower back pain. This is often the result of discogenic injury. Mundt et al[326] conducted a study of possible risk factors for herniated lumbar and cervical discs. The authors found a positive association between bowling and herniation at both the lumbar and cervical regions of the spine.

Bungee Jumping

There are two main categories of injury associated with bungee jumping, those secondary to equipment failure and those resulting from technical misjudgment. The hot air balloon-launching site is vulnerable to undetected changes in altitude, which can cause the cord length to be longer than the distance to the ground. The potential for fatality in this situation is obvious. When jumping from a balloon, there have been reports of the basket tumbling to the ground and the rebounding jumper striking the basket. Jumpers from fixed sites such as bridges have also struck their platforms on the rebound. Reports have occurred of jumpers becoming tangled in their cord, with the cord "lassoing" their neck.

Catastrophic mishaps have also occurred when the strap or harness attaching the jumper to the cord breaks. Harries[182] reported a similar fatal technical error when a carnival worker neglected to attach his cord to the platform before diving. One such occurrence, reported by Shapiro et al,[418] resulted in only minor injury because of an air cushion placed below the jump site for safety.

Neurological injuries associated with the sport range from peroneal nerve palsy and concussion to quadriplegia and death.[196,418,471] Injury is more common when the jumper attaches the cord to his/her ankles versus using a body harness. Hite et al[196] reported two cases of bungee-associated accidents that could have had fatal outcomes. In the first case, the cord became tightly wrapped around the jumper's neck shortly after the first rebound. This caused the victim to snap from a head-down position to upright, suspended by the cord. Fortunately, the jumper was able to interpose her hands between the cord and her neck, and avoided serious injury. She suffered only abrasions and ecchymosis of the neck. The authors suggested that the victim probably avoided severe injury from hanging due to her small size, the fact that she dropped only a short distance with the cord actually wrapped around her neck, and the elasticity of the bungee cord. The second case involved a reverse bungee jump. The participant was a veteran of the sport, having taken more than 100 standard jumps. When released, one side of his restraints failed, causing his head to violently jerk to the left. The patient suffered immediate pain in the cervical spine and decreased sensation from the sternum down. He was later found to have a sensory level of C6-7 with absent deep tendon reflexes in the lower extremities. Lateral cervical spine films revealed a 3-mm anterior subluxation of C6 on C7, with prevertebral soft-tissue swelling. Narrowing of the distance between the posterior spinous processes of C6-7 and unilaterally locked facets were suggested by posteroanterior cervical spine films. Computed tomography (CT) confirmed a left locked facet with rotary subluxation of C6-7. Following the accident, the patient remained quadriplegic. Louw et al[277] reported a 23-year-old man who developed gradual weakness and numbness of his limbs over 14 days following an uneventful jump. These symptoms remained stable for 2 months, then deteriorated into an asymmetric quadriparesis. Imaging revealed a severe midline disc herniation at C6-7, with significant spinal cord compression and posterior longitudinal ligament disruption. Following a three-level discectomy, the patient regained normal function.

Bungee Jumping: History

Residents of the Pentacost Island in the South Pacific are believed to be the first to jump from high wooden platforms, using elastic liana vines tied to their ankles to break the fall.[387] Modern thrill-seekers plunge off a fixed or mobile site such as a crane, platform, bridge, cliff, or hot air balloon, usually 200-400 feet from the ground, and break the fall with an elastic cord before contacting the ground. The cord may be attached to the ankles or, more commonly, to a body harness. The jumper may fall between 80 and 650 feet. The abrupt deceleration at the end of a jump can subject the body to a force 16 times that applied to the cervical spine by a hangman's noose.[277] Surprisingly, with all of the risks involved, it is still considered one of the safest activities of the "extreme sports."

Since 1988, when the first commercial bungee jumping facility opened, more than 1 million bungee jumps have been performed in the U.S. Reverse bungee jumping is also becoming popular. In this form of the popular sport, the participant is held to the ground while the cord is stretched upward. The person is released and is shot upward from the force of the cord.

Catastrophic Injury

In the U.S., at least seven fatalities and numerous severe injuries have been reported since the late 1980s in bungee jumpers and those using a hot air balloon. Most of these were the result of operator error.[181,275,276] Two of the fatalities were secondary to incorrect connections of the cord to the platform, three were the result of a hot air balloon basket falling to the ground, and two persons were killed when using a hot air balloon for a platform and not noticing a decrease in altitude (Finocchiaro C, personal communication).[444] In both of these cases, the jumper impacted the ground.

Peripheral Nerve Injury

Peroneal nerve palsy is a common peripheral neuropathy that results in foot drop. The foot drop secondary to this injury is the result of paralysis of the extensors and foot inversion from peroneal muscle paralysis. The lateral and anterior aspects of the lower leg and foot may also develop paresthesias and anesthesia with injury to this nerve.[133] The common peroneal nerve is vulnerable to injury from its origin in the upper popliteal fossa to its ending distal to the fibular tunnel. Peroneal neuropathy is usually secondary to external compression.[121,167,262] Less commonly, traumatic forces to the lower extremity can result in damage to this nerve.[23,439]

Torre et al[471] reported a case secondary to a bungee jump. The injury occurred in a man testing equipment for a bungee jumping company. He reportedly had performed more than 2000 jumps in a 6-month period, the majority with the cord attached by a harness to his ankles. He presented with a "dead foot," with paresthesias for approximately 6 weeks. This case of peroneal nerve palsy was likely the result of chronic shearing forces on the peroneal nerve from repeated stretching during bungee jumps.

Canoeing/Kayaking: History

Canoeing was recognized as a competitive sport in 1866, with the International Canoe Federation founded in 1924. At this time, canoeing was included in the Olympics Games as a demonstration sport. Sprint canoeing and kayaking were later recognized as official Olympic sports in 1936 in Berlin. The strongest national teams to compete in sprint canoeing and kayaking usually come from Germany, Sweden, Norway, Hungary, the former Yugoslavia, the former Union of Soviet Socialist Republics, France, and Italy. The U.S. has also been historically competitive in this activity.

Canoeing/Kayaking

Lower back pain and injury are the most frequent complaints of athletes who are injured while canoeing or kayaking.[495] As expected, these problems are more severe in those who undergo intense training. They also are more frequent in the over 25-year-old population. These injuries are usually responsive to conservative therapy. Kameyama et al[231] surveyed 821 active canoeists, members of the Japan Canoe Association, and performed a medical check of 63 top competitive canoeists. Of the 417 respondents, 94 canoeists (23%) reported that they experienced pain in the lower back and buttocks, 21% experienced shoulder pain, 4% elbow pain, and 11% wrist pain. On medical examination, back pain was found to be mainly of myofascial origin or due to spondylolysis. Impingement syndrome was also observed in four canoeists with shoulder problems.

Apparently, lower back pain in canoeists is not just a recent problem. A study of 373 Inuit skeletons from Alaska and Canada produced 16 examples of spondylolysis (eight from each area).[309] The majority were males between 18 and 20 years old. The sacral spondylolysis appeared to have resulted from stress fracturing that occurred while S1 was still unfused, and the high frequency observed in this population is attributed to the concentration of unusual stresses in the lower back of adolescent males due to such activities as kayak paddling and harpooning.

Catastrophic cervical spine injury in this population is a possibility. A kayaker recently presented to the authors' institution with a Jefferson fracture incurred while kayaking; this athlete was flipped in a section of rapids and hit her head on rocks under the water's surface, which resulted in extreme hyperflexion of the neck (Figure 3).

Participants may also suffer from medial nerve entrapment or secondary carpal tunnel syndrome. These conditions are secondary to the chronic torquing of the wrist that occurs while paddling.

Cycling

Participation in the sport of bicycling has been growing rapidly for the past two decades. It is estimated that cycling provides a dynamic form of aerobic and anaerobic fitness to nearly 100 million Americans. In 1987, more bicycles were purchased than automobiles.[90] One reason for this increase in popularity is the "Rails to Trails" program that is converting abandoned railroad tracks into bike trails across the U.S. A new form of the sport, off-road bicycling, has also become extremely popular.

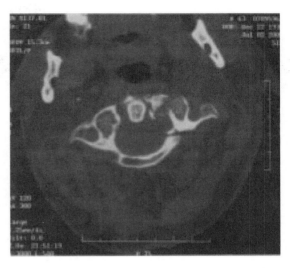

Figure 3: Jefferson fracture secondary to hyperflexion of the neck sustained while kayaking.

Epidemiology of Injury

Cycling injuries account for more than 600,000 emergency room visits and cost more than 1 billion healthcare dollars annually.[13,34,64] Injuries can be secondary to acute trauma or overuse. More than one half of the total injuries result from interactions with motor vehicles. Although the number of traffic fatalities has declined over the past 25 years, bicycling still accounts for 2% of fatalities. This figure is higher in Sweden, where cyclists contribute up to 15% of the traffic fatalities (National Center for Statistics and Analysis, 1991). These usually result from the vehicle driver failing to see the cyclist, and for obvious reasons occur with more frequency in the dawn and dusk hours.[16] A study of bicycle-related injuries sustained by 197 junior high school students aged 12 to 15 years found that nearly 40% of the accidents occurred between 3:00 PM and 7:00 PM and more than half of the accidents took place near street corners.[415] A study by Rivara et al[376] attempted to determine risk factors for serious injury to bicyclists. This risk was found to increase with motor-vehicle collisions, self-reported speed of less than 15 mph, and age younger than 6 years or older than 39 years. Kiburz et al[239] found that significant factors contributing to bicycle accidents include rider carelessness, cycle malfunction, environmental factors, turns, hills, and companion riders. Mechanical problems with the bicycle[21,119,120] and road surface imperfections such as potholes and damaged shoulders[239] are also common causes of injury.

According to the U.S. National Center for Health Statistics and the National Electronic Injury Surveillance System, between 1000 and 1300 participants die annually from bicycle-related activities (Centers for Disease Control, 1984-1988).[34] Children under 15 years old account for more than half of both bicycle-related deaths and nonfatal injuries. In this age group, bicycle-related accidents result in more emergency room visits than do injuries from sleds, skateboards, roller skates, and all other toys combined.[473] Injuries commonly occur to the head as well as the upper and lower extremities. Various peripheral nerve and genital injuries are related to the seat and handlebars. Unlike most sports, the cyclist is riding a vehicle that is capable of high rates of speed. This puts their entire body at risk of acute traumatic injury. A common cause of this type of injury is the cyclist being thrown from the vehicle when it comes to a rapid stop. This type of accident can be most serious if the front wheel is the first to stop, which is often the result of riding over a sewer opening or rain drainage grate. This scenario may create an angular acceleration of the cyclist that could increase their speed above that reached while riding. This can also result from a broken spoke becoming trapped in the structures surrounding it and causing the wheel to seize. Bicycle accidents that occur

Cycling: History

In 1869, the first competitive bicycle race was held in France. Today, competitive events include road races, track or Velodrome races, and youth BMX races. Off-road bicycling, also referred to as mountain biking, has become increasingly popular worldwide since its introduction in the late 1970s in the western U.S.

Although early mountain bicycles were similar to the versions used on the street, mountain bikes today typically include high-strength, lightweight frames, with a wide array of available suspension and braking systems. As the popularity of this type of cycling has increased, so too has the interest and level of participation in the competitive aspects of the sport. Currently, two organizations, the National Off-Road Bicycle Association and the Union Cycliste Internationale, hold major events within the U.S. and around the during racing are often the result of a punctured tire or hitting a stone and often cause a chain reaction of collisions. Riding in pace lines, done to decrease the effects of wind resistance, results in collisions from the bicyclists riding in close proximity to one another. Of note, off-road cyclists have far fewer serious injuries than other participants in the sport. They do, however, incur a higher proportion of injuries to their extremities. Rivara et al[377] found that mountain bikers are less likely to suffer head and face injuries than other cyclists and are more likely to wear helmets. Their lower incidence of severe injuries is believed to be secondary to helmet use, the slower speeds at which they travel, and the absence of motor vehicles.[91,209,350,521]

A new type of cycling-related injury is being observed secondary to the use of bicycle-towed trailers for transporting children and child seats mounted on adult bicycles. Powell and Tanz[358] conducted a retrospective analysis of data from the National Electronic Injury Surveillance System of the USCPSC for 1990 to 1998 and found 49 injuries during the 9-year study period, of which six were associated with the use of bicycle-towed trailers and 43 were related to the use of bicycle-mounted child seats. Of the injuries resulting from bicycle-towed trailers, one was the result of contact with a bicycle wheel or spokes, two were the result of collisions with a motor vehicle, and three were the result of falls. Of the bicycle-mounted child seat injuries, four were from motor-vehicle collisions, eight from contact with a bicycle wheel or spokes, and 31 the result of falls. The head or face accounted for 83% of injuries among those riding in bicycle-towed trailers and 49% of injuries among children in bicycle-mounted child seats. The authors recommended that bicycle helmets be worn by children riding in both types of transportation.

Head Injury

Injuries to the head are common in cycling accidents, with the majority of fatal accidents the result of head injuries. From 1984 to 1988, cycling resulted in 2985 fatalities related to head injury (62% of all bicycling-related deaths).[390] In the same period, a total of 905,752 head injuries related to cycling occurred. Forty-one percent of the head-injury fatalities and 76% of the total head injuries occurred in children under 15 years of age. Almost one fourth of all brain injuries in children under the age of 15 years are accounted for by bicycle accidents.[251] The rate of fatalities in children from bicycle accidents exceeds causes such as poisoning, falls, suffocation, and firearms injuries that have traditionally received much more attention.[505] Deaths from head injuries are almost always the result of intracranial hemorrhage, such as acute subdural hematoma. Few victims use helmets despite clear evidence that they are effective at preventing and reducing the severity of injuries. In fact, it is rare for a helmet user to suffer a head injury.[496,501,503,507] The U.S. Centers for Disease Control have calculated that if 50% of cyclists wore helmets, more than 300,000 head injuries would be prevented annually.[390]

Spinal Injury

Pain in the neck and back is extremely common in cyclists, occurring in up to 60% of participants.[506] The etiology is the combination of increased load on the arms and shoulders required to support the cyclist and hyperextension of the neck in the horizontal, bent-forward position of riding. If the bicycle is not properly fitted to the cyclist and he/she must reach forward to the handlebars, these stresses are aggravated by the resultant hyperextension of the neck and extreme flexion of the back. Wilber et al[511] analyzed overuse injuries among cyclists. The most common anatomical site for overuse injuries was the neck (49%); the back accounted for 30% of complaints. The odds of female cyclists developing neck and shoulder overuse problems have been reported to be 1.5

and 2.0 times more, respectively, than their male counterparts. Lower back pain in these athletes is partially the result of hyperextension of the pelvic/spine angle, which results in an increase in stress at the promontorium. Salai et al[392] found that, by simply adjusting the seat to an anterior inclining angle, more than 70% of a group of cyclists complaining of lower back pain reported a major improvement.

According to the NSCIDRC, the mean age of persons with a cycling-related SCI in 1980 and 1981 was 24 years (range 14-57) (K. Clarke, 1983). All of the injuries occurred in men, and 43% occurred in individuals considered adept at the sport. In 43%, the injury resulted in quadriplegia. In 86%, the injuries occurred to an individual not participating in an organized class or team. A study by Rivara et al[376] found that the risk of neck injury was increased in cyclists struck by motor vehicles or hospitalized for any injury.

Numerous authors have indicated that Scheuermann's disease is very common in the adolescent cyclist. In a group of cyclists studied by van Elegem,[485] 40% presented with signs of the disorder. Several theories exist regarding the high incidence of Scheuermann's disease. In young athletes, the vertebral endplates are still in a growth phase and the kyphotic posture assumed in cycling, along with contracted neck and back muscles, puts a significant amount of pressure on the vertebral bodies. While the posterior column of the vertebrae is less stressed and more mature, the increased anterior pressure can result in remodeling of the vertebrae that appears as anterior compression. Since the posterior column is under little pressure, growth occurs rapidly. In the anterior portion of the vertebral body, growth is slowed. A similar mechanism has been proposed for rowers with the condition.[229] A second theory is simply that the heavily flexed position of the cyclist and repetitive microtraumas cause fractures of the anterior portion of the vertebral endplate that result in wedging of the vertebrae. This is believed to be the cause of Scheuermann's disease in gymnasts.[316,448] The disorder does not appear to continue to progress into adulthood in the bicycling athlete.

An injury commonly seen in bicycling is pain and spasm of the left levator scapula and upper third of the left trapezius muscles. These injuries only occur where bicycles are driven on the right side of the road and result from the rider constantly turning to the left to look for approaching traffic. They have been shown to occur even when cyclists utilize mirrors on their helmets.

Peripheral Nerve Injury

Goldberg et al[161] reported two cases of damage to peripheral nerves following bicycle riding that represent the most common peripheral nerve deficits associated with the sport. The first patient had an injury of the ulnar nerve at the level of the wrist, which presented as hypesthesia of the two ulnar digits and paresis of the intrinsic muscles. The second case involved the pudendal nerves with numbness of the buttocks and genitalia, and with difficulty in achieving erection. After cycling was stopped for a few weeks, the symptoms in both patients disappeared spontaneously, without residual deficits.

Neuropathies with symptoms in the distributions of the pudendal and genitofemoral nerves are common in cyclists, with as many as half of male cyclists competing in long-distance day rides complaining of these symptoms.[50] Injury to the pudendal nerve can result from overuse or poor positioning of the seat. The injury presents as paresthesias of the scrotum and shaft of the penis. Injuries are commonly related to the bicycle seat and could be the result of poor position in terms of height, angle, and fore-and-aft position. Less frequently, the shape of the seat may be the culprit. The condition is the result of compression of the dorsal branch of the pudendal nerve against the pubic symphysis. The genital branch of the genitofemoral nerve is also often involved, resulting in scrotal anesthesia.[50] Male impotence has also been reported in cyclists. This is probably secondary to the previously mentioned pudendal neuropathy.[124] Electrophysiological findings suggest that reversible ischemic neuropathy of the dorsal (sensory) and cavernous (vasomotor) nerves of the penis are the cause.[59] Andersen and Bovim[14] assessed the frequency and duration of symptoms suggesting peripheral nerve compression after long-distance cycling. Of 160 participants in the study, 35 reported symptoms in the distribution of the pudendal or cavernous nerve and 33 had penile numbness or hypesthesia after cycling. The numbness lasted for more than 1 week in 10 subjects. Impotence was reported by 21 (13%) of the males, and lasted for more than a week in 11 and more than a month in three patients. Mechanical management of this condition includes re-adjustment of the seat and the use of padded bicycling shorts. A saddle pad may also be used, and the seat itself may be replaced.

Injury at the interface between the handlebars and the hand of the cyclist are the result of compression and chronic energy transfer. Frequent compression neuropathies of the ulnar nerve, and much less commonly the median nerve, are reported in cyclists. If promptly recognized and managed, they rarely result in permanent injury or deficit. Ulnar neuropathy occurs most frequently in competitive and long-distance cyclists. Destet first recognized this condition in cyclists more than 100 years ago.[149] Hoyt[204] reported 117 cases over a 4-year period. It is commonly referred to as cyclist's or handlebar palsy and results in the gradual development of paresthesias in the fourth and fifth fingers and weakness of the intrinsic muscles of the hand innervated by the affected nerve. While the majority of cases result in both motor and sensory symptoms, pure motor or sensory deficits do occur. This condition most commonly occurs during a protracted ride, often over rough terrain. Its resolution is variable and may take up to several months. The condition is caused by compression of the ulnar nerve at or about Guyon's canal and is related to wrist hyperextension.[130,516] The ulnar nerve enters the hand through the aforementioned canal, which is also commonly referred to as the ulnar tunnel. Because this pathway is more superficial than that through which the median nerve travels, the ulnar nerve is more vulnerable to external compression injuries.[225] This is compounded by the fact that the transverse carpal ligament, which covers Guyon's canal, is significantly thinner than the roofing of the carpal tunnel.[58]

The ulnar nerve is the largest branch of the medial cord of the brachial plexus. It carries fibers from both the eighth cervical and the first thoracic nerve root. The nerve gives off a branch, the dorsal cutaneous nerve, approximately 8 cm above the wrist. This branch is responsible for sensation in the dorsal ulnar area of the hand. As the nerve passes through its tunnel, it divides into a deep and a superficial branch. The palmaris brevis muscle is innervated by the superficial branch, which also gives sensory innervation to the ulnar section of the hypothenar eminence and the fourth and fifth digits. In the most severe cases of this condition, these fingers may begin to claw. The deep branch of the nerve innervates the intrinsic interosseous, the abductor and flexor digiti quinti, and the flexor pollicis brevis muscles.[417] The condition has been divided into three syndromes determined by the clinical presentation of the disorder,[417] which are the consequence of different sites of compression. Type I syndrome is a combination of motor and sensory loss. This results from compression just proximal to or in the ulnar tunnel, before the bifurcation. Because the ulnar nerve is intact proximal to the wrist, the dorsal ulnar area of the hand has intact sensation. The victim has sensory loss over the hypothenar eminence and the fourth and fifth digits, as well as weakness of the hand muscles innervated by the ulnar nerve. If the subject has only motor deficits, the syndrome is referred to as Type II. This is the result of injury solely to the deep motor branch of the nerve and can occur distal to where it exits the ulnar tunnel. The number of muscles affected is dependent on the exact location of injury, and this can be used to further subdivide the syndromes, as done by Wu et al.[523] This type of injury can also be the result of a stretch injury of the nerve as it courses around the hook of the hamate, caused by prolonged hyperextension of the wrist. If the subject has only sensory deficits, the syndrome is referred to as Type III, and the lesion affects the superficial sensory branch of the nerve. The victim experiences hyperesthesia over the hypothenar eminence as well as the volar ring and little finger. Because this branch courses superficially along the ulnar border of the hand, it is vulnerable to extended pressure. Of the varying types of injury, Type I appears to be the most prevalent.[327]

The cyclist can reduce the incidence of this condition by frequently changing hand positions and riding with unlocked elbows. Mechanical and medical management are effective in relieving symptoms and preventing recurrence. In a series of 117 patients, Hoyt[204] reported that all of the neuropathies resolved without recurrence simply by adjusting the bicycle and changing the riding technique. The use of padded gloves or handlebars may also be of benefit.

Although much less common than ulnar dysfunction, carpal tunnel syndrome secondary to compression of the medial nerve has also been observed in the cyclist.[58] Chan et al[81] attempted to detect median nerve lesions in 14 professional cyclists. Four cyclists (seven hands) had neurological symptoms related to median nerve and four (five hands) had abnormal electrodiagnostic examinations. This prevalence of median nerve lesions in cyclists was substantially higher than expected. Nonetheless, because the condition is uncommon in this population of athletes, other causes of the condition should be researched. Interestingly, both ulnar and medial compression can occur in the same athlete, and if a carpal tunnel release is performed, the ulnar dysfunction usually resolves spontaneously.[424] Impingement of the ulnar nerve has been reported in two triathletes using a new type of handlebars known as "aerobars."[352]

Several authors have reported paresthesias of the foot and metatarsalgias. The condition is fairly common in long-distance riders and is usually the result of tight toe straps or clips, improper foot position, and increased pedal pressure. The condition is treated mechanically by loosening toe straps, obtaining the proper size of toe clips, and changing the gear ratio to decrease pedal resistance.

Serious injuries to the fingers with permanent neurological deficits can occur from bicycle spokes.[172,252,399] These injuries are almost always the result of negligence, since the hands should be nowhere near the tires while they are spinning, often occurring when a cyclist attempts to adjust the cycle without stopping. The injuries have also occurred to passengers who get their heels caught in the back wheel.

The Use of Bicycle Helmets

Undoubtedly, the most important piece of safety equipment in bicycling is the helmet. Just as participants in football put on their helmets before entering a game, cyclists should consider the helmet a part of their required uniform. Thompson and Patterson[189,464] reported that the use of helmets is associated with a reduction in the risk of head injury by 85%, brain injury by 88%, and severe brain injury by at least 75%. In 1986, the U.S. Cycling Federation mandated helmet use in all sponsored races, and the equipment is currently required in most competitions. When New Zealand began requiring the mandatory use of helmets by all bicyclers, the use rate rose from approximately 20% for adults and teenagers, and 40% for younger children, to more than 90% in all age groups. This increased use of helmets resulted in a reduction of head injuries by between 24% and 32% in nonmotor-vehicle crashes and by 20% in motor-vehicle crashes.[357] Similar legislation requiring the use of helmets while bicycling has been passed in several areas of the U.S., including California, Florida, Maryland, Massachusetts, New Jersey, New York, Ohio, Pennsylvania, and the District of Columbia.[226] Borglund et al[52] studied the effectiveness of Florida's mandatory helmet law for children. Known helmet use rose from 6% to 21%, with children aged 10 to 12 years having the greatest increase in helmet use (27%). Puder et al[365] evaluated the effectiveness of three different bicycle helmet laws in three New York City suburbs. The first community's helmet law requires approved helmets for all cyclists regardless of age, the second requires cyclists younger than 14 years to wear helmets, and the third requires cyclists younger than 12 years to wear helmets when riding on highways. As expected, the first group's cyclists had the highest rate of helmet use (35%), followed by the second (24%) and third (14%) groups of cyclists. This study demonstrated that legislation with no age limits has the greatest benefit.

While legislation has proved effective at increasing the use of helmets, so have health promotion campaigns. A community-based bike helmet promotion campaign targeting children up to 14 years of age increased the use of helmets from 4% in 1990 to 67% in 1996.[508] This program also resulted in a decrease in the number of head-injury admissions from 46 in 1990 to 24 in 1996. Sacks et al[391] performed a national telephone survey to estimate ownership and use of bicycle helmets among children in the U.S. in 1994. The authors concluded that 27.7 million children between the ages of 5 and 14 years ride bicycles. Of these, one half own a helmet and one quarter always wear the helmet when cycling. The ownership of helmets appears to increase with income and educational level and decrease with age. As expected, regions of the country with the highest proportion of states with helmet laws also had the highest proportion of helmet use. Counseling by physicians during routine visits was effective at increasing helmet use, with 44% of those counseled using a helmet compared with 19% of those not so counseled.

The scientific evidence that bicycle helmets protect against head, brain, and facial injuries has been well established by numerous well-designed case-control studies and time-series studies in Australia and the U.S. Helmets have been found to provide substantial protection for cyclists of all ages who are involved in accidents ranging from falls to collisions with fixed and moving objects as well as with motor vehicles.[464] The structure of the helmet results in the absorption and distribution of impact forces. Most are constructed of high-density expanded polystyrene or polyurethane that crushes on impact. Therefore, it is important to replace helmets after a severe blow. While this increases the cost to the athlete, the use of resilient materials in helmets makes them less effective because they produce a rebound that can actually increase the force of the impact,[41] leading to contrecoup injury. It is also important to replace helmets every 5 years because some of the materials used in the construction of the helmet deteriorate with age, reducing their protective ability (Snell Memorial Foundation, 1990).

Modern helmets come in several varieties (see Chapter 16 for extensive data on the design of helmets for varying uses). The traditional form consists of a hard shell with a crushable foam liner. While its effectiveness is unequivocal, it can be heavy (weighing up to 1.5 lb) and somewhat bulky. Because of this, new forms of helmets have been developed. A no-shell helmet is available that consists only of a single layer of high-density expanded polystyrene covered with Lycra without a hard shell. While this form of helmet is lighter (approximately 7 ounces), it may create more sliding friction when it impacts the ground, predisposing the wearer to rotational injury of the neck.[451] Thompson and Patterson[464] found no significant differences in protection between these variations of helmet. The newest type of helmet is referred to as the "thin-shell," "micro-shell," or "mini-shell" helmet. A helmet that properly fits the head should contact the head at the crown, sides, forehead, and back. It should be worn squarely on the top of the head and cover the top of the forehead. Its design is similar to the no-shell helmet except that it has a thin, hard outer layer of semirigid plastic. For a helmet to be effective, it must remain on the head during a collision. Because of this, retention systems are as important as the helmet's effectiveness at dissipating impact.[65,66,451]

The American National Standards Institute (ANSI) and the Snell Memorial Foundation set safety standards based on impact protection and strap system strength for helmets in the U.S. Traditionally, the latter organization's standards have been more stringent. A seal of approval from either organization (a label on the equipment stating that it meets ANSI Z90.1 or Snell B-90 standards) ensures the athlete that the helmet can withstand 300 G of force.

Diving

The most catastrophic injuries associated with diving are to the cervical spine. They occur when the diver strikes the springboard or platform with his/her head during a dive or, more commonly, when a recreational athlete dives into water and there is head contact with the bottom of the surface. This results in an immediate halt of forward motion. The inertia of the body then causes the cervical spine to buckle, with disastrous results. Anterior cervical vertebral dislocation is commonly observed secondary to either hyperflexion of the neck or direct trauma to the vertex of the head.[409] Although in the U.S., football is the leading cause of cervical spine injury in organized sports, recreational sports injury to the neck is led by diving. Diving is the fourth leading cause of sports-related quadriplegia. According to the NSCIDRC (J. Young et al, 1982), 70% of neck injuries in sports that resulted in quadriplegia are due to a diving accident. This figure did not differentiate between formal competitive and informal recreational diving. Head and neck injuries are quite rare in competitive diving. The national governing body for organized diving, U.S. Diving, denies ever having a U.S. competitive diver incur an SCI in either practice or competition.[411] Thus, most injuries occur in an informal setting such as recreational swimming pools, ponds, and lakes. The NSCIDRC reported that the most common sites of diving injury to the spinal cord in 1980 and 1981 were lakes and rivers; 29% of accidents occurred in home pools and 17% in community pools. One half of the accidents involving home and community pools occurred with water depths of less than 4 feet. Carelessness and alcohol ingestion are factors in many of these cases. The presence of alcohol in victims has been noted in some studies (K. Clarke, 1983). Dives from roofs, balconies, water slides, and other innovative diving platforms often precede injury.

A study performed by Tator and Edmonds[459] demonstrated that the C5-6 level is most commonly injured in diving accidents (39%). In descending order of frequency, the next most common injury was to C4-5 (24%), C5 (16%), C6 (8%), C6-7 (8%), C7-T1 (3%), and T1-2 (3%). Posterior fracture/dislocation was observed in the majority of injuries. Other types of spinal injury included anterior fracture/dislocations, compression fractures, and burst fractures. Bailes et al[20] identified burst fractures in 52% of the patients they studied.

Equestrian Sports

In the U.S., an estimated 30 million people annually ride horses both competitively and for recreation (Centers for Disease Control, 1990). Horse-related injuries are recognized as a common but serious occurrence.[22,26,509] It is easy to imagine the potential for injury when you consider the weight of the horse (up to 1100 lb), the ability to travel at high speeds (up to 40 miles per hour), and the unpredictability of an animal with a rider perched as high as 10 feet above the ground.[180] The rate of serious injury per riding hour is higher for horseback riding than for motorcycle and automobile racing.[22,42] It is also higher than in either football or hockey.[337] The National Electronic Injury Surveillance

Diving: History

During the 1800s, a sport called plunging developed from diving head first into the water to swim. In 1904, the plunge became an official event of the Olympic Games in St. Louis, Missouri. Diving evolved when individuals attempted to plunge from greater and greater heights. At the beginning of the 19th century, the modern sport of diving began in Germany and Sweden. During that time, individuals began taking gymnastics equipment onto beaches for the summer months and would land in the water after they dismounted the various equipment. Eventually, the trapeze and rings were removed and diving from a platform or a springboard was left as the preferred piece of equipment.

In 1904, men's plain high diving became an official Olympic event. Four years later, springboard diving became an Olympic event as well. In 1912, men's fancy high diving and women's plain high diving became Olympic sports in Stockholm, Sweden. Women's springboard diving became an Olympic event in 1920 in Antwerp, Belgium. The International Olympic Committee introduced synchronized diving as a sport at the 2000 Olympic Games.

Equestrian Sports: History

The origins of equestrian sports dates back to the prehistoric tribesmen in Central Asia who domesticated the first horse in approximately 4500 BC. For thousands of years, equestrian sports were viewed as the activity of kings and the aristocracy. Today, people from various social classes can enjoy participating in or being a spectator at a variety of equestrian activities. The most popular equestrian sport today is the racing of mounted thoroughbred horses over even courses at distances of up to 2 miles.

Other types of modern equestrian sports include harness racing, steeplechase racing, and quarter horse racing. Horseracing is the second most widely attended U.S. spectator sport, after baseball. It is a professional sport in the U.S., Canada, Great Britain, Ireland, Australia, New Zealand, South Africa, South America, and Western Europe.

System in 1987 and 1988 recorded 92,763 emergency room visits resulting from horseback riding in the U.S. The next year, this figure rose (Centers for Disease Control, 1990). Nearly half of the injuries were to soft tissue and 20% were to the head or neck.[27,43,337] Of injuries to the nervous system, the brain is by far the most commonly involved. Approximately 3.5% of the injuries were concussions. Injury to the brain accounts for 17% of all horseback-riding injuries and more than 60% of equestrian-related fatalities, according to data compiled by the Brain Injury Association.[96,98]

Types of Injury

A case series by Hamilton and Tranmer[180] reviewed horseback-riding accidents occurring over a 6-year period. In this study, the average age of the patient was 25 years (range 1-72), and the ratio of male-to-female victims was close to equal. The series identified three basic patterns of equestrian injury: injuries to the head, the spinal cord, and the peripheral nerves. Head injury was clearly the most commonly suffered injury; 92% of patients suffered head injuries, usually consisting of cerebral contusions, concussions, or fractures of the skull. Fatal head injuries associated with horseback riding are more common in riders under the age of 21 years (USCPSC). The average age in the fatality group was 41 years (range 14-72). In 13% of patients, injury was to the spinal cord. SCIs were associated with head injuries in 40% of cases. Approximately 20% of injuries sustained in the young rider occur to the central nervous system.[32,60]

Peripheral Nerve Injury

Peripheral nerve injury was encountered in one person in the Hamilton and Tranmer study.[180] A wrist fracture caused the entrapment of the median nerve, requiring surgical release. This patient completely recovered from the injury. Generally, peripheral nerve injuries involving equestrian events are secondary to traction and are confined to the brachial and lumbosacral plexus. Prognosis with these injuries is usually good.[42]

In the Hamilton and Tranmer study,[180] 82% of the injuries were incurred while falling or being thrown from the horse. After the fall, 12 persons were kicked by the horse, four were crushed, and two were dragged. The primary mechanism of injury was a kick in fewer than 20% of accidents. These figures are corroborated by several other studies.[32,114,158,271] Grossman et al[176] prospectively studied 110 injured equestrians. They found no correlation between injury and age, sex, or experience. Equipment failure was shown to be a cause of several injuries. Fewer than 20% of the riders studied wore a protective helmet.

Head Injury

Of the 143 patients with head injuries in the Hamilton and Tranmer study,[180] 21 had basal skull fractures, 19 had linear skull fractures, and 17 had depressed skull fractures. CT identified cerebral contusions in 22 patients. Acute subdural hematoma was discovered in seven, epidural hematoma in six, and intracerebral hematoma in six. In 22 patients, surgery was required for head injury. The head injury was considered severe (Glasgow Coma Scale score of 8 or lower) in 18 patients, moderate (score of 9-12) in four, and minor (score 13-15) in 121. Outcomes in the head injury population were measured using the Glasgow Outcome Scale; good recovery was determined in 129 patients, moderate disability in two, severe disability in one, and 11 died. As expected, all of the deaths occurred in the severe head injury group. Of the deaths, six had bony head injury (three involved basal skull fractures, two had linear skull fractures, and one a depressed skull fracture). Acute subdural hematoma accounted for four deaths, intracerebral hematoma for three, and cerebral contusions for three. The risk of serious head injury is unaffected by the skill level or experience of the rider,[44,62] and serious head injuries more frequently occur during leisure activities than work or competition (G. Phillips, W. Stuckey, 1979).[62] More than 80% of the accidents in the study by Hamilton and Tranmer occurred during recreational activity. Work activities on a farm or ranch resulted in 10% of the injuries, and 7% were the result of rodeo mishaps. Only one injury occurred during an equestrian competition. Of the equestrian sports, horse racing has the most significant risk of catastrophic head injury.[22,24]

Spinal Injury

In 1997 and 1998, 465 SCIs related to equestrian sports were reported.[512] According to the NSCIDRC, equestrian sports accounted for 2% of all sports-related SCIs between 1973 and 1981. This represented less than 0.5% of all SCIs at the time (J. Young et al, 1982). The mean age of persons with equestrian sports-related SCI in 1980 and 1981 was found to be 28 years (range 19-42) (K. Clarke, 1983). All of the injuries occurred in men, and 80% occurred in persons considered adept at the sport; 60% resulted in quadriplegia and 60% occurred to an individual not participating in an organized class or team. In the study by Hamilton and Tranmer,[180] 19 received injuries to the spinal cord, which was associated with a head injury in nearly half of the cases. Fractures and dislocation of the cervical region occurred in six SCI patients; two of the patients required surgery for stabilization. Eleven injuries to the thoracic and lumbar spine occurred, with three incomplete cervical cord injuries, two spinal cord concussions, two cases of cauda equina syndrome, and one case of cervical radiculopathy. Outcome from the SCIs was also assessed using the Glasgow Outcome Scale; good outcome was determined in 16 patients and moderate disability was found in three.

The Use of Helmets

Headgear is readily available and effective at preventing severe head injury and even death. The proper use of a riding helmet has been associated with a marked decline in the occurrence of head injuries associated with this sport.[271] The compulsory use of helmets instituted by the U.S. Pony Club decreased the rate of concussions from 12% in 1980 to 9% in 1982.[338]

Despite the clear benefits, helmet use remains low. In the study by Hamilton and Tranmer[180] of 156 horse-related injuries to the central nervous system, only two of the victims wore helmets. The largest obstacle to their use appears to be social disdain.[42,60] This disdain is less prevalent in English-style riders, who use the commonly seen velvet-domed headgear. These are easily adapted to include a hard-shell helmet insert without significantly altering the traditional style.[338] Trail riders and western riders prefer the wide-brimmed Stetson hat. A respondent to a survey by Nelson et al[338] on helmet use explained his reluctance to change headgear with the statement "Roy Rogers, Hoot Gibson, and the Duke didn't wear helmets, so I see no need to wear one." Because of this attitude, a hard-shell helmet insert has been developed to fit inside a Stetson. A study by Condie et al[101] indicated that the main reasons for the nonuse of helmet were discomfort, expense, and inappropriateness for certain riding styles. Of the riders surveyed, 20% of riders wore helmets every time they rode and 40% never wore helmets. The survey revealed that helmet use increased with age. The sex of the rider did not appear to play a role. Peer-group pressure was a significant factor in the 14- to 17-year-old age group. The horse-riding population differs from the bicycling population in the reason why helmets are not always worn. While helmet use in both sports is proven to prevent injuries, many cyclists were unaware of this.[114] Equestrians, on the other hand, appear to recognize the safety advantage but avoid helmet use secondary to strong negative atti-

Golf: History

Some historians believe that golf originated in The Netherlands (the Dutch word "kolf" means club), but the Romans had a game played with a bent stick and a ball made of feathers that may have been the original source of the sport. It has been fairly well established, however, that the Scots actually devised the modern game in the 14th or 15th century. In 1457, James II of Scotland banned golf because it interfered with military training; therefore, we know that the sport has been around at least 500 years.

Today, it is estimated that more than 26 million Americans play golf. The popularity of golf has expanded from its core base of older professional men. Organizations such as the American Junior Golf Association have seen a remarkable increase in membership in the last 10 years, with a total of more than 4500 junior golfers from all 50 states and 25 foreign countries. Secondary to the game's increasing popularity, the more than 15,000 golf courses in the U.S. are more crowded now than ever before. It is estimated that 350 new courses are springing up yearly.[297]

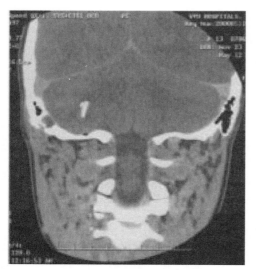

Figure 4: Image in a child impaled through the cerebellum when the shaft of a golf club broke off following impact with a rock. Note the bone fragment in the cerebellum.

tudes toward them. Many of the surveyed riders believed that they were not at risk because they were experienced riders, had a docile horse, or rode on flat ground at a moderate pace.[101]

Helmets for equestrian use have been available for the past 50 years. Because of the large number of head injuries associated with the sport, several equestrian organizations began requiring the use of approved helmets during competition. These included the American Horse Shows Association, U.S. Combined Training Association, the U.S. Equestrian Team, and the U.S. Pony Club.[12] Since the majority of head trauma occurs during recreational activities, riders must be cognizant of the importance of helmet use during all activities, not just during competition. Another obstacle to helmet use is the cost (approximately $100-$150). Because helmets are tightly fitted to the head, they are outgrown in the younger population and a helmet is usually required for every individual in the family.

Golf

Golf is perhaps considered one of the most benign sports. Despite this, professional golfers incur an average of two injuries a year, and it is estimated that between 10% and 30% of professional golfers are playing injured at any point in time.[294,297] The majority of these injuries are secondary to overuse and result from continual practice swings. Professionals often spend more than 8 hours a day practicing their swing. Injury to the lower back has been found to be the most common injury in both male professional and amateur golfers in several studies.[221,297] In the female golfer, injury to the wrist is the most common, followed by lower back injury.[295] Numerous freak injuries have been associated with the golf club itself, which appears to be a popular tool for hitting objects other than golf balls. In 1939, a golfer killed his caddie with an angry swing of the club following a missed shot. Another golfer broke his club on a tree, again after missing a shot, only to have it rebound and impale him. A similar incident occurred at the authors' institution involving a child hitting rocks with a golf club. The shaft of the club broke and the distal end entered the child's cerebellum (Figure 4). Everard[141] reported a player being struck in the head with a golf club thrown by his partner.

Golf-related fatalities are most often due to lightning, power lines, heart attack, and heat stroke. A lightning strike can cause death or various injuries to one or several players at once. Although the incidence of lightning-related deaths has decreased in the U.S. since the 1950s, lightning causes more deaths than hurricanes or tornadoes. The Centers for Disease Control's National Center for Health Statistics attributes 1318 deaths to lightning in the U.S. from 1980 through 1995.[264]

Back Injury/Pain

Injury to the back is commonly associated with golf and affects both the amateur and the professional. These injuries are often the result of poor conditioning, bad technique, and overuse. Extreme rotatory torque of the body occurs during the golf swing. The complex and intense loads generated on the lumbar spine can predispose the athlete to muscle strain, herniation of the nucleus pulposus, spondylolysis, facet arthropathy, and spinal stenosis.[5,241,510] The recreational golfers vastly outnumber the professional. The loads on the lumbar spine are magnified in these "weekend warriors" who play sporadically, often with less-than-perfect technique and conditioning for the extreme twisting action that the game requires.

Evolution of the golf swing has increased the stress generated on the back and appears to be the source of the high incidence of lower back injuries.[298,440] Unlike the classic flowing swing that originated in Scotland, today the entire body is used to generate torque, resulting in a more powerful swing.[199] Four types of forces are generated on the golfer's lower back during this swing: three axial and one rotational. Lateral bending force is developed in a lateral-lateral direction, a shear force is developed in an anterior and posterior direction, and a compressive force is generated craniocaudally. Rotational forces develop from the twisting of the vertebrae during the swing; along the axis of the spine. Hosea and Gatt[200] studied these forces in both the amateur and professional golfer and found that the amateur golfer created approximately 80% greater peak lateral bending and shear loads than the professional. They attributed this to the variability of the amateur's swing pattern. An amateur golfer generates a peak shear load of 560 N. In comparison, weightlifters doing squat lifts generate 867 N of peak shear load. These shear forces have been implicated as a cause of spondylolysis. Cadaveric testing by several authors revealed that mean peak shear loads in the range of 570±190 N can result in fractures of the pars interarticularis.[111,208] In the Hosea and Gatt study, golfers were producing compression loads of 6000-7500 N. A compression load of 5448 N was required, in a study by Adams and Hutton,[4] to produce disc disruption. It is easy to see how this continuous stress over time can cause damage to the vertebrae of the spine. The study also showed that the golf swing generated compression loads up to eight times the body weight in both the amateur and professional golfer. Torque at L3-4, which is associated with lower back pain and injury from the golf swing, averaged 85.2 N in amateurs and 56.8 N in the professional. This discrepancy is probably secondary to inferior technique.[5,142]

Lower back pain in the golfer can have numerous etiologies. It may be described as mechanical, discogenic, spondylogenic, or related to facet arthropathy.[234] Mechanical pain is commonly localized in the lumbar area, is associated with muscle spasms, and is often worsened with activity. Discogenic pain is often caused by herniation of the nucleus pulposus and results in irritation of the nerve root and sciatica. Pain is concentrated in the leg and is worsened by the Valsalva maneuver and sitting. It often presents with the victim witnessing a "pop" in the lower back followed in 1-2 days by lower-extremity pain and dermatomal deficits. L4 radiculopathy results in posterolateral thigh and anteromedial leg pain, which can be accompanied by weakened quadriceps and decreased deep tendon reflexes of the knee. L5 radiculopathy produces posterolateral thigh and anterolateral leg pain, with numbness of the lateral leg and the first dorsal web space. The anterior tibialis and extensor hallucis longus muscles may also be affected. The S1 nerve root is the most commonly affected. Radiculopathy results in posterolateral thigh and leg pain and decreased sensation of the lateral heel and foot. The deep tendon reflex of the ankle can be lost, and plantar flexion weakness is observed.[200] The straight-leg raising test is positive in discogenic pain. Spondylogenic pain is caused by a pars interarticularis defect. It is often the result of the repetitive loads placed on the lumbar spine during the swing.[111,208] It presents with lumbar back pain over the pars without sciatica or neurological deficits and is worsened by lumbar hyperextension. Facet joint arthropathy begins with degeneration of the synovial cartilage, progresses to the development of osteophytes and loose vertebral bodies, and is caused by repetitive trauma and the aging process. The chronic rotational and compressive forces of the golf swing are major factors in the development of this condition. The affected individual presents with nonlocalized back pain that is relieved by sitting and worsened with walking. The affected joints are tender to palpation.

Peripheral Nerve Injury

Golf-associated elbow injuries occur in 4% of professional and 24% of amateur golfers.[244] Most elbow injuries occur near or at the impact phase of the golf swing.[379] Symptoms of ulnar nerve involvement are frequently present; however, radial tunnel symptoms are very uncommon in this population. As many as 20% of players presenting with ulnar numbness are diagnosed with medial epicondylitis.

The repetitive nature of golf lends itself to the occurrence of carpal tunnel syndrome.[519] This is more common in the right hand of the right-handed golfer and the left hand of the left-handed golfer and is secondary to the greater range of motion of the dominant hand during the golf swing. The diagnosis is made clinically by tests such as Tinel's or Phalen's sign and a review of the medical history. The condition is treated by splinting and by restricting play for up to 6 weeks. Refractory cases may respond to surgical release of the carpal tunnel.

Morton's neuroma is a benign but annoying condition experienced by golfers. It is caused by entrapment of the common digital nerve between adjacent metatarsal heads and the transverse metatarsal ligament where it bifurcates into the proper digital nerve. This usually occurs in the third metatarsal interspace. Symptoms range from pain to anesthesia of the adjacent toes. Mulder's sign is the reproduction of symptoms by exerting pressure on the foot. Choosing shoes that are sufficiently wide so that they do not cause compression of the forefoot is the initial treatment for this condition. Injection with local anesthetic and surgical resection are also treatment options.

Gymnastics

The sport of gymnastics has become increasingly popular in the past 10 to 20 years and increased participation has exposed a greater number of athletes to both acute and chronic injuries. The overall injury rate is reportedly exceeded only by football, wrestling, and softball. The risk of injury is proportional to the skill level of the participant. This is likely the result of more hours of practice and greater exposure time as well as increased intensity during the workout. Some injuries appear to be specific to gymnastics. Certain activities such as vaulting and hyperextension cause particular impact loads that can result in repeated microtrauma injuries to the lower back. Snook[429] evaluated 70 participants in a 5-year study of women gymnasts and reported 66 major injuries (i.e., those brought to the attention of a physician and producing disability). Forty-seven of these athletes sustained injuries, and the author concluded that women's gymnastics should be recognized as a hazardous sport for the competitor. Pettrone and Ricciardelli[353] conducted a prospective analysis of club-level gymnastic injuries over one season. Among 542 competitive- and 2016 noncompetitive-level athletes, 62 injuries (51 acute and 11 chronic) were reported. This resulted in an overall rate of injury of 5.3 per 100 competitors and 0.7 per 100 beginners. The study demonstrated that certain activities were more prone to injury, with 21 injuries occurring during floor exercises, 13 on the beam, nine on the vault, six on the uneven parallel bars, and two on the springboard.

Lindner and Caine[266] compiled injury information on 178 competitive female gymnasts over a 3-year period. The overall injury rate was found to be 30 per 100 gymnasts per year, or 0.52 injuries per 1000 hours. "Missed moves" were the most frequently cited injury mechanisms, while somersaults and handsprings were the most injury-producing moves. The majority of injuries occurred with moves that were basic or moderately difficult and well established with the athlete. Kolt and Kirkby[245] conducted an 18-month prospective injury survey of 64 Australian elite and subelite female gymnasts. The authors reported 349 injuries. This resulted in a per-person injury rate of 6.29 for the elite and 4.95 for the subelite gymnasts over the 18-month study. The National Registry of Gymnastic Catastrophic Injury was established in 1978.[95] In the first 4 years, 20

Gymnastics: History

The origin of gymnastics dates back more than 2000 years. At that time, gymnastics was seen as an activity, not a sport. Gymnastics was introduced to the U.S. and its school systems in the 1830s. In 1881, the International Gymnastics Federation was formed, then called the Bureau of the European Gymnastics Federation, promoting international competition. In the U.S., the Amateur Athletic Union was established in 1833 to manage the sport of gymnastics, along with most other amateur sports. Prior to this time, gymnastic competitions were held by a variety of clubs and organizations. The first large-scale meeting of gymnasts occurred at the 1896 Olympics, when male athletes from five countries competed in gymnastic events (the horizontal bar, parallel bars, pommel horse, rings, and vault).

injuries of the cervical spine occurred. Of these, 17 gymnasts remained quadriplegic and three died secondary to the injury. Notably, most of the injuries occurred in experienced gymnasts during practice.

There is a relatively low incidence of injury to the brain in this sport. Catastrophic head injury is most commonly caused in this sport by the dismount in which an athlete lands on his/her head. Between 1982 and 1995, 0.43 annual head injuries per 100,000 high school gymnasts were reported. One fatality was recorded related to head trauma (F. Mueller and R. Cantu, 1996). Caine et al[72] reported one concussion during a study of injuries in young competitive gymnasts. This resulted in an incidence of fewer than 1% of all injuries related to the sport.

Spinal Injury

The back is an area of the body that is often injured by gymnasts. It is subject to any force that must be supported, which includes the body's weight itself, as well as the forces due to very high accelerations of body parts. Alexander[8] reported that gymnastics (along with weightlifting and football) is a sport with the greatest risk of back injury. The most common etiologies of back injury in this sport are the repeated hyperextensions of the back, which are compounded by impact loading from tumbling and landing from height.[494] Kolt and Kirkby[245] reported a back-injury rate of 15% in an 18-month study of elite and subelite female gymnasts. Goldstein et al[165] studied three groups of top-level female gymnasts of pre-elite, elite, national, and Olympic caliber for patterns of back injury. Of the gymnasts studied, 9% of pre-elite (one of 11), 43% of elite (six of 14), and 63% of Olympic-level (five of eight) had spine abnormalities. The authors concluded that the average hours of training per week and the participant's age are associated with abnormalities of the spine. Silver et al[423] reported 31 gymnastics-related spinal injuries between 1954 and 1984. Of these, 28 were in the cervical region and three in the thoracolumbar region.

Rhythmic gymnasts, who must combine gymnastics with dance, are at particular risk for lower back injury. A study of these athletes found that 86% of participants complained of back pain; the only injury recorded that required a period of nonparticipation in the sport was a low-back injury.[207] The etiologies of this pain ranged from muscle strains to complete fracture of the pars interarticularis (spondylolysis).

The young age of many participants can also play a role in injuries. Elite female gymnasts are more vulnerable to vertebral overload injuries during the pubertal growth phase. Young female athletes are going through periods of rapid growth, and intense training could provide for conditions where the gymnast is more injury prone. Magnetic resonance imaging (MRI) was performed by Tertti et al[463] on 35 young competitive gymnasts and 10 control subjects in order to detect the number of degenerated discs and other lumbar spinal disorders. All gymnasts who showed evidence of disc abnormality on MRI received lumbar radiographs. Three of the 35 gymnasts had evidence on MRI of degenerated discs associated with Scheuermann's manifestations and spondylolysis, which were confirmed by radiograph. The authors concluded that, despite the excessive range of motion and the strong axial loading of the lumbar spine associated with the sport, primary damage to the intervertebral discs is uncommon in young gymnasts during growth.

The lumbar spine is the only bony connection between the upper and lower body, and all forces must be transmitted via this structure. Female gymnasts display a higher than average incidence of stress-related injuries to this area. Garrick and Requa[154] reported that lumbar strains and sprains occur more frequently in this sport than in other women's interscholastic sports. Hall[178] evaluated lumbar hyperextension and impact forces of five commonly executed gymnastics skills. These skills were the front walkover, the back walkover, the front handspring, the back handspring, and the handspring vault. Of the skills examined, the handspring vault resulted in the highest vertical and lateral impact forces, and the back handspring and back walkover required the greatest amounts of lumbar hyperextension. Maximum lumbar hyperextension was found to occur near the time that either the hands or the feet sustained impact force during the front and back walkovers and the back handspring. Mackie and Taunton[280] studied injuries in 100 female gymnasts over 40 months and found five cases of lumbar hyperextension syndrome.

Spondylolysis is a relatively common injury in the gymnast. If the condition is not recognized early, it can evolve into spondylolisthesis. Letts et al[261] reported that stress fracture of the pars interarticularis is becoming an increasingly common cause of disability in highly competitive adolescent athletes. The authors have also documented this lesion in 14 adolescent athletes engaged in activities involving flexion/extension of the lumbar spine, and have found that gymnastics and hockey were the most common sports resulting in this lesion. The injury can be particularly troublesome. In four athletes, the lesions were bilateral and in 10 were unilateral. While the lesions healed with immobilization in a thoracolumbar brace in five athletes with unilateral lesions, none of the lesions in the nine other gymnasts healed in spite of 3 months of immobilization.

The effects of gymnastic spinal injury can reach into the athlete's life after ceasing participation in the sport. Konermann and Sell[246] examined 24 former female artistic gymnasts of the German national team for spinal deformities after the end of their athletic careers. Of 15 gymnasts who had complained of low back pain during their careers, seven had pain that persisted into retirement. Lumbar radiographs revealed bilateral spondylolysis at L5 in six athletes, scoliosis in six, degenerative changes of the intervertebral joints in five, spondylolisthesis at L5/S1 in three, retrolisthesis at L5/S1 in two, and unilateral spondylolysis in one. Wismach and Krause[518] studied 36 former competitive artistic female gymnasts and 10 female general gymnasts at least 3 years following their withdrawal from the sport, for any pathological changes in their vertebral column. In the artistic gymnast group, of the 64% who had complained of back pain during participation, 61% still had problems after having given up the sport. Radiographs showed degenerative changes of the vertebral bodies and the intervertebral joints in 51%, and a 31% incidence of spondylolysis was observed (2.5 times greater than the general population).

In 1997 and 1998, 325 SCIs related to gymnastics were reported.[512] According to the NSCIDRC, gymnastics accounted for 6% of all sports-related SCIs between 1973 and 1981 (J. Young et al, 1982). This represented 1% of all SCIs at the time. The mean age of gymnastics-related SCI in 1980 and 1981 was found to be 18 years (range 13-21). The injuries occurred in men in 88% and to an individual not participating in an organized class or team 88% of the time. Of those injured, 25% were considered skilled at gymnastics. Clarke,[97] in a study of quadriplegic injuries in high school and college athletes between 1973 and 1975, found gymnastics the only sport with female representatives.

Peripheral Nerve Injury

Injuries to the peripheral nerves of gymnasts are relatively uncommon. However, both ulnar neuropathies and femoral cutaneous nerve injuries have been reported.[194] Paralysis of the femoral nerve has also been reported secondary to gymnastic injuries. Takami et al[454] described two such cases secondary to traumatic rupture of the iliacus muscle and a resulting hematoma. Along with femoral nerve palsy, these patients usually present with groin pain, a tender mass in the iliac fossa, and flexion contracture of the hip. This condition occurs more frequently in subjects with bleeding disorders or who have a delayed onset of paralysis. Traumatic femoral neuropathy can also occur without the development of a hematoma. These cases are often the result of stretching of the affected nerve or hemorrhage into the nerve sheath and are frequently associated with the sudden flexion or extension of the hips.[61]

Hang Gliding

More than 30,000 people in the U.S. actively engage in hang gliding. The potential for catastrophic injury from this sport is not hard to imagine when you consider the idea of flying by attaching oneself to a very large kite and running down a steep hill or over a cliff. Despite these inherent risks, the sport continues to grow.

Between 1973 and 1975, there were 81 known fatalities from this sport in the U.S.; data are scarce on nonfatal injuries. A report by Tongue[465] in 1977 examined causes and types of injuries in a group of 144 injured pilots (the injuries were fatal in 37). Most of the injuries were the result of inflight errors in judgment versus equipment failure. Inflight errors were only slightly more common than preflight errors. Tongue estimated that 20% of all nonfatal accidents could have been avoided with proper preflight equipment checks, improved knowledge of micrometeorology, and better analysis of weather conditions. A common cause of injury in the inexperienced pilot is stalling the kite and attempting turns that cannot be completed and that result in high-speed downwind landings. The more experienced pilots tended to fly higher and farther and appeared to be the greater risk takers. Many of the injuries in the experienced pilots resulted when they attempted to alter seated harnesses into prone harnesses without a safety inspection. Only one death was related to a primary equipment failure. Of 37 fatal injuries, 20% involved alcohol. The greatest cause of injury was attempted inflight maneuvers, problems with equipment, and peer pressure (e.g., stunts and ingestion of alcohol). These injuries usually involved massive head, neck, and chest trauma, and included shattered skulls, ruptured aortas, heart lacerations, and pulmonary collapse. The majority arrived at the hospital deceased. The average age of victims of fatal injuries was 24 years.

Hang Gliding: History

The origin of gliding/flying dates back to the 1890s. At this time, German inventor Otto Lilienthal designed the first gliders made of wood. Orville and Wilbur Wright later modified the design of these gliders. These modifications produced the highly aerodynamic modern glider. Since the 1970s, hang gliding has been a popular form of flying. Hang gliders are crafts that are similar to kites. The flier is attached to a harness and is supported on a swing-like frame. Shifting the body weight allows the flier to steer the craft in various directions. Competitions are held at both the national and international levels.

Head, Neck, and Spinal Cord Injury

According to the NSCIDRC, the mean age of hang gliding-related SCI in 1980 and 1981 was 38 years (range 21-64). Seventy-five percent of injuries occurred in men. In all cases, injuries occurred to an individual not participating in an organized class or team. Of those injured, 75% were considered skilled at hang gliding and 25% resulted in quadriplegia (K. Clarke, 1983).

Of the 37 fatalities in the Tongue study,[465] three involved severe closed head injuries and two were the result of high cervical spine fracture/dislocations. Of these, three fell from just 30 feet above the ground. Only two of the victims were not wearing helmets. A severe scalp hemorrhage caused the death of a pilot suspended from a tree. It appears that experienced pilots are more at risk for fatal injury. This has also been shown to be true with skydiving. Nonfatal injuries commonly involve the upper extremities and spine. This is due in part to impact with the control bar.

Of the nonfatal injuries, 16% were to the head. This included facial injury as well as closed head trauma. Of nonfatal injuries, 17% involved the spine. Cervical spine injuries were more common with the pilot flying prone, while lumbosacral injuries were more frequent in seated pilots. Of the 24 spinal injuries examined, five resulted in paraplegia and one in quadriplegia. Because of the difference in landing trajectory between skydiving and hang gliding, parachutists incurred three times the number of lower-extremity injuries as hang-glider pilots.[187] The inexperienced pilot has the greatest risk of nonfatal injury.[253,465]

Hurling

A major difference between hurling and other "stick" games is that the majority of the play during hurling is above the participants' heads in the air. As a result, injuries to the head and face are common. Injuries are usually a result of impact with the ball or the stick. Crowley and Condon[108] found 34 of 94 hurling injuries to be to the head or face, and Cuddihy and Hurley[112] reported that 141 of 350 injuries related to hurling were to this area. Over the past 20 years, helmets and faceguards have been introduced to the sport, and a resulting decrease in injuries is apparent. However, many players resist their use, with the greatest resistance seen in the senior players.

Watson[502] conducted a prospective study of hurling injuries in 74 players over the 8 months of one season. There were 92 match- and 43 training-related injuries, giving 342.47 injuries per 10,000 hours of matches and 43.83 injuries per 10,000 hours of training. Overall, there were 107 injuries per 10,000 hours of participation and 2.74 injuries per player over a 12-month period. The most common type of injury was muscle strain, usually to the hamstring (24% of the 135 total injuries). The sites traditionally associated with the sport (i.e., the fingers, head, and face) accounted for 27% of the total injuries. The injuries were to the back in 11% and to the head in 9%. Concussions accounted for 3% of the total injuries. As in most sports, the majority of injuries occurred during competition.[18] Watson found no relationship between the position of the player and the injuries. Importantly, 41% of the injuries were attributed to foul play. The study also evaluated the use of protective equipment in participants. In 74 players, the majority used no safety equipment; 19 of the players wore helmets only and six wore helmets with visors. Mouthguards were worn by three players. The study by Watson suggested that the incidence of injuries in hurling is high and may be attributed to poor conditioning, poor protection, and lack of enforcement of the rules.

Lacrosse

Lacrosse is a game played in close contact at a fast pace, using swinging sticks to propel a hard projectile at high speed. Five mechanisms of head and neck injury exist. A player can be injured by being struck by another player, the ball, a stick, or an inanimate object such as a bench. Injuries can also occur from falls. In a study by Webster et al,[504] 89% of injuries were caused by sticks or balls. Goldenberg and Hossler[163] reported a rate of 91%. According to the NSCIDRC, in 1980 and 1981 all injuries occurred in men and in individuals considered adept at the sport (K. Clarke, 1983).

Men's lacrosse is considered a contact sport and women's lacrosse is a noncontact sport. Perhaps because of this, the use of protective equipment in the women's game is used only occasionally or not at all. There are even reports of some organizations that required the use of protective equipment to be shifting away from this requirement.[388] This has led to an increase in both eye and head injuries in the women's game. The NCAA reports that the incidence of head and face injury in the women is actually higher than in the men.[334,335] In college women's lacrosse, the rate of head and neck injuries has been reported as 0.6 per 1000 exposures;[335] scholastic women's lacrosse has even higher rates of head and face injury at 1.1 per 1000.[163] Webster et al[504] examined the incidence of head and face injuries in 700 female lacrosse players (aged 13-18 years) and reported an injury rate of 0.71 per 1000 exposures. Goldenberg and Hossler[163] found similar rates of injury to the head and face. Exposures included both games and practices. Injuries were three times more common in games, probably due to the more aggressive play spawned by competition. Goldenberg and Hossler also examined the effectiveness of protective goggles in decreasing injuries. They found that the overall injury rate of players wearing the goggles fell by 17%. When only game injuries were analyzed, the injury rate fell by 51%.

Head injuries are frequent and can be catastrophic.[259,260,270,292] Rimel et al[372] reported an acute epidural hematoma resulting from a strike to the head from a lacrosse stick. A study of 586 college players revealed six concussions.[325] Kuland et al[256] discovered three concussions in a study of 58 summer league players. In men's lacrosse, most head injuries are superficial, probably due to the requirement of helmets with facemasks.

Martial Arts

An estimated 1.5 to 2 million people practice the martial arts in the U.S. Of these, 20% are children.[40] The male-to-female ratio of participants is approximately five to one. Participants become involved for various reasons. Some are interested in competition or developing self-defense skills, while others hope to increase their cardiovascular fitness, flexibility, or self-esteem. Martial art participants usually practice 2-4 times a week. Sparring usually involves no contact to the head, back, legs, or groin. Although to spectators the sport may appear violent, severe injuries are rare. Oler et al,[345] analyzing data from national computer surveillance of emergency rooms, discovered no fatalities or weapon injuries related to the martial arts. Any fatalities reported in the martial arts are usually the result of impacts to the head or chest. Wilkerson[514] reported three fatalities from anterior chest trauma.

Older martial art participants appear to have a higher overall injury rate.[70] Advanced students were also at a higher risk of injury. In one study, the injury rate for karate was calculated to be 2.7 per 1000 hours of practice. This falls within the lower-injury range for various sports.[425,487,514] It has been reported that the martial arts are safer than golf, soccer, or gymnastics. The overall incidence of martial arts injury is 1/20th that of American football.[39,462] Head injuries are uncommon and are usually minor concussions.

Injuries occur at higher rates during tournaments. A survey by Birrer and Birrer[37] of more than 6000 athletes found that 59% of injuries occurred during tournament competition. These authors also found that the experience of the athlete is inversely proportional to the injury rate.[38,216,345] This conclusion was supported in studies by Stricevic et al.[441] They also reported that punches have a higher injury ratio versus kicks and that protective gear used on the head, hands, chest, and limbs decreases the morbidity associated with the sport. McLatchie et al[304] described injuries sustained in the first European Knock-down Karate Championships in 1978. In this competition, no protective equipment other than foot and shin pads and groin guards was allowed. Of 70 competitors, 37 sustained injuries; 15 of the injuries were potentially serious. Eleven injuries occurred to the head or face, including two concussions resulting from high kicks to the head. An earlier report by McLatchie and Morris[303] demonstrated a significant reduction in injuries when padding is used.

Pieter and Zemper[354] studied the rates of injuries sustained during junior taekwondo competitions involving 3341 boys and 917 girls. The authors found little difference in the rates of injury between boys and girls (58 and 56 per 1000 exposures, respectively). Most injuries occurred to the lower extremities. In the study, participants used head and chest protection, arm and shin pads, and groin cups. Head and neck injuries were the second most injured body parts and occurred at a rate of 21 per 1000 exposures in boys and 23 per 1000 exposures in girls.

Martial Arts: History

The sports that are referred to as martial arts have their origins mainly in Japan (Okinawa), Korea, and China. *Karate* originated in Okinawa, Japan and is known as "the way of the empty hand." It consists of an equal use of the hands and the feet. In tournaments, competitors wear no chest protection, and footpads are optional. *Taekwondo* began in Korea and is known as "the foot and hand way." It is thought of as a sport more than a form of self-defense. High kicks and stylistic techniques are common. The use of the feet is much more common than the hands. Taekwondo has become an Olympic sport. Participants in tournaments wear chest protectors along with foot pads and a head protector.

Kung fu, meaning skill and art, originated in China. It consists of flowing circular movements that appear quite graceful. The hand and foot are utilized equally, and open-handed pushing techniques are often used. Kung fu is considered one of the soft forms of martial arts. *Aikido*, the way of harmony, attempts to redirect the attacker's energy against himself. It has become well known as the style of the actor Steven Segal. Throws and joint-pressure techniques are perfected. Injuries are often due to falls or joint sprains. *Jujitsu* is similar in many respects to aikido and is referred to as compliance techniques. It also depends on joint manipulation to control an opponent. Jujitsu has, however, a more aggressive style. Injuries in Jujitsu, as in aikido, are usually due to falls and joint injuries. *Judo* is also known as "the compliant way" and relies on throwing the opponent and often resembles wrestling. *Hapkido* is a Korean form of martial arts. Hapkido closely resembles aikido, and consists of kicks and hand strikes.

Head Injury

In karate and taekwondo tournaments, kicks to the head are legal. Punches to the head are usually prohibited and, if allowed, the contact must be controlled. The use of headgear in the sport is controversial. Opponents claim that it actually increases the number of shear-force impacts to the brain because the athletes feel "protected" and attack the head more often and with more force. Shearing injury to the neurons of the brain results from the blunt trauma caused by blows to the head. The degree of injury is proportional to the degree of head acceleration. Impacts to the side of the head cause greater accelerative forces than those to the front. Comparisons of peak accelerations of blows to the head with and without headgear have been performed. The blows to the front and sides of the head were performed with bare hands, hand protectors, and 10-ounce boxing gloves. Kicks were also examined to the head with and without headgear using either bare feet or safety kick padding. Greater acceleration was achieved with kicks to the front of the head versus punches. In all cases, safety equipment and headgear did not lower peak accelerations.[2,103,414] Impacts to the chin can produce the maximum forces. This is secondary to the chin acting as a lever transmitting energy to the cranium.[414] Aside from direct damage to neurons, shearing forces can injure blood vessels, causing intracranial bleeding, most commonly resulting in subdural or intracerebral hematoma.

Poirier (personal communication, 1990) noted that head and neck injury accounted for 70% of injuries in young adult male and female participants in a semicontact karate competition. In this study, lower-extremity injuries accounted for 10% of the total. Poirier found a definite correlation between the weight of competitors and injury rate. This has also been observed in youth football, wrestling, and soccer.[160,274,296] Injuries most commonly resulted from unblocked attacks followed by attacking with a kick. Cerebral concussions occurred in 9% of the boys and 8% of the girls. Oler et al[345] studied injuries at a senior and junior U.S. National Taekwondo championship. In this study, head injuries made up 54% of all injuries. Upper extremities were involved in 14% of injuries and lower extremities in 13%. Concussions accounted for almost 10% of reported injuries, with 1% resulting in a loss of consciousness.

It has been shown that repeated concussive or subconcussive forces to the brain result in characteristic patterns of brain injury.[40] It is important to consider the effects of repeated blows to the head as cumulative. Dementia pugilistica is a syndrome resulting from traumatic encephalopathy. While first described in professional boxers, they are not the only athletes at risk.[109] Participants in American football, Rugby, soccer, and wrestling have been reported to face this hazard, which can occur in any person subjected to repeated impacts to the head.[2] The syndrome causes an increasingly euphoric personality with emotional lability. Both speech and the thought process are slowed, and the victim's memory is affected. The affected athlete usually has little insight into their mental deterioration.

Vertebral Artery Dissection

Crepin-Leblond et al[106] reported a case of vertebral artery dissection involving an 11-year-old judo participant following minor cervical trauma sustained during practice. When the injury occurred, the boy complained of immediate lateral cervical pain, which is the first symptom in approximately 80% of cases. Vertebral artery dissection is a rare but life-threatening injury in sports. It occurs most frequently following cervical trauma when the layers of the arterial wall are separated by blood flow. It has been reported in situations where the head is turned to the extreme, such as ceiling painting, driving backward, yoga, gymnastics, and chiropractic manipulation. Flexion or extension of less than 45° with a tilt of 30° is all that is needed to decrease vertebral artery flow.[466] This is secondary to the numerous bony structures in the neck, including the third atlantoaxial segment to which the vertebral artery is adjacent. It occurs more frequently in females, with an average age of approximately 40 years.

Injuries to the cervical spine are rare, as are head injuries, and they appear to be more common during tournament competitions.[39,354,479] Along with injuries related to falls and throws, the sport of judo allows some "choke holds" and can be hard on the cervical spine. The holds cut off blood flow through the carotid arteries, depriving the brain of blood and leading to loss of consciousness.[348,382]

Risks

Many injuries are the result of the spinning back kick or back hook kick, which are difficult to control. Kicks thrown slowly are easily countered, and the thrower's visibility is limited through much of the kick. A fatality caused by a spinning back kick to the face was reported by Oler et al.[345] Following the blow, the victim fell backward onto a hardwood floor and died within 24 hours. He was found to have incurred an occipital skull fracture, bilateral acute subdural hematomas, contusions of the frontal and temporal lobes, and secondary brainstem herniation.

Wood breaking is often a part of martial arts competition. To advance, the competitor must be able to break increasing thicknesses of wood using various parts of the body. Nieman and Swann[340] reported a student of karate developing weakness and wasting of the hypothenar eminence secondary to traumatic neurapraxia resulting from repeatedly impacting of hard objects with his hands.

Parachuting/Sky Diving

The conditions of the sport parachuting are quite different than those of the military. Sports descents are often from 3000 to 10,000 feet. There are also long intervals between jumpers. In contrast, military parachutists jump at a much lower altitude (800 to 1000 feet), carry a heavy load of equipment, and may leave the plane as quickly as half-second intervals apart. Obviously, these jumps have a significantly higher rate of injury. The U.S. Parachuting Association noted that in North America approximately 30 parachuting-related fatalities occur annually. This calculates into 1.2 deaths for every 100,000 jumps. Ellitsgaard[136] reported a rate of serious injury in sports parachutists of 0.14%. This figure was for jumpers of all skill levels. If only experienced parachutists are examined, the rate of serious injury declines to 0.13%.[10] Hallel and Naggan[179] reported a rate of serious injury of 0.156 for parachutists training in the military. When compared to bungee jumping, a parachuter has five times the risk of serious or fatal injury.[444] Approximately 10% of skydivers suffer injuries requiring medical attention, 1000 times the rate of injury for bungee jumping.[253] Most serious injuries and deaths are the result of two parachuters colliding while in descent. The frequency of injury is higher in the novice jumper.[10]

Types of Injury

Because of the difference in landing trajectory between skydiving and hang gliding, parachutists incurred three times the number of lower-extremity injuries as hang-glider pilots.[253] Parachutists and hang-glider pilots with more than 200 flights or jumps have higher risks of fatal mishaps versus the inexperienced jumper or pilot.[253] Lowdon and Wetherill[278] analyzed 205 injuries in 51,828 military parachute jumps over a 6-year

Parachuting/Sky Diving: History

The origin of parachuting is believed to date back to the 1100s, when individuals in China may have used parachutes and inventors such as Leonardo da Vinci of Italy designed plans for parachute-like devices. However, French inventor Andre-Jacques Garnerin is known as the first parachutist, making his first jump in 1797. During World War II, military forces relied heavily on parachutists, and after the war surplus parachutes were plentiful. In the mid-1960s, sport parachutes started to replace the old military-style systems as parachutists began calling the sport skydiving and calling themselves skydivers. Design changes enhanced the ability to open the parachute and made it more maneuverable. During the 1970s and 1980s, sport skydivers continued to test improved designs and materials that would enable participants to fly great distances with more maneuverability. Two-person and four-person tandem jumping equipment were also developed, allowing the novice a rapid introduction into the sport. After the late 1980s, skydiving continued to grow in popularity around the world because of the ease of use and reliability of the equipment.

period. They found a serious-injury rate of 0.22 per 100 descents and four fatalities. This rate of injury is lower than that reported for sports parachutists. Head injuries occurred in 14 jumpers (0.027%), and spinal fractures in 16 (0.031%). These rates are similar to those reported by Binns and Potter.[35] While the majority of injuries resulted from hard or awkward landings, most serious injuries occurred either from entanglement in another parachute or air steal. Entanglements and air steal accounted for four spinal fractures, three multiple injuries, and two fatalities. These injuries are similar to those reported by numerous other authors.[10,136,140,179]

Rodeo: History

The origin of the rodeo dates back to the mid 19th century. During the early days of the American cattle industry, events would be held at various market centers once or twice a year in order to celebrate the cattle round up. At these market centers, competitions would be held to demonstrate the skills of the cowboys. It is not known where the first official rodeo competition was held. However, it most likely took place in Cheyenne, Wyoming in 1872. Rodeos are popular attractions in the U.S., especially in the southern and western parts of the country. Events include saddle bronco riding, steer wrestling, team roping, bareback bronco riding, calf roping, and bull riding. Women's events are limited and often involve barrel racing, goat-tying, or breakaway roping.

Rodeo

The potential for serious injury is obvious when one considers the size and brute strength of the athlete's opponent. There is no question that rough-stock riding, which consists of bull riding, bareback bronco riding, and saddle bronco riding, is high on the list of dangerous sports. It involves contact, collision, and repetitive forces. The bull rider appears to be the most at risk, sustaining 37% of all rodeo-related injuries.[63] While many injuries occur, there are few fatalities. Ferrer[144] found only one rodeo-related death in the period from 1970 to 1978. During 1994 and 1995, the Louisiana Central Nervous System Injury Registry identified five cases of central nervous system trauma associated with bull riding in rodeo events.[63] A series by Hamilton and Tranmer[180] analyzed nervous system injuries in 156 horse-related accidents. Of these, 7% (11) occurred during rodeo activities. According to the NSCIDRC, rodeo sports accounted for 1% of all sports-related SCIs between 1973 and 1981 (J. Young et al, 1982). This represented fewer than 0.5% of all SCIs at the time.

Studies have been performed on rodeo competition at varying levels. In 1987 and 1988, members of the National Intercollegiate Rodeo Association Southern Region were observed for injuries during a 7-month (10-rodeo) season. Of 156 athletes, 62 sustained a total of 138 acute injuries resulting from 3292 exposures. These figures suggest that rodeo athletes face an 89% potential for injury per season. In comparison, the injury potential for college football players is 47%, as reported by Canale et al.[74] Of the total injuries in rodeo, 92% occurred in the rough-stock riding and steer-wrestling events and 8% occurred in roping events by female athletes. Most injuries were to the upper body (66%); of these, 25% involved the head and neck. While the majority of the injuries were contusions, 14% of the total injuries were concussions. All of the concussions were Grade 1 or 2 and had no neurological sequelae. Of the head injuries incurred by the steer wrestlers, 75% were dental or maxillofacial trauma secondary to contact with the animal's horns. There was one case of a seizure occurring secondary to lumbosacral trauma. Of the ropers, there was one back injury. The injuries occurred during the completion of an athlete's ride in 23% and were attributed to equipment mishaps in 21%. Interestingly, 40% of all injuries occurred during the preliminary performance and 34% during the final performance.[311] Butterwick et al,[71] in a prospective cohort study, documented injury rates and treatment during one competitive season of Canadian professional rodeo. The competitors were from several countries, including Australia, Brazil, New Zealand, the U.S., and Canada. The group reported that 94 athletes were injured during 3882 individual competitor exposures, resulting in a composite injury rate of 2.3 per 100 competitor exposures, lower than that often reported in contact sports. Bareback riders and bull riders were found to have the highest injury rates (4.6 and 3.6 per 100 competitor exposures, respectively). The knee and ankle were the most frequently injured parts of the body, followed by the shoulder, elbow, and lower back.

Griffin et al[171] evaluated injuries sustained at the elite professional level of rodeo competition over a 6-year period. Of the 738 participants, 12% sustained injuries. This rate is very low compared with rates reported by others at state-level competitions (33% and 20%). As expected, the majority were incurred during rough-stock riding events, accounting for 86% of the injuries. Bull riders had the highest percentage of injuries per exposure at 8%, and account for 41% of the injured participants. Both the controlled and uncontrolled dismounts from the animal were often associated with injury. Other causes of injury were found to be from equipment (rigging) failure. In the bull ride, concussions were reported secondary to being "hooked" by the bull. There were also reports of cervical and lumbar sprain and acute torticollis secondary to being thrown. Being thrown from a horse in both saddle and bareback bronco riding frequently resulted in a concussion. There was also a report of cervicothoracic strain secondary to missing the animal in the steer-wrestling competition. Only eight of 90 injuries were deemed serious enough to prevent the contestant from continuing in the competition, and no fatalities occurred. The safest event was roping. Nebergall et al[336] concluded that at the elite professional level, the risk of injury is much lower than at the state or college competition level. This is likely secondary to more experience, better physical conditioning, and greater athletic ability, as well as the fact that many athletes more prone to injury were "weeded out" before reaching this high level of competition.

Rowing

Rowing is a taxing sport that has a significant injury rate among competitive participants. Boland and Hosea[51] reported that the back and knees are the most common areas of injury. The sport requires both strength and aerobic conditioning. Because of this, competitive athletes often train year round and are more likely to suffer overuse injuries. The act of rowing places a large amount of stress on the back. Karlson[232] described this movement as being similar to an incomplete dead lift. In 1980, Stallard[436] reported that a technique known as sweep rowing, in which the athlete's back is slightly twisted during the stroke to increase its effectiveness, increases the incidence of back pain.

Injuries can range from spondylolysis to disc disease. Pain in the lower back that is exacerbated by extension suggests spondylolysis resulting from stresses to the pars interarticularis during the stroke. Soler and Calderon[430] found a 17% incidence of spondylolysis in high-level rowers. This is significantly greater than that of the general population, which varies between 3% and 7%. They concluded that sports with elements of torsion against resistance, lumbar hyperextension, and rotation have a greater risk for this condition. At the beginning of the stroke, the back is in a flexed position, which increases the stress to the vertebral discs. Disc disease in the rower has been reported to frequently present without the usual symptoms of pain radiating to the legs.[232] This is believed to be due to central disc disease, which does not compress the nerve roots of the spinal cord.

Injuries to the peripheral nerves are usually the result of improper techniques or poorly fitting equipment. Rowers are at risk for carpal tunnel syndrome secondary to entrapment of the median nerve. This is the result of the constant grip that the athlete must maintain on the oar. Rowers who hold the equipment too tightly increase the risk of this injury. Injury to the sciatic nerve of the athlete is also a threat. This is commonly secondary to pressure from an improperly fitted seat. Karlson[232] described a ridge on the front of the seat that can place direct pressure on this nerve.

Rowing: History

The sport of competitive rowing dates back centuries to the galleys of ancient Rome and Egypt. The oldest modern rowing contest began in 1715 and is still held annually between Oxford and Cambridge University. Collegiate rowing became firmly established in 1895, when several colleges joined together and founded the Intercollegiate Rowing Association. It was adopted by the modern Olympics in 1900, and became a formal part of the Olympic Games in 1908. Currently, there is increasing participation with recreational rowing machines. Some of these machines actually use a computer to generate a competitor, making aspects of the sport available to those who have never been in a boat.

Shooting Sports: History

Shooting was introduced as an Olympic sport in 1896 and has been in each of the modern Olympiads except the Games of 1904 and 1928. It has evolved from a leisurely, more aristocratic European tradition of shooting to a strict discipline of uniform courses of fire and strict regulations governing clothing, equipment, and firearms. Olympic competition consists of 13 shooting events encompassing disciplines in the small-bore and air-powered rifle, handgun, and shotgun. Seven of these events are for men and four for women; two events involving the shotgun are open to both men and women. The popularity of shooting sports in the U.S. is evident in the more than 12,000 shooting events sponsored each year by the National Rifle Association, the national governing body for competitive shooting sports in this country.

Shooting Sports

Back Injury/Pain

The most common musculoskeletal complaint of the competitive shooter is lower back pain. A study by Volski et al[493] found that nearly 80% of shooters experience back pain during a competition and 63% suffer back pain after a competition. This is likely secondary to the prolonged hyperextension and rotation of the spine required while aiming. Back pain could also be the result of ilioband tightness.

Peripheral Nerve Injury

Injuries to the long thoracic nerve in shooters often cause paralysis of the serratus anterior muscle. This is usually the result of traction to the nerve secondary to the positional stress of the shooting position. Woodhead[520] reported this injury in a world-class marksman. Full recovery usually occurs in an average of 9 months and may take up to 2 years. The injury often presents with spontaneous severe pain in the region of the shoulder followed about 2 weeks later by weakness of the serratus anterior and a winged scapula deformity associated with its loss of function.[147]

Hearing

Injury to hearing is a common complaint among shooters. The right ear is more significantly affected than the left ear due to the position of the rifle in most right-handed shooters. Charakorn and Amatyakul[84] found that 9% of studied subjects were suffering from hearing impairment at the level of 3000-8000 Hertz. The authors also found a correlation between hearing deficits and the length of shooting exposure.

Neurological Toxicity Associated with Lead Exposure

Lead absorption and intoxication in users of indoor small-bore rifle ranges can be a significant problem. Svensson et al[447] found increased blood lead levels in 22 marksmen during an indoor shooting season (median level: before 106, after 138). George et al[157] found that the average red cell lead level of male shooters was 2.4 times normal and is comparable to the levels found in many occupationally exposed groups. Maximum air lead levels in facilities studied were 210 mg/m^3, more than twice the workplace exposure standard of the U.S. Department of Labor. Both Novotny et al[342] and Fischbein et al[146] reported central nervous system symptoms correlating with the blood lead and zinc protoporphyrin levels in shooters. High levels of lead absorption are known to cause symptomatic neuropathy. Landrigan et al[258] found slowing of motor and sensory nerve conduction velocity secondary to lead poisoning among instructors at an indoor pistol range. He et al[186] studied subclinical neuropathy due to low levels of occupational lead exposure by electroneurographic studies. Statistically significant differences in lead-exposed subjects were demonstrated in 11 electroneurographic parameters, including motor nerve conduction velocity and distal latency of median, ulnar, and peroneal nerves as well as sensory nerve conduction velocity and distal latency of median, ulnar, and sural nerves. Indoor ranges are not the only shooting environments with a risk of lead toxicity. Goldberg et al[162] reported that significant lead exposure and absorption could occur even at outdoor firing ranges. The authors also suggested that the use of copper-jacketed ammunition might decrease airborne lead levels and lead absorption. Tripathi et al[476] concluded that the use of totally copper-jacketed bullets significantly reduced airborne lead levels by a factor of 21 in the personal breathing zone samples and by a factor of 7.5 in the general area air samples.

Skiing

Skiing is a high-speed sport with an associated high risk of injury to the nervous system that can result in quadriplegia or death. Nonetheless, it attracts more than 200 million participants annually.[205] The overall rate of injury is approximately 2.5 injuries per 1000 skier-days.[222] This has decreased substantially from the 1950s, when the injury rate was reported to be 10 injuries per 1000 skier-days.[139] This is secondary to improvements in equipment, such as release bindings and ski brakes. Injuries to the head and spine account for between 8% and 11% of skiing injuries.[223,267]

Catastrophic Injury

Morrow et al[324] reported a rate of one fatality per 1.5 million skier-days in a 7-year study of deaths related to skiing. A common cause of serious injury is traveling at a high rate of speed in an uncontrolled manner. Recreational skiers can easily reach speeds of 40 miles per hour when traveling down a slope, and injuries similar to those seen in automobile accidents can result. Collisions are also common etiologies of catastrophic injury. In a retrospective study of skiers categorized as severely injured, 31% were injured by colliding at considerable speed with either a moving object (such as a skier, snow cat, or ski lift) or a fixed object (such as a tree or rock). The most severe injuries were the result of collisions with fixed objects.[139] A 5-year study by Myles et al[328] analyzed 145 downhill skiers who suffered injury to the nervous system or spine resulting in five fatalities. These injuries were three times more common in men than in women, and the mean age of the victims was 24 years. The authors reported that 88 skiers sustained a head injury, 25 had spinal fractures, 20 had spinal cord or nerve root injury, and 12 had peripheral nerve injury. The injuries were most commonly the result of a fall, followed in frequency by collision with a tree. Collisions were more frequently associated with more serious injuries. Factors in the accidents included reckless skiing, the design of ski runs, and the use of man-made snow.

Second-impact syndrome has been reported by McQuillen et al,[307] in the case of an 18-year-old downhill skier who remained in a persistent vegetative state following a fall. This occurs when an athlete suffers a head injury such as a concussion and has a second head injury before the symptoms of the first assault have resolved. In this syndrome, the second injury can be remarkably minor.[77,79]

Head Injury

Between 1982 and 1995, 15.11 annual head injuries per 100,000 college skiers were reported; one fatality was recorded related to head trauma (F. Mueller and R. Cantu, 1996). A study by Morrow et al[324] found that of 16 skiing-related fatalities reported in the state of Vermont over a 7-year period, 14 were secondary to injuries of the head and neck and 13 victims had skull fractures. These data suggest a rate of 0.25 head injuries per 1000 skier-days. Interestingly, the Morrow data demonstrated that occipital fractures often lead to a rapid demise of the patient, while parietotemporal and basal fractures led to survival for a longer period. These injuries are more frequent in the young male athlete. Experienced participants more commonly suffer serious injuries to this area of the body. In a review of 258 head injuries, Lindsjo et al[267] found the most common type to be a contusion with open wounds (44% of cases); contusions with concussions accounted for 33%. They also reported one fatality secondary to a basal skull fracture. Harris[183] reported 82 skull fractures in 347 skiing-related neurological injuries. Of these, the frontal bone was the most commonly affected, followed by basal and parietal fractures. The recreational skiing population has not widely accepted the use of helmets, despite their proven ability to decrease the risk of head injury.[481]

Penetrating craniocerebral injuries during alpine skiing have also been reported. Takakuwa et al[453] described a 25-year-old woman whose calvarium was impaled with a ski pole in the anterior part of the orbital roof following a collision with another skier. The injury resulted in a small intracerebral hematoma. The authors also described a 9-year-old boy who collided with a tree and had a twig penetrate his left maxillary sinus. CT revealed a round low-density area from the anterior lobe to the caudate nucleus (the tract of the twig).

Spinal Injury

Injuries to the spine have been reported to account for 3% of skiing-related injuries (Figure 5).[222] Data collected by Morrow et al[324] suggested a spinal injury rate of 0.075 per 1000 skier-days. More recently, Tarazi et al[457] demonstrated a spinal injury rate of 0.01 per 1000 skier-days. These injuries are more often a consequence of falls than a collision. Injuries to the cervical spine are the most common and are often accompanied by head trauma. Kip and Hunter[240] conducted a 5-year review of alpine skiing injuries and reported cervical fractures in 16 men and two women; avulsion injuries of the spinous processes occurred in six persons. The authors estimated that cervical fractures represented approximately 0.1% of all skiing injuries.

Peripheral Nerve Injury

Various peripheral nerve injuries, usually the result of acute trauma, have been reported in the skier. Lacerations to the palmar surface of the hand can result in damage to the median nerve; this injury may be caused by the sharp outer edge of the ski. Belanger and Akelman[30] reported a 20-year-old expert skier who sustained ulnar arterial, median nerve, and multiple flexor tendon injury. Damage to the radial nerve can occur secondary to a transverse fracture of the humerus.

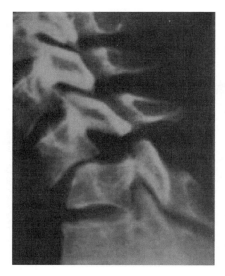

Figure 5: Radiograph showing cervical fracture/dislocation following a skiing accident.

Cross-Country Skiing

Cross-country skiing is a relatively low-risk sport that can be enjoyed by persons of all ages. Injury rates range from 0.2 to 1.5 per 1000 skier-days.[54,224] Although not common in this type of skiing, injuries to the nervous system do occur. Traveling down hills is the most risky part of this activity because the participant can develop significant kinetic energy. Boyle et al[54] reported both a concussion and a fracture of the sacrum in a cross-country skier. Because these athletes usually fall on their buttocks, they are also at risk for compression fractures. This is especially true in the older participant. Repetitive hyperextension motion during the kick phase and recurring spinal flexion and extension during the double-poling phase of the activity can lead to lower back pain. Renstrom and Johnson[370] found this complaint to be more common in skiers 16 to 21 years of age versus similarly aged nonskiers.

Ski Jumping

Ski jumpers can attain speeds of 60 miles per hour on the in-run and 90 miles per hour in the air. Participants are most frequently injured following a fall on the in-run. Wright[522] reported injury rates of 4.3 per 1000 skier-days during training and 1.2 per 1000 skier-days during World Cup and Olympic competitions. When injuries occur in this type of skiing, they commonly involve the head and neck. Weather conditions can contribute to the risk of injury during flight. High winds can make the jumper unstable in the air, and soft snow at the landing site can cause the participant to be thrown forward.

Freestyle Skiing

The new Olympic sport of freestyle skiing combines skiing with acrobatics and carries a high risk of injury to the cervical spine. Because of this risk, the U.S. Ski Association banned inverted aerial maneuvers in 1975; under tighter regulations, the maneuvers were reinstated in 1980. Dowling[128] reported an injury rate of 4.7 per 1000 skier-days prior to this ban, with injuries to the head and neck accounting for 46%. With stricter control, this rate appears to have decreased significantly. Athletes in this sport are also at risk of repetitive mild trauma to the head as a result of commonly occurring "slapbacks." These occur when the athlete overrotates a backward somersault and hits the back of his/her head on the ground. This has been reported to have an incidence of more than 16% and raises the concern of second-impact syndrome and repetitive brain trauma.[308]

Snowboarding

Snowboarding is one of the fastest growing winter sports in the world, with participation increasing at a rate of 17% a year.[15] Ski resorts that once disdained them, now report that snowboarders account for up to three fourths of their business.[362] It is estimated that there are currently 1.8 million snowboarders in the U.S.[362] The typical participant is young and male, which is also the group known for the greatest amount of risk taking. The average age of an injured snowboarder is 20-21 years, approximately 8 years younger than the injured skier.[89,116] The majority learn the sport on their own or through friends, and many have no prior skiing experience.[243] Abu-Laban[1] found that 36% of surveyed snowboarders were first-time participants. The USCPSC reported a 42% increase in snowboarding accidents between 1993 and 1994.[497] Fatalities are few, but have been reported.[73,150,243,323]

While snowboarders make up an estimated one quarter of participants on the slope, some claim that they account for nearly half of the emergency room trips from the slopes.[89] Other studies report an equal rate of injury compared to skiing, ranging from two to four injuries per 1000 snowboarder-days.[45,48,152,419] McLennan and McLennan[305] reported the injury rate to be 1.7 per 1000 snowboarder-days. One fifth of these injuries occurred in participants with little instruction. Ganong et al[152] reported injury rates of two per 1000 snowboarder-days and also suggested that novices are the most prone to injury.

In snowboarding, the most common injuries are to the upper extremities, particularly the wrist.[89] The lower extremities are spared because the legs are fixed into position on the board, which limits the torsional stresses applied from the hips down to the ankles. Since the legs are fixed, the snowboarder reaches out using the arms to break the fall, resulting in upper-extremity injury.[356] Although uncommon, head and spinal cord injuries do occur. Chow et al,[89] in a study of 390 snowboarding injuries, reported that nearly 14% were to the head and 7% to the spine. The most common types of head

Snowboarding: History

While the exact origin of snowboarding is hard to determine, Sherman Popper is often credited with making the first major strides in the progression of this sport. In 1965, Popper, an inventor, saw his daughter attempting to stand on her sled while sliding down a hill. This prompted him to attach two child-sized skis to each other. Popper named his invention the "Snurfer," and in 1966, it became the first mass-produced snowboard.

injury reported were cerebral concussions, and the most common spinal injury was a strain.

Injuries in this sport are usually the result of collisions or falls. Collisions occur with other snowboarders, skiers, or stationary objects such as trees, ski lifts, or snowmaking machines. Injuries to the head and spine are commonly associated with the athlete attempting an aerial maneuver, also known as "catching air." There have been reports of snowboarders being found buried head-first in the snow.[243] High-speed collisions are another significant cause of severe injuries and fatalities. In a report by Chow et al,[89] two injured snowboarders collided with inanimate objects at high speed. One of these accidents resulted in a skull fracture with cerebral bleeding. Collision rates of 6% to 15% have been reported.[1,152] In a study by Prall et al,[362] the rate was significantly higher because this study involved only severely injured snowboarders. Collisions with fixed objects causing blunt head and spine trauma are also frequently reported.[324,419,472]

A Comparison of Snowboarding with Skiing

Numerous studies have examined differences in snowboarding injuries compared to alpine skiing. Snowboarders tend to fall backward more frequently than skiers, resulting in more impacts to the occiput of the head. This tendency is a result of the participant always facing sideways with both feet in a fixed position, causing greater ventrodorsal instability in the snowboarder. There is also an opposite-edge phenomenon in snowboarding.[445] Catching snow with the valley-side edge of the board can cause strong rotational acceleration, resulting in forward or backward falls. If a snowboarder falls forward, extending the hands for protection, there is a greater risk of upper-extremity injury. If the fall is backward, there is a greater likelihood of injuring the head. Chow et al[89] compared the types and frequencies of injuries between snowboarders and skiers. The mean age of injured snowboarders was 19 years (range 10-48). Ski injury victims, on the other hand, tended to be older with a mean age of 28 years. This demographic is similar to that reported by Prall et al[362] in a study of serious injuries related to snowboarding and skiing. More than 80% of injured snowboarders were male. This has more to do with the epidemiology of participation versus risks of the subgroups. Novice snowboarders are at a higher risk of injury than novice skiers; almost one quarter of reported injuries are sustained the first time that snowboarding is attempted.[300,355,446] Several reports also suggest that the majority of serious snowboarding injuries occur in athletes with more than a year of experience. The condition of the snow does not appear to have an affect on the frequency or type of injury. Alcohol and drug use is a contributing factor in a small percentage of injuries.[89] Most injuries occur in the afternoon.[1] This is believed to be due to fatigue and the subsequent errors in judgment and decreased performance. The distribution by month of injuries between snowboarders and skiers varies. The majority of skiing accidents occur in February or March, while the majority of snowboarding injuries have been reported to occur in January.

O'Neill and McGlone,[347] in a study of injury patterns in first-time snowboarders and skiers, found that 4% of both groups sustained injury. As observed in other studies, snowboarders had a higher number of upper-extremity injuries (53%), while skiers had more lower-extremity injuries (63%). The snowboarder was found to be at a higher risk of injury requiring emergent care such as concussions. Of the snowboarding injuries, 42% were considered emergent, while the rate was 16% in skiing injuries.

Head Injury

The risk of head injury during snowboarding has been variably reported between 2% and 21%.[1,45,46,73,330,527] In a report by Nakaguchi et al[330] examining 559 snowboard-related injuries, 143 (26%) were to the head. In comparison, the same resort reported 749 skiers with injuries, of which 158 (21%) were to the head. The incidence of snowboard-related head injury was found to be 6.5 per 100,000 visits to the resort studied, significantly higher than the 3.8 per 100,000 incidence for skiers. None of the patients was wearing a helmet at the time of injury. Of 11 total severe head injuries, nine were to snowboarders (6.3% of snowboarding injuries) and two to skiers (1.3%); the injuries included contusion hematoma in five, acute subdural hematoma in two, subarachnoid hemorrhage in two, putaminal hemorrhage in one, and epidural hematoma in one. None was the result of collision. The injuries were from simple falls or falls while attempting jumps; 91% were from occiput impact. Eight of the nine severe head injuries in snowboarders were in novices, while both severe skiing head injuries were to intermediate athletes. Also noteworthy was that five of the six severe head injuries caused by simple falls occurred on slopes designed for beginners. Eight of nine cases were also secondary to falling backward. The study also found that novice snowboarders were at greater risk of injury than their skiing counterparts. Major head injuries were also more common in the snowboarding population (6%) than the skiing population (1%). The most frequent causes of head injury in snowboarding were falls during jumps, falling backward, and occipital impact.

High incidences of concussions in snowboarders have been reported by several authors. O'Neill and McGlone[347] reported a concussion incidence of 15% of all injuries. Prall et al[362] examined 37 consecutive patients with severe snowboard-related injuries; mild closed head injuries comprised more than half. Five patients suffered intracranial hemorrhages and two had skull fractures. The rate of serious injury while snowboarding was determined to be 0.03 injuries per 1000 snowboarder-days. While the rates of serious injury were similar in snowboarders versus skiers, concussions were more common. Spinal injury occurred more frequently in skiers (24%) than in snowboarders (5%). No fatalities occurred to snowboarders, while skiers had a mortality rate of 2%. Ganong et al[152] reported three concussions in a study of 415 snowboarding injuries. Abu-Laban[1] reported one skull fracture among 115 injured snowboarders. Shorter et al[421] reported a depressed skull fracture from a collision with a skier and a basilar skull fracture from impact with a tree.

Spinal Injury

Shorter et al[421] studied snowboarding injuries in children and adolescents. Of 28 patients, 19 were injured in falls, six collided with immobile objects, and one collided with a skier; there were two lumbar burst fractures. It was suggested that the occurrence of two burst fractures in the studied population might represent a predisposition of snowboarders to this type of injury. Abu-Laban[1] and Sacco et al[389] also reported a high incidence of spinal injuries. Ferrera et al[145] reported a high incidence of vertebral column fractures (11% of injuries), which could be secondary to the preponderance of backward falls in which the energy is taken directly by the buttocks and absorbed by the spinal column.[1,46] In contrast, reports by Chow et al[89] show an overall incidence of 2% of spinal injuries, Ganong et al[152] reported three vertebral fractures in 415 injuries, and Pigozzi et al[355] noted two cases in 106 injuries.

Risks

The most important preventable risk factors for severe head and spinal injury in snowboarding are the performance of aerial maneuvers and traveling at high speeds. Jumping with the snowboard is a very popular activity, and results in a substantial number of injuries. Shorter et al[421] reported that at least 25% of the falls were the result of attempting a jump. These activities should be reserved for the experienced athlete and avoided altogether in crowded conditions. Potentially the most serious injuries in the sport are related to backward falls with impact of the head. Helmets to protect the occipital region would decrease this risk. Release bindings may also be of benefit, and are currently being tested. Since a large percentage of the injuries occur to the novice snowboarder, lessons during the first year of the sport should be encouraged.

Soccer: History

The origin of soccer dates back as early as 200 BC. There are reports that the Chinese played a type of soccer that they used in military training. An unusual element found in this early game was that a player needed to dribble the ball. Greeks and Romans also played a type of soccer that permitted them to carry the ball. During the 1300s, this sport gained popularity in England. Records indicate that soldiers often played football games to celebrate a military victory, and there are even reports that the first official soccer game was played using the skull of an enemy as the ball. In 1365, King Edward III banned the game of soccer because there were almost no rules and the game had become a mob scene. The game had become so popular, however, that participation grew despite a succession of royal bans.

At the second modern Olympic Games, held in Paris in 1900, soccer was represented, not as an official Olympic event, but as a demonstration sport. In 1904, the initial meeting of the Federation International de Football was held in Paris, and attended by representatives of seven nations, including Belgium, Denmark, France, The Netherlands, Spain, Sweden, and Switzerland. This became the world governing body for the sport. The first world championship tournament was organized by the association in 1930.

Soccer

Soccer has been the most popular participant sport in the world since the codification of its rules in Great Britain in 1863, and has exploded worldwide in recent years with an estimated 200 million players.[203] The Soccer Industry Council of America estimated that more than 6 million children under 12 years old played on soccer teams in 1990. Over the past 10 years, the number of soccer-related injuries has increased, secondary to its increasing popularity. In Europe, it has been estimated that one half of the sports injuries are soccer related.[283] Nilsson and Roaas[341] found the overall injury rate of the Norwegian Cup Tournament soccer players between the ages of 11 and 18 years to be 14 per 1000 hours exposure for boys and 32 per 1000 hours exposure for girls. These rates are higher than those reported by most other studies, which can be explained by the way the authors defined the term injury. They included minor injuries such as blisters. The study was repeated in 1984, with resulting injury exposure rates of 8.9 for boys and 17.6 for girls. The study used the same definition of injury.[282] Ekstrand and Gillquist[131] studied injury rates in young (average age 25 years) male soccer players. They found an injury rate of 7.6 per 1000 hours of practice and 16.9 per 1000 hours of game play.[339] A study of injuries in male elite soccer players by Engstrom et al[137] found an injury rate of 1.3 per player per season. A study of elite Swedish players reported an incidence of five injuries per 1000 hours. A long-standing problem with the interpretation of injury data has been the variability of the definition of an injury. In 1986, the European Council formally adopted the definition of injury as "acquired during a game or practice, causing one or more of the following: reduction of activity, the need for treatment or medical advice, and/or negative social and economic consequences."[410] Schmidt-Olsen et al[410] performed a study on 12- to 18-year-old soccer players using the newly accepted injury definition and reported an injury exposure rate of 3.7. As in other studies, these authors noted a higher injury rate among older adolescents.

Sullivan et al[443] reported on injuries during an adolescent soccer season and found an injury exposure rate of 0.5 for boys and 1.1 for girls per 1000 hours played using an injury definition of medical conditions that prevented play. They also noted an increase in injury rates among goalkeepers versus midfielders. It is believed that the elite soccer players are at an increased risk of injury secondary to a higher training intensity and increased participation in competitive games. At all levels of play, the injury rates have been shown to be 3 to 4 times higher in game play than in practice. At the elite levels of play, the overall injury rate ranged from 5 to 50 injuries per 1000 hours of exposure.[132,137,138,339] The Nilsson and Roaas[341] study of Norwegian Cup Tournament soccer players at the elite level found the most common injuries to be to the lower extremities. They also reported that the older players were at more risk of injury. The majority of studies demonstrated no difference in injury risk based on the position of the player. Up to 70% of adult soccer injuries are minor. They are more frequent at higher skill levels and during games.[235,339] Eighty-five percent of these injuries occur to the lower extremies.[131] In youth soccer, up to 85% of injuries are minor. Young players have an increased incidence of head and face injury.[381]

Heading the Ball

Soccer is one of the few sports where the head is purposely used to direct the ball. This practice is known as "heading the ball" and involves the repetitive and intentional direct contact of the ball with the participant's head. The average player heads the ball up to 10 times every game (the degree of heading is much less in indoor soccer).[227] The concern that this could result in long-term neurological sequelae has gained a significant amount of media attention due to the large numbers of youths involved in the sport. An article by Matthews[289] in 1972 described several cases of migraine headaches secondary to heading a soccer ball (or football). This caused researchers to study the effects of repetitive, low-impact forces on the brain incurred while participating in the sport. There was concern that the soccer player could develop a syndrome similar to dementia pugilistica, a chronic and progressive traumatic encephalopathy, that had been identified in up to 25% of professional boxers.[177,384] Although this syndrome's etiology is unknown, several risk factors for its occurrence have been identified, including the length of the athlete's career, the age of exposure, and genetics. A study by Jordan et al[228] demonstrated that boxers with longer exposures to fighting and a particular genotype (apolipoprotein E epsilon4) had an increased risk of neurological deficits. There is the possibility that, over the course of a career, an accumulation of subconcussive insults, sometimes combined with frank concussions, may result in a similar syndrome in the soccer player. However, when comparing the sport's risk, it should be noted that the force of a boxer's punch is far greater than those incurred by heading, and a boxer receives many more impacts than a soccer player.[371]

Early studies of the relationship of chronic low-impact forces on the brain from soccer to neurological deficits did show a significant correlation. However, these studies lacked adequate control populations and did not account for the actual concussions incurred during a game. Tysvaer et al,[480] in 1989, found both acute and chronic electroencephalography (EEG) changes in soccer athletes versus a matched control set of track athletes. In 1995, an abstract was presented at a meeting of the American Psychological Society reporting that heading the ball during soccer caused a decrease in the IQ scores of participants (A. Witol and F. Webbe). Although the study involved only a relatively small number of players (n=60) and contained numerous flaws, it became the focus of media attention for a period of time. Concerned parents worried that their children would suffer long-term sequelae from the sport. The study's control group consisted of only 12 subjects, with no consideration given to sports activity or to prior acute head injuries. The participants completed a battery of six neuropsychiatric tests. Only two of these, the Trail Making Test and the Shipley Test of IQ, showed differing results for the soccer players versus the controls. As acknowledged by the authors of the article, the Shipley IQ Test is a poor test of brain injury. The study also did not find a consistent pattern of increasing deficits based on the frequency that a player headed the ball during games, which should be evident if this activity were the cause of the problem.

Jordan[227] compared members of the U.S. National Soccer Team with track athletes of similar age and found an increased incidence of neurological symptoms in the soccer players. They also compared MRIs and responses to questionnaires between the two groups. No differences were found between the groups with respect to brain MRIs.

There was a significant difference in responses on the head-injury questionnaires between soccer players who had suffered acute head injury and those who had not. This same trend occurred among the track athletes, although it was not statistically significant. These results point to acute TBIs such as concussions as being the major contributors to chronic brain differences in soccer players, and not the chronic, repetitive, subconcussive forces of heading. If this conclusion is accurate, the consequences of repetitive, subconcussive forces on a brain that has suffered a concussion are still unknown.[169] Theoretically, this situation could result in the catastrophic second-impact syndrome that has been seen in sports such as boxing and football. This syndrome usually occurs when a player suffers an acute brain injury such as a concussion and returns to play before he/she is completely recovered. A second, usually minor, trauma to the brain results in catastrophic brain injury. While the cause of this syndrome is unknown, it could be the result of a concussion temporarily paralyzing the vascular autoregulation of the brain.[79] No incidence of this syndrome has been reported in soccer.

Haglund and Eriksson[177] compared amateur boxers, track athletes, and soccer players by neuropsychiatric testing and radiological and EEG studies. The study found no difference between the three groups of athletes throughout their careers. The results of EEG did suggest an increased risk of closed head injuries in the older population of soccer players, most likely the result of acute traumatic episodes versus the repetitive trauma of heading the ball. These injuries were not demonstrated to result in long-term neurological sequelae.[227,480]

Aside from the serious side effects of heading, the activity has also been reported to cause headaches in participants. A study during the U.S. Olympic Festival found that headaches were associated with improper heading techniques in 32% of male and 43% of female athletes.[25] Some of the participants attributed their headaches to overinflated balls. Migraine attacks have been associated with heading the ball and provoked by facial impacts in other sports.

Head Injury

Head injuries in soccer are a significant cause of morbidity. The NCAA has recorded the number of injuries in all sports as the number per 1000 exposures. The NCAA reports an incidence of 0.15 concussions per 1000 hours of participation for college athletes in general. They found no difference in risk between men and women.[398] The overall concussion rates in college soccer between 1991 and 1996 were found to average 0.31 for men and 0.33 for women.[320] A rate as high as 0.31 per 1000 athlete exposures has been reported and constitutes a significant risk of concussion over the span of an athlete's career. Between 1982 and 1995, 0.14 annual head injuries per 100,000 high school soccer players were reported, including two fatalities related to head trauma (F. Mueller and R. Cantu, 1996). The rate of concussion in both men's and women's NCAA soccer has been increasing steadily since 1991.[320] Green and Jordan[169] reviewed participants at the 1995 Major League Soccer Combine who reportedly had an average of 18 years playing the game, equating to approximately 4000 exposures. They reported that 21% had suffered at least one soccer-related concussion. Barnes et al[25] questioned soccer players at the 1993 U.S. Olympic Sports Festival about concussions. Amazingly, 89% of the men and 43% of the women claimed to have suffered an acute head injury at some point in their careers. Putukian et al[366] conducted a prospective study of soccer injuries resulting from a 3-day indoor tournament; they reported that concussions represented 5% of the total injuries incurred by the nearly 1000 participants. Various studies report that between 7% and 24% of soccer injuries are concussions.[168] NCAA data from 1991 to 1996 report that concussions are the fifth most common injury in men's and women's soccer.[168] The NCAA Injury Surveillance System from 1991 to 1996 reported that concussions accounted for 4.5% of all soccer-related injuries. This figure is similar to that of gridiron football, with 5% of all injuries being concussions.

Frenguelli et al[148] studied the mechanisms of soccer-related head injuries. The group reported that 96% were the result of collision with another player. A small percentage resulted from colliding with the goalpost (2.5%) or impact with the ground (1.5%). Although goalpost collisions occur relatively infrequently, they can have serious consequences.[169] A study by Barnes et al[25] used soccer players participating in the 1993 U.S. Olympic Sports Festival to evaluate the causes of concussions (not just head injuries) and found the most frequent cause of head injury to be collision with another player (65% of the males studied and 78% of the females). According to data compiled by the Brain Injury Association, approximately 5% of soccer players incur an injury to the brain. This is usually caused by head-to-head contact, head-to-ball contact, or falls. Numerous studies of soccer players receiving multiple head injuries have reported observable neuropsychological and behavioral changes.[75,76,126]

Surfing

"When the surf is up and the waves ideal for riding, there may be as many as 60 surfboard riders variously riding the waves, going out, or waiting for the right wave along the 360 meters beach front that extends half a kilometer out to sea."[9] This quote from an author in the 1970s aptly describes the crowded conditions that are possible on a beach front ideal for surfing. Heavy use often leads to surfers going back out into the ocean in the path of incoming wave riders.

Allen et al[9] reviewed 35 patients injured while boardsurfing and bodysurfing. Bodysurfing is riding waves without any equipment. The skill involved is to catch the wave at the right time using the wave's energy to propel the participant. The average age of the injured body/boardsurfer was 20 years (range 3-38). Forty-nine percent of the injuries involved inexperienced surfers, 45% intermediate, and 6% experts. The injuries to experts occurred only to bodysurfers. The risk of injury in both types of surfing is relatively low compared to other sports. For example, the risk of injury in the study by Allen et al was one per 17,500 surfer-days. Two causes of injury predominate. The surfer can be hit by a loose board or can impact with the bottom of the ocean. The former predominates in the boardsurfer and carries a higher risk of head injury, while the latter is more associated with the bodysurfer and can lead to serious spinal injury.

Head Injury

Head injuries often result from being struck by a surfboard. Surfers are frequently hit by their own board when, after falling, the board is flung into the air by the surf and comes down on the surfacing victim. Injuries to the head include basilar and parietotemporal fractures and cerebral concussions. Other injuries include maxillofacial and ophthalmic injuries from impacts with loose boards, ruptured tympanic membranes, and various soft-tissue injuries. One reported fatality was the result of the keel of a loose surfboard severing the carotid artery of a surfer. The sport can also have risks for bystanders. Numerous injuries have been reported to bystanders struck by loose boards drifting to shore. Surfing straps can be used to tether the board to the surfer; although this decreases injuries to others by loose boards, the risk of impact to the surfer with his/her own board is higher. As surfboards became lighter, the risk of head injury decreased. However, there has been a recent trend back to the traditional "longboards"

Surfing: History

Surfing is an ancient sport believed to have originated in Polynesia or Micronesia as far back as 1500 AD In 1778, British explorer James Cook was the first European to have witnessed he'e nalu, the Hawaiian word for the sport. In 1907, it was introduced to the U.S. when a California land developer named Henry Huntington asked George Freeth to give a surfing demonstration at the opening of the Redondo-Los Angeles railroad at Redondo beach. This demonstration ignited a revolution and the California shores soon became the staging area for the sport's expansion.

Currently, there are more than 1.7 million surfers in the U.S. and more than 18 million surfers world-wide.[284] The sport has not yet become an Olympic game, mainly due to its dependence on an ocean or machine that will produce "surfable" waves. It was a demonstration sport at the 2000 Summer Olympics.

that can weigh up to 35 pounds. Injury may be prevented by avoiding crowded sites and not paddling out in the path of incoming surfers. Covering the head with both arms and surfacing with one arm extended can help avoid impacts to the head. Avoiding reefs and shorebreaks can decrease the risk of impact with the bottom. As with any aquatic activity, surfing is safer if done with a companion.

Spinal Injury

Craniospinal injuries occurred in 34% of the injured surfers. The majority of these were spinal injuries occurring when the surfer was thrown into the sand at the end of a run. Cervical injuries were the most common, and resulted in quadriplegia in one victim; high thoracic and lumbodorsal injuries were also observed. Empirically, bodysurfing carries a higher risk of central nervous system injury than boardsurfing. The majority of spinal injuries occur while bodysurfing, since it is ideal in shallow water and thus results in greater risk of injury. The risk increases the closer to the shore that the waves break. Injury usually occurs when the surfer misses a wave and tumbles or impacts his/her head into the sand. Scher[401] reported three patients paralyzed due to an injury suffered while bodysurfing and compared this population to persons paralyzed from diving into shallow water. The bodysurfing victims were significantly older (mean age 46 years). No fractures or dislocations were observed, but radiological evidence of osteoarthrosis was present in all. Scher[408] observed a pattern of incomplete paralysis consistent with central cord syndrome. Central cord syndrome is caused by hemorrhage into the central gray matter of the spinal cord. The syndrome also involves the white matter to varying degrees that can damage central arm and leg tracts. Anterior horn cells are damaged for several segments, which causes lower motor neuron paralysis of the hands and arms. Urinary incontinence or retention is common, and the white matter damage causes weakness and spasticity of the legs.[412] Forced hyperextension of the head and neck secondary to the surfer being driven into the sand appeared to be the mechanism of injury. The subarachnoid space around the cervical spine is narrowest in the C3-6 levels, making this area the most vulnerable to injury. This space is decreased further with extension. Increased narrowing of this area by osteophytes and ligamentum flavum could predispose the older population with osteoarthritic changes to these injuries. Older bodysurfers should be aware that pre-existing osteoarthrosis can increase their risk of injury. Cheng et al[87] also described a series of patients injured during bodysurfing with similar neurological deficits, age, and the absence of fractures or dislocations.

Swimming: History

The origin of swimming dates back thousands of years. One of the earliest records of swimming is a scene depicted on an ancient Egyptian wall that illustrates soldiers of Pharaoh Ramses II pursuing their enemies by swimming across the Orontes River. In ancient Rome and Greece, swimming was viewed as an excellent way to condition warriors.

In Japan, swimming competitions were held as early as the 1st century BC. In the late 19th century, amateur swimming clubs began holding competitions in the U.S. and Britain, and in 1896 swimming became an official Olympic event in Athens, Greece.

Swimming

The sport of swimming appears to be one of the safest with regard to the nervous system. It has a low incidence of injury to the head, back, spine, and peripheral nerves. However, catastrophic injuries have been reported to the cervical spine. These usually occur when the participant's head contacts the wall or bottom of the pool. This often results when a participant dives into the water at the start of a race. Some of these racing-start dives, such as the scoop, have been shown to require at least 4 feet of water, even when practiced by trained divers.[47] Cervical wedge and compression fractures are most commonly found in this type of injury. Marinella and Barsan[285] reported a case of a spontaneous cervical epidural hematoma that developed while swimming. This occurred in a healthy 60-year-old woman who presented with transient hemiparesis and recovered with conservative treatment. Most patients with this condition present with paraparesis or tetraparesis. While most lower and middle back pain is due to musculoskeletal injury, acute and chronic injuries to the bony structures of the spine do occur. Goldstein et al[165] compared national-caliber female swimmers to top-level female gymnasts in a study of spinal injuries and found that 16% of the swimmers had spine abnormalities. The average hours of training per week and the participants' age were found to be associated with an increased incidence of abnormalities. An increased intensity and length of training also correlated with spinal injuries.

Tennis

Tennis is played by more than 14 million people annually and involves persons of all ages.[248] The sport has been characterized as one in which the participant must deal with a continuous series of emergencies to which there must be a response.[175] These responses include rapid changes of direction, stopping and starting, and sprinting. These tasks repetitively strain the bony and ligamentous structures of the athlete's body. Chard and Lachmann[85] conducted an 8-year retrospective study of 631 injuries resulting from racquet sports. Of these injuries, tennis accounted for 21%.

Posterior Interosseous Nerve Compression Syndrome/ Radial Tunnel Syndrome

Compression of the posterior interosseous nerve can result in both radial tunnel syndrome and posterior interosseous nerve compression syndrome. These injuries can be mistaken for lateral epicondylitis (tennis elbow). Neuropathy of the radial nerve results from compression of the nerve at any point along its course between the radial head and the supinator muscle. Patients with this condition present with an aching pain of the extensor or supinator muscles of the proximal forearm. This pain frequently radiates into the distal arm and forearm. The condition is often differentiated from lateral epicondylitis by the character and location of associated discomfort. Pain from radial tunnel syndrome is most intense distal to the leading edge of the supinator muscle and is characteristically more diffuse (and often described as an "ache"). Discomfort from tennis elbow, on the other hand, is usually maximum directly over or slightly anterior to the lateral epicondyle. Interestingly, Kalb et al[230] found that 52% of their patients who underwent surgery because of posterior interosseous nerve compression suffered from tennis elbow as well. The authors proposed that radial tunnel syndrome is a specific form of tennis elbow. Lateral epicondylitis occurs in more than 50% of athletes using overhead arm motions and is characterized by pain in the area where the common extensor muscles meet the lateral humeral epicondyle.

Ulnar Neuropathy

While medial elbow pain in the tennis player is often caused by medial epicondylitis, it can be the result of ulnar neuropathy. This condition usually follows overuse. The etiology of this injury can be traction, compression, or trauma to the nerve. Because an injured and unstable elbow can open with valgus stress, traction injuries to the ulnar nerve are possible. Compression is often secondary to scar-tissue formation and other degenerative elbow joint changes. This condition usually presents with numbness and paresthesias of the fourth and fifth digits of the affected upper extremity. The athlete may also complain of medial elbow discomfort that radiates into the forearm. The site of injury to the nerve can be in either the ulnar groove or distally as the nerve pierces the flexor carpi ulnaris. This condition is often recalcitrant to conservative therapy and requires surgical correction.

Other peripheral neuropathies have also been reported in tennis players. Kuhn and Hawkins[255] reported injuries to the axillary, long thoracic, and suprascapular nerves. Iatrogenic injuries to the ulnar nerve were reported by Stahl and Kaufman,[435] who described damage of the ulnar nerve at the elbow following steroid injection for medial epicondylitis in a patient with undetected recurrent dislocation of the nerve.

Head and Spine Injury

Fortunately, head injuries are extremely rare in this sport. Between 1982 and 1995, no fatalities were recorded in high school or college tennis players related to head trauma (F. Mueller and R. Cantu, 1996).

Pain in the lower back is a common complaint of the tennis player. A study by Marks et al[286] reported that 38% of the male professional tennis players studied missed a tournament secondary to this condition. Of 148 players, 43 reported chronic low back pain, and of 38 players who suffered an acute injury, 11 did so to the lumbosacral spine. Chard and Lachmann[85] reported a high incidence of lumbar disc prolapse in an 8-year retrospective study of 631 racquet sports injuries. Tennis players are at an increased risk of lumbar disc disease from rotational and hyperextension shearing forces incurred during play. In a study of 30 elite tennis players between the ages of 17 and 25 years, 15 had a history of thoracolumbar back pain that lasted at least 1 week.[450] The stroke that appears to cause the most stress to the spine is the serve;[286] it involves hyperextension and rotation of the lumbar spine and lateral flexion of the trunk. Injuries can include lumbar strain, discogenic disease, facet impingement, and piriformis syndrome.

Trampoline: History

While their use is believed to be as old as man, modern trampolines have only been evolving over the last 50 years. In 1936, George Nissen's trampoline design set the trend for the past 30 years. Uses of the trampoline vary. In the 1960s, trampoline entertainment centers opened across the country, with the devices positioned in open areas. Notably, little protective padding or supervision was used. Both the U.S. Air Force and the space agencies used trampolines to train both pilots and astronauts.

In medicine, the use of the trampoline in working with individuals with handicaps has demonstrated benefits. Trampolining is a sport in which multiple somersaults and twists at a height of up to 25 feet necessitate a superior technique. Competitions have increased in recent years, and trampolining was introduced as an Olympic event in 2000.

Trampoline

The use of trampolines has been found to carry a great risk for catastrophic injuries. Thirty-two of 50 instances of SCI in gymnastics reported by the NSCIDRC between 1973 and 1981 involved trampolines (J. Young et al, 1982). Ellis et al[134] reported five cases of SCI involving trampolines as far back as 1960. Three of the cases resulted in quadriplegia, and the injuries in four were the result of an incorrectly attempted somersault. In 1977, the American Academy of Pediatrics formally advocated a ban of trampolines in schools and colleges. They determined that "next to football, trampolines were found to be the highest cause of permanent paralysis." This ban was rescinded several years later with the organization still emphasizing the importance of supervision.[100] In 1978, the American Alliance for Health, Physical Education, and Recreation adopted guidelines for the controlled use of trampolines and minitramps, including the supervised absence of somersaults in basic physical education programs and locking up the devices when unattended. The NCAA adopted similar guidelines, allowing for the controlled use of the trampoline to develop competitive skills (1978).

Most injuries involving trampolines occur on the apparatus and are not the result of falls. This heightens the importance of proper training and good technique so that the athlete maintains control during maneuvers. It is important to note that the trampoline itself is considered an injury-prevention device by gymnasts. With the trampoline, the athlete can practice advanced maneuvers under controlled conditions.

Weightlifting

Weight training is an increasingly popular exercise technique, competitive sport, and recreational activity among all age groups. Neurological injuries range from chronic overuse syndromes to acute quadriplegia, and include spondylolysis, spondylolisthesis, intervertebral disc herniation, and various peripheral nerve injuries. Powell et al[361] found a 30-day prevalence of injury in approximately 1%-3% of weightlifters. Brady et al[57] examined 80 young athletes with weight training-related injuries. In 43 of these athletes, there was a direct causal relationship to weight training. In 37 other athletes, injuries were also experienced, but it was difficult to pinpoint the cause because they participated in other sports. In 29, lumbosacral pain developed; of these, seven required hospitalization and four required surgical treatment. Anterior iliac spine avulsion occurred in six athletes, and a cervical sprain developed in four. Konig and Biener[247] reported a 21% incidence of back injury related to weightlifting. Goertzen et al,[159] in a study of 358 body-builders and 60 powerlifters, found the upper extremity (particularly the shoulder and elbow joint) to have the highest injury rate, with more than 40% of all injuries occurring in this area. In powerlifting, the injury rate was twice as high as in bodybuilding. Injuries occur much more frequently when using free weights versus weight machines. The rate of injury appears to be lowest in prepubescent and older athletes.[293]

Spinal Injury/Pain

The lumbar area of the spine is often injured by weightlifters. Alexander[8] reported that weightlifting, along with gymnastics and football, were sports with the greater risk of lower back injury. These injuries are most commonly muscle strains, ligament sprains, lumbar vertebral fractures, disc injuries, and neural arch fractures. The most common serious injury to the lower back is a neural arch fracture at the pars interarticularis, known as spondylolysis. Defects in the pars interarticularis of one side of the verte-brae and a bilateral defect in the pars interarticularis, known as spondylolisthesis, can also occur. These injuries are often accompanied by forward displacement of the verte-bral body. Rossi and Dragoni[385] found a high percentage of spondylolysis associated with weightlifting (23%) in a population of 3132 competitive athletes. The Northeast Collab-orative Group on Low Back Pain[326] studied the association between participation in sev-eral specific sports, use of free weights, and use of weightlifting equipment and herniated lumbar or cervical intervertebral discs. The study included 287 patients with lumbar disc herniation and 63 with cervical disc herniation. The authors found that herniated lum-bar or cervical discs were not associated with the use of weightlifting machines, although a possible association was indicated between the use of free weights and cervical hernia-tion (relative risk 2%, confidence interval 0.74 to 4.74). Chen et al[86] presented a patient who suffered three episodes of upper-back pain of sudden onset followed by sensory and motor dysfunction after weightlifting. While neurological deficits in the first two episodes recovered spontaneously and completely, paraplegia persisted even after emer-gency surgery in the last episode. Serial studies with CT myelography and MRI demon-strated a spontaneous spinal epidural hematoma.

Peripheral Nerve Injury

Nerve injuries in a variety of anatomical locations are common in this sport. Long thoracic neuropathy can develop and usually presents with shoulder pain or dysfunction and scapular winging consistent with serratus anterior weakness. The injury is usually the result of stretching the nerve and responds well to conservative management. Rossi

Weightlifting: History

The origin of weightlifting dates to the beginning of recorded history where man's natural interest with the human physic can be found among many ancient writings. Ancient Greek sculp-tures represent acts of lifting, and the weights were usually stones. These stones would later be replaced by dumb-bells. The origin of the word "dumbbells" actually comes from the practice of removing a clapper from a bell, making them soundless during lifting.

In 1896, weightlifting was included as an official sport of the Olympic Games. Although weightlifting did not appear in the 1900 Olympics, it returned in the games of 1904. Weightlifting became a regular Olympic event in 1920. Three lifts were standard by 1932: the press (which was subse-quently eliminated in 1972), the snatch, and the clean-and-jerk. Women com-peted in the weightlifting event in the 2000 Olympics for the first time.

et al[386] reported progressive bilateral medial pectoral neuropathy in a bodybuilder. This type of injury is believed to result from intramuscular entrapment of the medial pectoral nerves secondary to pectoralis minor hypertrophy. Musculocutaneous nerve injury has also been associated with weight training. The condition typically presents following vigorous upper-extremity resistive exercise as painless weakness of the biceps brachii and brachialis muscles and sensory loss in the distal volar forearm. The problem usually resolves with rest.[56] Suprascapular nerve palsy associated with weightlifting has been reported. The condition usually presents with atrophy of the infraspinatus muscle on the involved side and decreased strength of shoulder abduction and external rotation, and is often the result of scarring, entrapment, tethering, or kinking at the suprascapular notch. Exercises that involve shoulder abduction appear to increase the incidence of this condition.[6,33,528] Meralgia paraesthetica, or injury of the lateral cutaneous nerve of the thigh, is another condition not uncommon to bodybuilders.[452] Exposing the wrist to repetitive movements and heavy weights may cause carpal tunnel syndrome. Mauer et al[291] found a clear positive correlation between the estimated total duration of training and the distal motor latency of the median nerve.

Wrestling: History

Wrestling is perhaps mankind's oldest and most basic form of recreational combat, tracing its origins back to the dawn of civilization. Its origin dates back over 15,000 years, when cave drawings in France depicting this sport are believed to have been completed.

The sport was one of the most popular events in the ancient Greek Olympics. The first national competition in the U.S. was conducted in 1887, and the Amateur Athletic Union formally sanctioned its first national tournament in 1888. Interestingly, despite its long history, wrestling did not become an official sport in the modern Olympics until 1904.

Wrestling

Wrestling is one of the most physically demanding sports in high school and college athletics and a significant number of injuries are incurred during participation. During the 1980 NCAA Wrestling Championships, 110 injuries requiring the attention of a physician and/or an athletic trainer occurred among the 353 participating athletes. The overall injury rate per athlete was found to be 31%, with no relationship to weight classification. Only six of the injured athletes (5%) had to withdraw from the tournament.[237] Jarret et al[220] evaluated NCAA Injury Surveillance System data on wrestling during an 11-year period. Most injuries occurred during takedowns and sparring, with areas of concern being rotation about a planted foot and contact with environmental objects. Illegal action accounted for 5% of injuries in competition. As often seen in other sports, the rate of injury is significantly higher during competition than practice. The authors found no significant differences in injury patterns among weight classes. Several studies have shown that certain parts of the wrestlers' anatomy are more prone to injury. An overall injury rate of 13% was reported in two wrestling tournaments involving 1742 participants, aged 6 to 16 years.[274] Primary areas of injury were the upper extremity (33%) and the head and neck (30%). The time-loss injury rate was reported to be 5.63 per 1000 exposures.

Head Injury

Catastrophic injuries related to head trauma are unusual in weightlifting. Between 1982 and 1995, no fatalities were recorded in either high school or college wrestling related to this type of injury (F. Mueller and R. Cantu, 1996). Less severe head injuries, however, are quite common. Powell and Barber-Foss[360] found wrestlers to account for 11% (n=128) of 1219 mild TBIs suffered in 10 sports studied over a 3-year period. The injury rate for wrestling was found to be 1.58 per 100 player-seasons.

Spinal Injury

According to the NSCIDRC, wrestling accounted for 3% of all sports-related SCIs between 1973 and 1981 (J. Young et al, 1982). The mean age of wrestling-related SCI in

1980 and 1981 was 20 years (range 17-22). All injuries occurred in men and all resulted in quadriplegia (Figure 6) (K. Clarke, 1983).

The sport of wrestling has been associated with severe trauma to the cervical spine and spinal cord. While certain head-holds with a higher risk of these injuries (such as the full nelson) have been made illegal, this problem persists. Currently, the most common cause of these injuries in wrestling is landing with the body twisted on the head and neck. This is because while the intervertebral discs, joints, and ligaments are resistant to compression stresses, they are very susceptible to injury by rotational and shearing forces.[378] Bailes et al[19] analyzed 63 patients who sustained cervical spinal injuries while participating in organized sporting events; 45 patients suffered permanent injury to the vertebral column and/or spinal cord and 18 suffered transient spinal cord symptoms. Wrestling accounted for the second highest number of injuries, preceded only by football. Leidholt[263] studied sports injuries, excluding football, over a 1-year period at the Air Force Academy. They reported a total of 31 SCIs, of which 11 were related to wrestling. Wu and Lewis[524] reported on three young athletes suffering quadriparesis and quadriplegia. The first athlete's injury was a fracture/dislocation of the C5-6 vertebrae secondary to a full nelson applied during high school wrestling practice. The second athlete was injured during a regulation high school wrestling match when he was thrown and landed on the right side of his neck in a twisted position; he immediately became quadriplegic with a sensory level of C4. Radiography revealed a fracture/dislocation of C3 anteriorly onto C4. The third athlete was also injured by being thrown during a regulation match. He landed in a twisted configuration on his head, neck, and shoulders. The injury was less acute and he did not lose significant leg strength until 48 hours after the injury. Although radiography revealed no bony deformities, myelography revealed a block at C7-T1. An emergent laminectomy was performed revealing petechial hemorrhage and edema of the epidural fat. The spinal concussion gradually improved and in 7 months the wrestler was able to walk without assistance. All of the athletes in this series regained function, probably secondary to incomplete lesions.

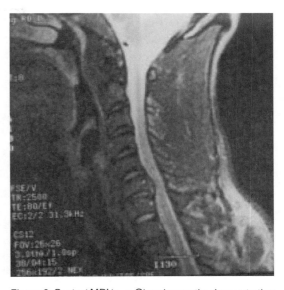

Figure 6: Sagittal MRI in an Olympic wrestler demonstrating a large C6/7 disc herniation.

Various combinations of radiological abnormalities of the thoracolumbar spine have been found to be more prevalent in wrestlers versus other athletes and the general population.[188] Spondylolysis is a common occurrence in the competitive wrestler. Rossi and Dragoni[385] reported 390 cases of spondylolysis found in 3132 randomly selected competitive athletes. This prevalence is much higher than found in the general public. Slightly more than 29% of wrestlers have been shown to suffer this condition, making wrestling one of the highest risk athletic activities for this injury.

Peripheral Nerve Injury

Although primarily a football injury, burners have been reported in wrestling secondary to acute head, neck, and/or shoulder trauma. The condition is usually self-limiting. There is, however the chance of permanent neurological deficits. Injury to the spinal accessory cranial nerve has been reported in a wrestler by Cohn et al.[99]

Sudden Death

Rontoyannis et al[383] described the sudden death of a young healthy wrestler during a match secondary to acute ischemia of the brainstem. This was the result of the interruption of blood flow to the vertebral-basal system. This injury was incurred during a legal maneuver when the head was improperly positioned (trapped between the mat and the wrestler's own forearm) while the athlete was in the inferior disadvantaged position and the wrestler's opponent was attempting to overthrow him. This resulted in the overflexion and rotation of the head and injury/rupture of the vertebral blood vessels.

Maxillofacial/Ocular Trauma

Ocular sports trauma is responsible for more than 100,000 preventable eye injuries each year and is a leading cause of permanent vision loss in the U.S.[491] Injuries range from abrasions to optic nerve avulsions. In the late 1960s, the popular professional baseball player Tony Conigliaro was struck in the face with a pitch. The resultant eye injury was devastating and ended his career. This incident prompted a closer look at eye injuries in sports. A study by Grin et al[173] of 278 eye injuries found baseball to be one of the sports most commonly involved. A retrospective review of Rugby players who had claimed financial compensation for permanent injury from 1978 to 1994 reported 26 players suffering some form of permanent vision loss.[260] The International Federation of Sports Medicine considers basketball a high-risk sport for eye injury,[490,492] and the Consumer Product Safety Commission in 1982 ranked basketball second only to baseball in sport-related eye injuries. Zagelbaum et al[525] found an incidence of eye injuries in National Basketball Association players to be 1.44 per 1000 game exposures. Ocular complications of bungee jumping usually involve hemorrhage of intraocular or extraocular tissue,[488] and cases of serious ocular injury causing permanent vision loss have been reported.[210] The most common cause of ocular injuries in cycling is from flying debris such as rocks and insects. The use of eye protection could prevent many of these injuries. State-of-the-art eye protective devices use lenses made of highly impact-resistant optical material, usually polycarbonate, in sturdy frames.

An estimated 4% to 18% of all sports injuries involve the maxillofacial region. Tanaka et al[456] investigated the number and type of maxillofacial fractures caused by various athletic activities. In 98 patients treated between 1977 and 1993, sports-related injury accounted for 10% of all patients with facial bone fractures. Rugby and skiing were the most commonly involved sports, followed by baseball and soccer. The ratio of males to females was 5.5:1, and most patients were between 10 and 29 years of age. In another study of 137 patients with sports-related facial fractures, Australian Rules football was the causative sport in 53%. Orbitozygomatic fractures were most common, occurring in 58% of these injuries.[265] Gymnastics has also been considered to be a high-risk discipline for this type of injury.[29] In a study by Kvittem et al,[257] 72% of wrestlers had at least one orofacial injury per athlete in a season. Orofacial injuries are common in Rugby players, especially in younger players. Kvittem et al determined the incidence of at least one orofacial injury per athlete in a season to be 55% in basketball. While the majority of injuries to the cyclist's face are abrasions and lacerations, facial bone fractures do occur. The most common bony injuries to this area are mandibular fractures. These fractures are usually of the condyle of the mandible, which differs from fractures to this bone from other causes. The next most common type of maxillofacial injuries are fractures of the maxilla that usually involves the middle third of the zygoma.[375] Mountain bikers appear to be particularly prone to severe facial trauma.

Conclusion

Although neurological injuries are less common in the traditionally "noncollision" sports, they do occur and result in substantial morbidity and mortality. Prevention is the most important method of decreasing the severity and frequency of these mishaps. Proper protective equipment is essential, as is the development of skills that minimize neurological injury. Participants should understand the epidemiology of neurological injury in their chosen activity. A study by Goldhaber[164] revealed that 8% of parents in the study associated concussion as an injury concern in their child's sport. This study was performed with the parents of football players, so undoubtedly the percentage is much lower with activities of a more benign nature.

Proper diagnosis and rapid treatment should also be a high priority. Guidelines should be followed regarding when an athlete may return to competition following a head injury, keeping in mind that an athlete who sustains a concussion has up to a four-fold greater risk of a second head injury versus a person who has never had an injury.[513] To prevent second-impact syndrome, an athlete who has suffered a head injury should not return to competition until all symptoms have resolved. This rule should cross the boundaries of various sports seasons. For example, an athlete suffering a concussion during wrestling season in the winter should not participate in spring Rugby until all symptoms have resolved. It is also important to remember that repeated minor traumas to the nervous system have additive effects on an athlete's cognitive abilities. Finally, the rules of the game are designed to protect the player and should be enforced by the official or umpire.

References

1. Abu-Laban RB: Snowboarding injuries: an analysis and comparison with alpine skiing injuries. **Can Med Assoc J** 145:1097-1103, 1991
2. Adams CW, Burton CJ: The cerebral vasculature in dementia pugilistica. **J Neurol Neurosurg Psychiatry** 52:600-604, 1989
3. Adams ID: Rugby football injuries. **Br J Sports Med** 11:4-6, 1977
4. Adams M, Hutton W: Mechanics of the intervertebral discs, in Ghosh P (ed): **The Biology of the Intervertebral Disc.** Boca Raton, Fla: CRC Press, 1988, pp 39-71
5. Adams M, Hutton W: The relevance of torsion to the mechanical derangement of the lumbar spine. **Spine** 6:241-248, 1981
6. Agre JC, Ash N, Cameron MC, et al: Suprascapular neuropathy after intensive progressive resistive exercise: case report. **Arch Phys Med Rehabil** 68:236-238, 1987
7. Akpata T: Spinal injuries in U.S. Rugby. **Rugby**, 1990, pp 14-15
8. Alexander MJ: Biomechanical aspects of lumbar spine injuries in athletes: a review. **Can J Appl Sport Sci** 10:1-20, 1985
9. Allen RH, Eiseman B, Straehley CJ, et al: Surfing injuries at Waikiki. **JAMA** 237:668-670, 1977
10. Amamilo S, Samuel A, Hesketh K, et al: A prospective study of parachute injuries of civilians. **J Bone Joint Surg (Br)** 69:17-19, 1987
11. American Academy of Orthopedic Surgeons: **Orthopedic Knowledge Update 3: Lumbar Spine.** Park Ridge, Ill: American Academy of Orthopedic Surgeons, 1990
12. American Academy of Pediatrics Committee on Sports Medicine and Fitness: Horseback riding and head injuries. **Pediatrics** 89:512, 1992
13. Amundson L, Mellion M: Common skin problems in athletes, in Mellion M (ed): **Office Management of Sports Injuries and Athletic Problems.** Philadelphia, Pa: Hanley & Belfus, 1988, pp 146-159
14. Andersen KV, Bovim G: Impotence and nerve entrapment in long distance amateur cyclists. **Acta Neurol Scand** 95:233-240, 1997
15. Anonymous: **Ski Magazine,** Vol 61, 1993
16. Armson CJ, Pollard CW: Child cyclist injuries: a prospective study. **Med J Aust** 144:144-146, 1986
17. Ashworth B: Migraine, head trauma and sport. **Scot Med J** 30:240-242, 1985
18. Backx F: in Institute of Sports and Healthcare, University of Utrecht, Oosterbeek, Netherlands, 1991
19. Bailes JE, Hadley MN, Quigley MR, et al: Management of athletic injuries of the cervical spine and spinal cord. **Neurosurgery** 29:491-497, 1991
20. Bailes JE, Herman JM, Quigley MR, et al: Diving injuries of the cervical spine. **Surg Neurol** 34:155-158, 1990
21. Ballham A, Absoud EM, Kotecha MB, et al: A study of bicycle accidents. **Injury** 16:405-408, 1985
22. Barber H: Survey of accidents with horses. **Br Med J** 3:532-534, 1973
23. Barbour P, Levitt L: Tennis foot drop. **J Sports Med** 23:427-428, 1983
24. Barclay W: Equestrian sports. **JAMA** 240:1892-1893, 1978
25. Barnes BC, Cooper L, Kirkendall DT, et al: Concussion history in elite male and female soccer players. **Am J Sports Med** 26:433-438, 1998
26. Barone G, Rodgers B: Pediatric equestrian injuries: a 14 year review. **J Trauma** 29:245-247, 1989
27. Barrentine SW, Fleisig GS, Whiteside JA, et al: Biomechanics of windmill softball pitching with implications about injury mechanisms at the shoulder and elbow. **J Orthop Sports Phys Ther** 28:405-415, 1998
28. Barton S, Margolis M: Rotational obstruction of the vertebral artery at the atlantoaxial joint. **Neuroradiology** 9:117-120, 1975
29. Bayliss T, Bedi R: Oral, maxillofacial and general injuries in gymnasts. **Injury** 27:353-354, 1996
30. Belanger MJ, Akelman E: Median nerve injury in an expert skier: a case report. **Am J Orthop** 28:648-649, 1999
31. Bennett DR, Fuenning SI, Sullivan G, et al: Migraine precipitated by head trauma in athletes. **Am J Sports Med** 8:202-205, 1980
32. Bernhang A, Winslet G: Equestrian injuries. **Phys Sportsmed** 11:90-97, 1983
33. Berry H, Kong K, Hudson A, et al: Isolated suprascapular nerve palsy: a review of nine cases. **Can J Neurol Sci** 22:301-304, 1995
34. Bicycle-related injuries: data from the National Electronic Injury Surveillance System. **MMWR Morbid Mortal Wkly Rep** 36:269-271, 1987
35. Binns J, Potter J: Head injuries in military parachutists. **Injury** 3:133-134, 1971
36. Bird YN, Waller AE, Marshall SW, et al: The New Zealand Rugby Injury and Performance Project: V. Epidemiology of a season of Rugby injury. **Br J Sports Med** 32:319-325, 1998
37. Birrer R, Birrer C: Martial arts injuries. **Phys Sportsmed** 10:103-108, 1982
38. Birrer R, Birrer C, Son D, et al: Injuries in Taekwon-Do. **Phys Sportsmed** 9:97-103, 1981
39. Birrer RB: Trauma epidemiology in the martial arts. The results of an eighteen-year international survey. **Am J Sports Med** 24 (Suppl): S72-S79, 1996
40. Birrer RB, Halbrook SP: Martial arts injuries. The results of a five year national survey. **Am J Sports Med** 16:408-410, 1988
41. Bishop PJ, Briard BD: Impact performance of bicycle helmets. **Can J Appl Sport Sci** 9:94-101, 1984
42. Bixby-Hammet D, Brooks W: Neurological injuries in equestrian sports, in Jordan B (ed): **Sports Neurology.** Rockville, Md: Aspen Pub-

lications, 1989, pp 229-234

43. Bixby-Hammett D, Brooks WH: Common injuries in horseback riding. A review. **Sports Med** 9:36-47, 1990

44. Bixby-Hammett DM: Accidents in equestrian sports. **Am Fam Phys** 36:209-214, 1987

45. Bladin C, Giddings P, Robinson M: Australian snowboard injury data base study. A four-year prospective study. **Am J Sports Med** 21:701-704, 1993

46. Bladin C, McCrory P: Snowboarding injuries. An overview. **Sports Med** 19:358-364, 1995

47. Blanksby BA, Wearne FK, Elliott BC, et al: Aetiology and occurrence of diving injuries. A review of diving safety. **Sports Med** 23:228-246, 1997

48. Blitzer CM, Johnson RJ, Ettlinger CF, et al: Downhill skiing injuries in children. **Am J Sports Med** 12:142-147, 1984

49. Blumenthal S, Roach J, Herring J, et al: Lumbar Scheuermann's: a clinical series and classification. **Spine** 12:929-932, 1987

50. Bohlmann T: Injuries in competitive cycling. **Phys Sportsmed** 9:118, 1981

51. Boland AL, Hosea TM: Rowing and sculling and the older athlete. **Clin Sports Med** 10:245-256, 1991

52. Borglund ST, Hayes JS, Eckes JM: Florida's bicycle helmet law and a bicycle safety educational program: did they help? **J Emerg Nurs** 25:496-500, 1999

53. Bowling A: Injuries to dancers: prevalence, treatment, and perceptions of causes. **Br Med J** 298:731-734, 1989

54. Boyle H, Johnson R, Pope M, et al: **Proceedings of Skiing Trauma and Safety: Fifth International Symposium**, pp 411-422

55. Braakman R, Penning L: **Injuries of the Cervical Spine**. Amsterdam: Excerpta Medica, 1971

56. Braddom RL, Wolfe C: Musculocutaneous nerve injury after heavy exercise. **Arch Phys Med Rehabil** 59:290-293, 1978

57. Brady TA, Cahill BR, Bodnar LM: Weight training-related injuries in the high school athlete. **Am J Sports Med** 10:1-5, 1982

58. Braithwaite I: Bilateral median nerve palsy in a cyclist. **Br J Sports Med** 26:27-28, 1992

59. Brogger-Jensen T, Hvass I, Bugge S: Injuries at the BMX Cycling European Championship, 1989. **Br J Sports Med** 24:269-270, 1990

60. Brooks W, Bixby-Hammett D: Prevention of neurologic injuries in equestrian sports. **Phys Sportsmed** 16:84-95, 1988

61. Brozin IH, Martfel J, Goldberg I, et al: Traumatic closed femoral nerve neuropathy. **J Trauma** 22:158-160, 1982

62. Buckley S, Chaimers D, Langley J: Falls from horses resulting in death and hospitalization: descriptive epidemiology. University of Otago Medical School, New Zealand, 1990

63. Bull riding-related brain and spinal cord injuries—Louisiana, 1994-1995. **MMWR Morbid Mortal Wkly Rep** 45:796-798, 1996

64. Buntain W: in **Proceedings of the 29th Annual Meeting of the American Association for Automative Medicine, Washington, DC, 1985**

65. Burke E: Hard hats. **Sportcare Fitness** 2:50-52, 1989

66. Burke E: Safety standards for bicycle helmets. **Phys Sportsmed** 16:148-153, 1988

67. Burry H, Calcinai C: The need to make Rugby safer. **Br Med J** 296:149-150, 1988

68. Burry H, Gowland H: Cervical injury in Rugby football—a New Zealand survey. **Br J Sports Med** 15:56-59, 1981

69. Busby J: Injuries in short track asphalt racing. **Am Fam Phys** 18:137-140, 1978

70. Buschbacher RM, Shay T: Martial arts. **Phys Med Rehabil Clin North Am** 10(6):35-47, 1999

71. Butterwick DJ, Nelson DS, LaFave MR, et al: Epidemiological analysis of injury in one year of Canadian professional rodeo. **Clin J Sport Med** 6:171-177, 1996

72. Caine D, Cochrane B, Caine C, et al: An epidemiologic investigation of injuries affecting young competitive female gymnasts. **Am J Sports Med** 17:811-820, 1989

73. Calle S, Evans J: Snowboarding trauma. **J Pediatr Surg** 30:791-794, 1995

74. Canale ST, Cantler ED Jr, Sisk TD, et al: A chronicle of injuries of an American intercollegiate football team. **Am J Sports Med** 9:384-389, 1981

75. Cantu RC: Cerebral concussion in sport. Management and prevention. **Sports Med** 14:64-74, 1992

76. Cantu RC: Head and spine injuries in youth sports. **Clin Sports Med** 14:517-532, 1995

77. Cantu RC: Second-impact syndrome: immediate management. **Phys Sportsmed** 20:55, 1992

78. Cantu RC, Mueller FO: Catastrophic spine injuries in football (1977-1989). **J Spinal Disord** 3:227-231, 1990

79. Cantu RC, Voy R: Second impact syndrome: a risk in any contact sport. **Phys Sportsmed** 23(6):27-34, 1995

80. Caveness LS: Ocular and facial injuries in baseball. **Int Ophthalmol Clin** 28:238-241, 1988

81. Chan RC, Chiu JW, Chou CL, et al: [Median nerve lesions at wrist in cyclists]. **Chung Hua I Hsueh Tsa Chih (Taipei)** 48:121-124, 1991 (Chin)

82. Chandy T, Grana W: Secondary school athletic injury in boys and girls: a three year comparison. **Phys Sportsmed** 13:106-111, 1985

83. Chapman M, Oni J: Motor racing accidents at Brands Hatch. **Br J Sports Med** 3:121-123, 1991

84. Charakorn C, Amatyakul P: Hearing impairment in Thais due to sport shooting: a preliminary report. **J Med Assoc Thai** 81:344-351, 1998

85. Chard MD, Lachmann SM: Racquet sports—patterns of injury presenting to a sports injury clinic. **Br J Sports Med** 21:150-153, 1987

86. Chen C, Fang W, Chen C, et al: Spontaneous spinal epidural hematomas with repeated remission and relapse. **Neuroradiology** 39:737-740, 1997

87. Cheng CL, Wolf AL, Mirvis S, et al: Bodysurfing accidents resulting in cervical spinal injuries. **Spine** 17:257-260, 1992

88. Cheng TL, Fields CB, Brenner RA, et al: Sports injuries: an important cause of morbidity in urban youth. District of Columbia Child/Adolescent Injury Research Network. **Pediatrics** 105:E32, 2000

89. Chow TK, Corbett SW, Farstad DJ: Spectrum of injuries from snowboarding. **J Trauma** 41:321-325, 1996

90. Cinque C: Bicycle safety: a balancing act. **Phys Sportsmed** 17:177-183, 1989

91. Cinque C: Mountain biking: does rough terrain make rugged riders? **Phys Sportsmed** 15:184-190, 1987

92. Clancy W, Shelbourne K, Zoellner G, et al: Treatment of knee joint instability secondary to rupture of the posterior cruciate ligament. **J Bone Joint Surg (Am)** 65:310-322, 1983

93. Clark CR, O'Hanlon AP, Wright MJ, et al: Event-related potential measurement of deficits in information processing following moderate to severe closed head injury. **Brain Inj** 6:509-520, 1992

94. Clark JE: Apophyseal fracture of the lumbar spine in adolescence. **Orthop Rev** 20:512-516, 1991

95. Clarke K: An epidemiological view, in Torg JS (ed): **Athletic Injuries to the Head, Neck and Face**. St Louis, Mo: Mosby-Yearbook, 1991, pp 19-21

96. Clarke K: Premises and pitfalls of athletic injury surveillance. **J Sports Med** 3:292-295, 1975

97. Clarke K: Spinal cord injuries in organized sports. **SCI Digest** 16, 1980

98. Clarke KS, Braslow A: Football fatalities in actuarial perspective. **Med Sci Sports** 10 (2):94-96, 1978

99. Cohn BT, Brahms MA, Cohn M: Injury to the eleventh cranial nerve in a high school wrestler. **Orthop Rev** 15:590-595, 1986

100. Committee on Accident and Poison Prevention and Committee on Pediatric Aspects of Physical Fitness, Recreation, and Sports: Trampolines II. **Pediatrics** 67:438, 1981

101. Condie C, Rivara FP, Bergman AB: Strategies of a successful campaign to promote the use of equestrian helmets. **Publ Health Rep** 108:121-126, 1993

102. Coonley-Hoganson R, Sachs N, Desai B, et al: Sequelae associated with head injuries in patients who are not hospitalized: a follow-up survey. **Neurosurgery** 14:315-317, 1984

103. Corsellis J, Brutan C, Freeman-Brouse D: The aftermath of boxing. **Psychol Med** 3:270-303, 1975

104. Crapo R, Morris A: Standardize single breath normal values for carbon monoxide diffusing capacity. **Am Rev Respir Dis** 123:185-190, 1981

105. Cremona-Meteyard SL, Geffen GM: Persistent visuospatial attention deficits following mild head injury in Australian Rules football players. **Neuropsychologia** 32:649-662, 1994 [erratum in **Neuropsychologia** 33:659, 1995]

106. Crepin-Leblond T, Moulin T, Chopard L, et al: Dissection of the verte-

bral artery: a study of 23 patients. **Cerebrovasc Dis 2**:230, 1992

107. Crites B, Moorman C: Spine injuries associated with falls from hunting tree stands. **J South Orthop Assoc 7**:241-245, 1998

108. Crowley PJ, Condon KC: Analysis of hurling and camogie injuries. **Br J Sports Med 23**:183-185, 1989

109. Cruikshank JK, Higgens CS, Gray JR: Two cases of acute intracranial haemorrhage in young amateur boxers. **Lancet 1**:626-627, 1980

110. Cruz M, Arpa J: Carpal tunnel syndrome in childhood: study of six cases. **Electroencephalogr Clin Neurophysiol 109**:304-308, 1998

111. Cryon B, Hutton W: The fatigue strength of the lumbar neural arch in spondylolysis. **J Bone Joint Surg (Br) 60**:234-238, 1978

112. Cuddihy B, Hurley M: Contact sports and injury. **Irish Med J 83**: 98-100, 1990

113. Daneshmend T, Hewer R, Bradshaw J: Acute brain stem stroke during neck manipulation. **Br Med J 288**:189, 1984

114. Danielsson L, Westlin N: Riding accidents. **Acta Orthop Scand 44**: 597-603, 1973

115. Datti R, Gentile SL, Pisani R: Acute intracranial epidural haematoma in a basketball player: a case report. **Br J Sports Med 29**:95-96, 1995

116. Davidson TM, Laliotis AT: Snowboarding injuries, a four-year study with comparison with alpine ski injuries. **West J Med 164**:231-237, 1996

117. Davies JE, Gibson T: Injuries in Rugby Union football. **Br Med J 2**: 1759-1761, 1978

118. Davis J: Anaerobic threshold: review of the concept and directions for future research. **Med Sci Sports Exer 17**:6-17, 1985

119. Davis MW, Litman T: Figure skater's foot. **Minn Med 62**:647-648, 1979

120. Davis MW, Litman T, Crenshaw R, et al: Bicycling injuries. **Phys Sportsmed 8**:88-96, 1980

121. Dawson D, Hallet M, Millander L (eds): **Entrapment Neuropathies.** Boston, Mass: Little, Brown, & Co, 1990

122. Delaney JS, Lacroix VJ, Leclerc S, et al: Concussions during the 1997 Canadian Football League season. **Clin J Sport Med 10**:9-14, 2000

123. DeOrio J, Bianco A: Lumbar disc excision in children and adolescents. **J Bone Joint Surg (Am) 64**:991-995, 1982

124. Desai K, Gingell J: Hazards of long distance cycling. **Br Med J 298**: 1072-1073, 1989

125. Deutsch F: Isolated lumbar strengthening in the rehabilitation of chronic low back pain. **J Manip Physiol Ther 19**:124-133, 1996

126. Dikmen S, McLean A, Temkin N: Neuropsychological and psychosocial consequences of mild head injury. **J Neurol Neurosurg Psychiatry 49**:227-232, 1986

127. Dobyns J, O'Brien E, Linschied R, et al: Bowler's thumb—diagnosis and treatment: a review of 17 cases. **J Bone Joint Surg (Am) 54**: 751-755, 1972

128. Dowling PA: Prospective study of injuries in United States Ski Association freestyle skiing—1976-77 to 1979-80. **Am J Sports Med 10**: 268-275, 1982

129. Duda M: News briefs: chest pads advised in youth baseball. **Phys Sportsmed 15**:21-35, 1987

130. Eckman P, Perlstein G, Altrocchi P: Ulnar neuropathy in bicycle riders. **Arch Neurol 32** 130-131, 1975

131. Ekstrand J, Gillquist J: Soccer injuries and their mechanisms: a prospective study. **Med Sci Sports Exerc 15**:267-270, 1983

132. Ekstrand J, Gillquist J, Moller M, et al: Incidence of soccer injuries and their relation to training and team success. **Am J Sports Med 11**:63-67, 1983

133. Ellis H: **Clinical Anatomy.** Oxford: Blackwell Scientific, 1977

134. Ellis W, Green D, Holzaepfel N, et al: The trampoline and the serious neurologic injuries. **JAMA 174**:1673-1676, 1960

135. Ellison A (ed): **Training and Sports Medicine.** Chicago, Ill: American Academy of Orthopedic Surgeons, 1984

136. Ellitsgaard N: Parachuting injuries: a study of 110,000 sports jumps. **Br J Sports Med 21**:13-17, 1987

137. Engstrom B, Forssblad M, Johansson C, et al: Does a major knee injury definitely sideline an elite soccer player? **Am J Sports Med 18**: 101-105, 1990

138. Engstrom B, Johansson C, Tornkvist H: Soccer injuries among elite female players. **Am J Sports Med 19**:372-375, 1991

139. Erhart S, Furrer M, Frutiger A, et al: [Blessings of technology? The severely injured skier—a result of technical equipment on the ski slope]. **Z Unfallchir Versicherungsmed 87**:22-26, 1994 (Ger)

140. Essex-Lopresti P: The hazards of parachuting. **Br J Surg 34**:1-13, 1946

141. Everard A: Golf. **JR Coll Gen Pract 19**:293-295, 1970

142. Farfan HF, Cossette JW, Robertson GH, et al: The effects of torsion on the lumbar intervertebral joints: the role of torsion in the production of disc degeneration. **J Bone Joint Surg 52**:468-497, 1970

143. Feinberg J, Nadler S, Krivickas L: Peripheral nerve injuries in the athlete. **Sports Med 24**:385-408, 1997

144. Ferrer MI: Sports hazards. **J Am Med Womens Assoc 35**:62, 1980 (Editorial)

145. Ferrera PC, McKenna DP, Gilman EA: Injury patterns with snowboarding. **Am J Emerg Med 17**:575-577, 1999

146. Fischbein A, Rice C, Sarkozi L, et al: Exposure to lead in firing ranges. **JAMA 241**:1141-1144, 1979

147. Foo C, Swann M: Isolated paralysis of the serratus anterior. **J Bone Joint Surg (Br) 65**:552-556, 1983

148. Frenguelli A, Ruscito P, Bicciolo G, et al: Head and neck trauma in sporting activities. Review of 208 cases. **J Craniomaxillofac Surg 19**: 178-181, 1991

149. Frontera W: Cyclist palsy: clinical and electrodiagnostic findings. **Br J Sports Med 17**:91-93, 1983

150. Gabl M, Lang T, Pechlaner S, et al: [Snowboarding injuries]. **Sportverletz Sportschaden 5**:172-174, 1991 (Ger)

151. Gainor BJ, Piotrowski G, Puhl J, et al: The throw: biomechanics and acute injury. **Am J Sports Med 8**:114-118, 1980

152. Ganong R, Heneveld E, Beranek S, et al: Snowboarding injuries: a report on 415 patients. **Phys Sportsmed 20**:114, 1992

153. Garrick JG, Requa RK: Ballet injuries. An analysis of epidemiology and financial outcome. **Am J Sports Med 21**:586-590, 1993

154. Garrick JG, Requa RK: Epidemiology of women's gymnastics injuries. **Am J Sports Med 8**:261-264, 1980

155. Garth WP Jr, Van Patten PK: Fractures of the lumbar lamina with epidural hematoma simulating herniation of a disc. A case report. **J Bone Joint Surg (Am) 71**:771-772, 1989

156. Gennarelli T: Cerebral concussion and diffuse brain injuries, in Cooper P (ed): **Head Injuries.** Baltimore, Md: Williams & Wilkins, 1987, pp 108-124

157. George P, Walmsley T, Currie D, et al: Lead exposure during recreational use of small bore rifle ranges. **NZ Med J 106**:422-424, 1993

158. Gierup J, Larsson M, Lennquist S: Incidence and nature of horse-riding injuries. **Acta Chir Scand 142**:57-61, 1976

159. Goertzen M, Schoppe K, Lange G, et al: [Injuries and damage caused by excess stress in body building and power lifting]. **Sportverletz Sportschaden 3**:32-36, 1989 (Ger)

160. Goldberg B, Rosenthal PP, Robertson LS, et al: Injuries in youth football. **Pediatrics 81**:255-261, 1988

161. Goldberg I, Peylan J, Amit S: [Nerve injuries in bicycle riders]. **Harefuah 121**:159-161, 1991 (Hebr)

162. Goldberg R, Hicks A, O'Leary L, et al: Lead exposure at uncovered outdoor firing ranges. **J Occup Med 33**:718-719, 1991

163. Goldenberg M, Hossler P: Head and facial injuries in interscholastic women's lacrosse. **J Athletic Training 30**:37-42, 1995

164. Goldhaber G: A national survey about parent awareness of the risk of severe brain injury from playing football. **J Athletic Training 28**: 306-311, 1993

165. Goldstein JD, Berger PE, Windler GE, et al: Spine injuries in gymnasts and swimmers. An epidemiologic investigation. **Am J Sports Med 19**: 463-468, 1991

166. Gomez E, DeLee JC, Farney WC: Incidence of injury in Texas girls' high school basketball. **Am J Sports Med 24**:684-687, 1996

167. Graling P, Colvin D: The lithotomy position in colon surgery. **AORN J 55**:1029-1039, 1992

168. Green G, Jordan S: Chronic head and neck injuries, in Garrett W, Kirkendall D, Contiguglia S (eds): **The U.S. Soccer Sports Medicine Book.** Baltimore, Md: Williams & Wilkins, 1996, pp 191-204

169. Green GA, Jordan SE: Are brain injuries a significant problem in soccer? **Clin Sports Med 17**:795-809, 1998

170. Gregg J, Labosky D, Harty M: Serratus anterior paralysis in the young athlete. **J Bone Joint Surg (Am) 61**:825-832, 1979

171. Griffin R, Peterson K, Halseth J, et al: Injuries in professional rodeo: an update. **Phys Sportsmed 15**:104-115, 1987

172. Griffiths DM, MacKellar A: Bicycle-spoke and "doubling" injuries. **Med J Aust 149**:618-619, 1988

173. Grin TR, Nelson LB, Jeffers JB: Eye injuries in childhood. **Pediatrics**

80:13-17, 1987

174. Grogan J, Hemminghytt S, Williams A, et al: Spondylolysis studied by computer tomography. **Radiology 145**:737-742, 1982
175. Groppel J: The biomechanics of tennis: an overview. **Int J Sports Biomechan 2**:141-155, 1986
176. Grossman JA, Kulund DN, Miller CW, et al: Equestrian injuries. Results of a prospective study. **JAMA 240**:1881-1882, 1978
177. Haglund Y, Eriksson E: Does amateur boxing lead to chronic brain damage? A review of some recent investigations. **Am J Sports Med 21**: 97-109, 1993
178. Hall SJ: Mechanical contribution to lumbar stress injuries in female gymnasts. **Med Sci Sports Exerc 18**:599-602, 1986
179. Hallel T, Naggan L: Parachuting injuries: a retrospective study of 83,718 jumps. **J Trauma 15**:14-19, 1975
180. Hamilton M, Tranmer B: Nervous injuries in horseback-riding accidents. **J Trauma 34**:227-231, 1993
181. Hanbury PH: Bungy jumping. **Aust NZ J Ophthalmol 18**:229, 1990
182. Harries M: The ups and downs of bungee jumping. **Br Med J 305**: 1520, 1992
183. Harris J: Neurologic injuries in skiing and winter sports in America, in Jordan BJ, Tsairis PT, Warren RF (eds): **Sports Neurology**. Rockville, Md: Aspen Publications, 1989, pp 295-304
184. Hart EJ: Little League baseball and head injury. **Pediatrics 89**:520-521, 1992 (Letter)
185. Hashimoto K, Oda K, Kuroda Y, et al: Case of suprascapular nerve palsy manifesting as selective atrophy of the infraspinatus muscle in an archery player. **Rinsho Shinkeigaku 23**:970-973, 1983
186. He FS, Zhang SL, Li G, et al: An electroneurographic assessment of subclinical lead neurotoxicity. **Int Arch Occup Environ Health 61**: 141-146, 1988
187. Heaton N: Review of accident causes. **Parachutist**, 1968, pp 9-11
188. Hellstrom M, Jacobsson B, Sward L, et al: Radiologic abnormalities of the thoraco-lumbar spine in athletes. **Acta Radiol 31**:127-132, 1990
189. Helmets cut injury risk even in bike-auto crashes. **Am Med News**, Jan 6, 1997
190. Henry J, Lareau B, Neigut D: The injury rate in professional basketball. **Am J Sports Med 1**:16-18, 1982
191. Hensinger R: Back pain and vertebral changes simulating Scheuermann's disease. **Orthop Trans 6**:1, 1982
192. Hickey GJ, Fricker PA, McDonald WA: Injuries of young elite female basketball players over a six-year period. **Clin J Sport Med 7**:252-256, 1997
193. Hinton-Bayre AD, Geffen GM, Geffen LB, et al: Concussion in contact sports: reliable change indices of impairment and recovery. **J Clin Exp Neuropsychol 21**:70-86, 1999
194. Hirasawa Y, Sakakida K: Sports and peripheral nerve injury. **Am J Sports Med 11**:420-426, 1983
195. Hirish D, Inglemark B, Miller M: The anatomical basis of low back pain. **Acta Orthop Scand 33**:1, 1963
196. Hite P, Greene K, Levy D, et al: Injury resulting from bungee cord jumping. **Ann Emerg Med 22**:1060-1063, 1993
197. Hochschuler S (ed): **The Spine Sports**. Philadelphia, Pa: Hanley & Belfus, 1990
198. Holley J, Butler J, Mahoney J: Carbon monoxide poisoning in racing car drivers. **J Sports Med Phys Fitness 39**:20-23, 1999
199. Hosea T, Gatt C, Gertner E: Biomechanical analysis of the golfers back, in Stover C, McCarroll J, Mallon W (eds): **Feeling Up to Par: Medicine from Tee to Green**. Philadelphia, Pa: FA Davis, 1994
200. Hosea TM, Gatt CJ Jr: Back pain in golf. **Clin Sports Med 15**:37-53, 1996
201. Hosey R, Puffer J: Baseball and softball sliding injuries. Incidence and the effect of technique in collegiate baseball and softball players. **Am J Sports Med 28**:360-363, 2000
202. Howse C: Wrist injuries in sport. **Sports Med 17**:163-175, 1994
203. Hoy K, Lindblad BE, Terkelsen CJ, et al: European soccer injuries. A prospective epidemiologic and socioeconomic study. **Am J Sports Med 20**:318-322, 1992
204. Hoyt C: Ulnar neuropathy in bicycle riders. **Arch Neurol 33**:372, 1976 (Letter)
205. Hunter RE: Skiing injuries. **Am J Sports Med 27**:381-389, 1999
206. Husni E, Bell H, Storer J: Mechanical occlusion of the vertebral artery: a new concept. **JAMA 196**:475-478, 1966
207. Hutchinson MR: Low back pain in elite rhythmic gymnasts. **Med Sci**

Sports Exerc 31:1686-1688, 1999

208. Hutton W, Stott J, Cyron B: Is spondylolysis a fatigue or fracture. **Spine 2**:202-209, 1977
209. Illingworth CM: Injuries to children riding BMX bikes. **Br Med J (Clin Res Ed) 289**:956-957, 1984
210. Innocenti E, Bell TA: Ocular injury resulting from bungee-cord jumping. **Eye 8**:710-711, 1994 (Letter)
211. Ireland M, Micheli L: Bilateral stress fractures of the lumbar pedicles in a ballet dancer: a case report. **J Bone Joint Surg (Am) 67**:140-142, 1987
212. Itoh Y, Wakano K, Takeda T, et al: Circulatory disturbances in the throwing hand of baseball pitchers. **Am J Sports Med 15**:264-269, 1987
213. Jackson D, Mannarino F: Lumbar spine in athletes, in Scott W (ed): **Principles of Sports Medicine**. Baltimore, Md: Williams & Wilkins, 1984, pp 212-215
214. Jackson D, Wiltse L: Low back pain in athletes. **Phys Sportsmed 2**:53, 1983
215. Jacome D: Ritual relieved axial dystonia triggered by gaze-evoked amaurosis. **Am J Med Sci 314**:348-350, 1997
216. Jaffe L, Minkoff J: Martial arts: a perspective on their evolution, injuries, and training formats. **Orthop Rev 17**:208-209, 213-215, 220-221, 1988
217. Janda D, Viano D, Andrezejak D, et al: An analysis of preventive methods for baseball-induced chest impact injuries. **Clin J Sport Med 2**:172-179, 1992
218. Janda DH, Hankin FM, Wojtys EM: Softball injuries: cost, cause and prevention. **Am Fam Phys 33**:143-144, 1986
219. Janda DH, Wojtys EM, Hankin FM, et al: A three-phase analysis of the prevention of recreational softball injuries. **Am J Sports Med 18**: 632-635, 1990
220. Jarret GJ, Orwin JF, Dick RW: Injuries in collegiate wrestling. **Am J Sports Med 26**:674-680, 1998
221. Jobe F, Yocum L: The dark side of practice. **Golf 30**:22, 1988
222. Johnson R, Ettinger C, Shealy J: **Proceedings of Skiing Trauma and Safety: Fifth International Symposium**, pp 144-156
223. Johnson R, Incavo S: Alpine skiing injuries, in Casey M, et al (eds): **Winter Sports Medicine**. Philadelphia, Pa: FA Davis, 1990, pp 351-358
224. Johnson R, Incavo S: Cross country ski injuries, in Casey M, et al (eds): **Winter Sports Medicine**. Philadelphia, Pa: FA Davis, 1990, pp 302-307
225. Jones J: Ulnar tunnel syndrome. **Am Fam Phys 44**:497-502, 1991
226. Jones S: Safe bicycling is good for all. **Bicycle USA 28**:12-13, 1992
227. Jordan BD: Acute and chronic brain injury in United States National Team Soccer Players. **Am J Sports Med 24**:704-705, 1996 (Letter)
228. Jordan BD, Relkin NR, Ravdin LD, et al: Apolipoprotein E epsilon4 associated with chronic traumatic brain injury in boxing. **JAMA 278**:136-140, 1997
229. Judet H: Micro-traumatique et inflammatoire, in Judet H, Porte G (eds): **Medecine du Cyclisme**. Paris: Masson, 1983, p 106
230. Kalb K, Gruber P, Landsleitner B: Compression syndrome of the radial nerve in the area of the supinator groove. Experiences with 110 patients. **Handchir Mikrochir Plast Chir 31**:303-310, 1999
231. Kameyama O, Shibano K, Kawakita H, et al: Medical check of competitive canoeists. **J Orthop Sci 4**:243-249, 1999
232. Karlson K: Rowing injuries. **Phys Sportsmed 28**:40-50, 2000
233. Kassirer M, Manon N: Head banger's whiplash. **Clin J Pain 9**:138-141, 1993
234. Keim H, Kirkaldy-Willis W: Low back pain. **Clin Symp 32**:1-32, 1980
235. Keller CS, Noyes FR, Buncher CR: The medical aspects of soccer injury epidemiology. **Am J Sports Med 15**:230-237, 1987
236. Keller TM, Holland MC: Chronic subdural haematoma, an unusual injury from playing basketball. **Br J Sports Med 32**:338-339, 1998
237. Kersey RD, Rowan L: Injury account during the 1980 NCAA wrestling championships. **Am J Sports Med 11**:147-151, 1983
238. Kew T, Noakes T, Scher A, et al: A retrospective study of spinal cord injuries in Cape Province Rugby players. **S Afr Med J 80**:127-133, 1991
239. Kiburz D, Jacobs R, Reckling F, et al: Bicycle accidents and injuries among adult cyclists. **Am J Sports Med 14**:416-419, 1986
240. Kip P, Hunter RE: Cervical spinal fractures in Alpine skiers. **Orthopedics 18**:737-741, 1995
241. Kirkaldy-Willis W, Wedge J, Yong-Hing K, et al: Pathology and pathogenesis of lumbar spondylosis and stenosis. **Spine 3**:319-328, 1978

242. Kitagawa T, Kimura S, Ogata H: [Fatigue fracture]. **Seikei Geka** **17**:564-546, 1966 (Jpn)

243. Kizer K, MacQuarrie M, Kuhn B, et al: Deep snow immersion deaths, a snowboarding danger. **Phys Sportsmed 22**:49-61, 1994

244. Kohn HS: Prevention and treatment of elbow injuries in golf. **Clin Sports Med 15**:65-83, 1996

245. Kolt GS, Kirkby RJ: Epidemiology of injury in elite and subelite female gymnasts: a comparison of retrospective and prospective findings. **Br J Sports Med 33**:312-318, 1999

246. Konermann W, Sell S: [The spine—a problem area in high performance artistic gymnastics. A retrospective analysis of 24 former artistic gymnasts of the German A team]. **Sportverletz Sportschaden 6**:156-160, 1992 (Ger)

247. Konig M, Biener K: [Sport-specific injuries in weight lifting]. **Schweiz Z Sportsmed 38**:25-30, 1990 (Ger)

248. Koplan JP, Siscovick DS, Goldbaum GM: The risks of exercise: a public health view of injuries and hazards. **Publ Health Rep 100**:189-195, 1985

249. Koutedakis Y, Frischknecht R, Murthy M: Knee flexion to extension peak torque ratios and low-back injuries in highly active individuals. **Int J Sports Med 18**:290-295, 1997

250. Kovac D, Negovetic L, Vukic M, et al: [Surgical treatment of lumbar disc hernias in athletes]. **Reumatizam 46**:35-41, 1998 (Roman)

251. Kraus J, Fife O, Cox P, et al: Incidence, severity, and external causes of pediatric brain injury. **Am J Dis Child 140**:687-693, 1986

252. Kravitz H: Preventing injuries from bicycle spokes. **Pediatric Ann 6**:713-716, 1977

253. Krissoff WB, Eiseman B: Injuries associated with hang gliding. **JAMA 233**:158-160, 1975

254. Krueger B, Okazaki H: Vertebral-basilar distribution infarction following chiropractic cervical manipulation. **Mayo Clin Proc 55**:322-332, 1980

255. Kuhn JE, Hawkins RJ: Surgical treatment of shoulder injuries in tennis players. **Clin Sports Med 14**:139-161, 1995

256. Kuland D, Schildwachter T, McCue F: Lacrosse injuries. **Phys Sportsmed 7**:83-90, 1979

257. Kvittem B, Hardie NA, Roettger M, et al: Incidence of orofacial injuries in high school sports. **J Publ Health Dent 58**:288-293, 1998

258. Landrigan P, McKinney A, Hopkins L, et al: Result of poor ventilation in an indoor pistol range. **JAMA 234**:394-397, 1975

259. Lapidus CS, Nelson LB, Jeffers JB, et al: Eye injuries in lacrosse: women need their vision less than men? **J Trauma 32**:555-556, 1992

260. Lawson JS, Rotem T, Wilson SF: Catastrophic injuries to the eyes and testicles in footballers. **Med J Aust 163**:242-244, 1995

261. Letts M, Smallman T, Afanasiev R, et al: Fracture of the pars interarticularis in adolescent athletes: a clinical-biomechanical analysis. **J Pediatr Orthop 6**:40-46, 1986

262. Lieblich S: Peripheral nerve injury during anesthesia. **Anesth Prog 37**:258-260, 1990

263. Liedholt J: Spine injuries to athletes: be prepared. **Orthop Clin North Am 4**:691-707, 1973

264. Lightning-associated deaths—United States, 1980-1995. **MMWR Morbid Mortal Wkly Rep 47**: 391-394, 1998

265. Lim LH, Moore MH, Trott JA, et al: Sports-related facial fractures: a review of 137 patients. **Aust NZ J Surg 63**:784-789, 1993

266. Lindner KJ, Caine DJ: Injury patterns of female competitive club gymnasts. **Can J Sport Sci 15**:254-261, 1990

267. Lindsjo U, Hellquist E, Engkuist O, et al: **Proceedings of Skiing Trauma and Safety: Fifth International Symposium**, pp 375-381

268. Link MS, Wang PJ, Pandian NG, et al: An experimental model of sudden death due to low-energy chest-wall impact (commotio cordis). **N Engl J Med 338**:1805-1811, 1998

269. The Little League way; making youth baseball safer. **Athletic Business,** 1984

270. Livingston L: Mandatory ocular protection in women's field lacrosse. **Sports Vision 1**:18-21, 1997

271. Lloyd RG: Riding and other equestrian injuries: considerable severity. **Br J Sports Med 21**:22-24, 1987

272. Lo YP, Hsu YC, Chan KM: Epidemiology of shoulder impingement in upper arm sports events. **Br J Sports Med 24**:173-177, 1990

273. Long RR, Sargent JC, Pappas AM, et al: Pitcher's arm: an electrodiagnostic enigma. **Muscle Nerve 19**:1276-1281, 1996

274. Lorish TR, Rizzo TD Jr, Ilstrup DM, et al: Injuries in adolescent and

275. preadolescent boys at two large wrestling tournaments. **Am J Sports Med 20**:199-202, 1992

275. Los Angeles Times, 1991, B9

276. Los Angeles Times, 1993, H6

277. Louw D, Reddy KK, Lauryssen C, et al: Pitfalls of bungee jumping. Case report and review of the literature. **J Neurosurg 89**:1040-1042, 1998

278. Lowdon IM, Wetherill MH: Parachuting injuries during training descents. **Injury 20**:257-258, 1989

279. Lowrey CW, Chadwick RO, Waltman EN: Digital vessel trauma from repetitive impact in baseball catchers. **J Hand Surg (Am) 1**:236-238, 1976

280. Mackie S, Taunton J: Injuries in female gymnasts. Trends suggest prevention tactics. **Phys Sportsmed 22**:40-45, 1994

281. Maddocks D, Saling M: Neuropsychological deficits following concussion. **Brain Inj 10**:99-103, 1996

282. Maehlum S: Frequency of injuries in a youth soccer tournament. **Phys Sportsmed 12**:114-117, 1984

283. Maehlum S, Daljord OA: Football injuries in Oslo: a one-year study. **Br J Sports Med 18**:186-190, 1984

284. Marcus B: The future is now: demographics. **Surfer Mag 37**:70, 1996

285. Marinella MA, Barsan WG: Spontaneously resolving cervical epidural hematoma presenting with hemiparesis. **Ann Emerg Med 27**:514-517, 1996

286. Marks MR, Haas SS, Wiesel SW: Low back pain in the competitive tennis player. **Clin Sports Med 7**:277-287, 1988

287. Maron BJ, Link MS, Wang PJ, et al: Clinical profile of commotio cordis: an under-appreciated cause of sudden death in the young during sports and other activities. **J Cardiovasc Electrophysiol 10:** 114-120, 1999

288. Maron BJ, Poliac LC, Kaplan JA, et al: Blunt impact to the chest leading to sudden death from cardiac arrest during sports activities. **N Engl J Med 333**:337-342, 1995

289. Matthews WB: Footballer's migraine. **Br Med J 2**:326-327, 1972

290. Mauch F, Bauer G: Traumatic dislocation of the long fingers at the metacarpophalangeal joint while bowling—case report of an extremely rare injury. **Sportverletz Sportschaden 13**:76-78, 1999

291. Mauer UM, Lotspeich E, Klein HJ, et al: [Body building—effect on neural conduction velocity of the median nerve in the carpal tunnel]. **Z Orthop Ihre Grenzgeb 129**:319-321, 1991 (Ger)

292. Mayer N, Kenney J, Edlich R, et al: Fractures in women lacrosse players: preventable injuries. **J Emerg Med 5**:177-180, 1987

293. Mazur LJ, Yetman RJ, Risser WL: Weight-training injuries. Common injuries and preventative methods. **Sports Med 16**:57-63, 1993

294. McCarroll J, Gioe T: Professional golfers and the price they pay. **Phys Sportsmed 10**:54-70, 1982

295. McCarroll J, Mallon W: Epidemiology of golf injuries, in Stover C, Mallon W (eds): **Feeling Up to Par: Medicine from Tee to Green.** Philadelphia, Pa: FA Davis, 1994

296. McCarroll J, Meaney C, Seibert J: Profile of youth soccer injuries. **Phys Sportsmed 12**:113, 1984

297. McCarroll J, Rettig A, Shelbourbe K: Injuries in the amateur golfer. **Phys Sportsmed 18**:125, 1990

298. McCleery P: Bad back: how to avoid an old hang up. **Golf Digest 35**:58, 1984

299. McCoy G, Piggot J, Macafee A, et al: Injuries of the cervical spine in schoolboy Rugby football. **J Bone Joint Surg (Br) 66**:500-503, 1984

300. McCrory P, Bladin C: Fractures of the lateral process of the talus: a clinical review. "Snowboarder's ankle." **Clin J Sport Med 6**:124-128, 1996

301. McCrory PR, Berkovic SF, Cordner SM: Deaths due to brain injury among footballers in Victoria, 1968-1999. **Med J Aust 172**:217-219, 2000

302. McFarland EG, Wasik M: Epidemiology of collegiate baseball injuries. **Clin J Sport Med 8** (1):10-13, 1998

303. McLatchie G, Morris E: Prevention of karate injuries—a progress report. **Br J Sports Med 11**:78-82, 1977

304. McLatchie GR, Davies JE, Culley JH: Injuries in karate—a case for medical control. **J Trauma 20**:956-958, 1980

305. McLennan J, McLennan J: Snowboarding: what injuries to expect in this rapidly growing sport. **J Musculoskeletal Med 8**:75-89, 1991

306. McNeil S, Spruill W, Langley R, et al: Multiple subdural hematomas associated with breakdancing. **Ann Emerg Med 16**:114-116, 1987

307. McQuillen JB, McQuillen EN, Morrow P: Trauma, sport, and malignant cerebral edema. Am J Forensic Med Pathol 9:12-15, 1988

308. Mecham M, Greenwald R, Macintyre J, et al: in Proceedings of the Second World Congress on Sports Trauma, AOSSM 22nd Annual Meeting, 1996

309. Merbs C: Spondylolysis of the sacrum in Alaskan and Canadian Inuit skeletons. Am J Phys Anthropol 101:357-367, 1996

310. Messina DF, Farney WC, DeLee JC: The incidence of injury in Texas high school basketball. A prospective study among male and female athletes. Am J Sports Med 27:294-299, 1999

311. Meyers MC, Elledge JR, Sterling JC, et al: Injuries in intercollegiate rodeo athletes. Am J Sports Med 18:87-91, 1990

312. Micheli L: Back injuries in dancers. Clin Sports Med 2:473, 1983

313. Micheli L: Low back pain in adolescents: differential diagnosis. Am J Sports Med 7:362-364, 1979

314. Micheli L, Hall J, Miller E: Use of modified Boston brace for back injuries in athletes. Am J Sports Med 8:351, 1980

315. Micheli L, Wood R: Back pain in young athletes. Arch Pediatr Med 149:15-18, 1995

316. Micheli LJ: Back injuries in gymnastics. Clin Sports Med 4:85-93, 1985

317. Micheli LJ: in Proceedings of the National Youth Foundation for the Prevention of Athletic Injuries, Boston, Mass, 1984

318. Milan K: Injury in ballet: a review of relevant topics for the physical therapist. J Orthop Sports Phys Ther 19:121-129, 1994

319. Miller E, Benedict F: Stretch of the femoral nerve in a dancer. J Bone Joint Surg (Am) 67:315-317, 1985

320. Mishra D, Friden J, Schmitz M, et al: Anti-inflammatory medication after muscle injury. A treatment resulting in short-term improvement but subsequent loss of muscle function. J Bone Joint Surg (Am) 77: 1510-1519, 1995

321. Mooney V, Robertson J: The facet syndrome. Clin Orthop 115: 149-156, 1976

322. Moretz J, Grana W: High school basketball injuries. Phys Sportsmed 6:92-95, 1978

323. Morrow PL, Adesina A: Ski fatalities in Vermont. J Trauma 31:150, 1991 (Letter)

324. Morrow PL, McQuillen EN, Eaton LA Jr, et al: Downhill ski fatalities: the Vermont experience. J Trauma 28:95-100, 1988 [erratum, J Trauma 28:561, 1988]

325. Mueller F, Blyth C: A survey of 1981 college lacrosse injuries. Phys Sportsmed 10:87-93, 1982

326. Mundt DJ, Kelsey JL, Golden AL, et al: An epidemiologic study of sports and weight lifting as possible risk factors for herniated lumbar and cervical discs. The Northeast Collaborative Group on Low Back Pain. Am J Sports Med 21:854-860, 1993

327. Munnings F: Cyclist's palsy. Phys Sportsmed 19:113-119, 1991

328. Myles ST, Mohtadi NG, Schnittker J: Injuries to the nervous system and spine in downhill skiing. Can J Surg 35:643-648, 1992

329. Nadeau MT, Brown T, Boatman J, et al: The prevention of softball injuries: the experience at Yokota. Milit Med 155:3-5, 1990

330. Nakaguchi H, Fujimaki T, Ueki K, et al: Snowboard head injury: prospective study in Chino, Nagano, for two seasons from 1995 to 1997. J Trauma 46:1066-1069, 1999

331. Naraen A, Giannikas KA, Livesley PJ: Overuse epiphyseal injury of the coracoid process as a result of archery. Int J Sports Med 20:53-55, 1999

332. Nathan N, Goedeke R: The incidence and nature of Rugby injuries experienced at one school during the 1982 Rugby season. S Afr Med J 64:132-137, 1983

333. National Basketball Trainers Association: Injury Reporting System: National Basketball Association, New York, 1991

334. National Collegiate Athletic Association: Injury Surveillance System: women's lacrosse 1992-93. Overland Park, Kan: National Collegiate Athletic Association, 1993

335. National Collegiate Athletic Association: Injury Surveillance System: women's lacrosse 1994-95. Overland Park, Kan: National Collegiate Athletic Association, 1995

336. Nebergall R, Bauer J, Eimen R: Rough rides: how much risk in rodeo? Phys Sportsmed 20:85-92, 1992

337. Nelson DE, Bixby-Hammett D: Equestrian injuries in children and young adults. Am J Dis Child 146:611-614, 1992

338. Nelson DE, Rivara FP, Condie C: Helmets and horseback riders. Am J Prev Med 10:15-19, 1994

339. Nielsen AB, Yde J: Epidemiology and traumatology of injuries in soccer. Am J Sports Med 17:803-807, 1989

340. Nieman E, Swann P: Karate injuries. Br Med J 1:233, 1971

341. Nilsson S, Roaas A: Soccer injuries in adolescents. Am J Sports Med 6: 358-361, 1978

342. Novotny T, Cook M, Hughes J, et al: Lead exposure in a firing range. Am J Publ Health 77:1225-1226, 1987

343. O'Carrol P, Sheehan J, Gregg T: Cervical spine injuries in Rugby football. Irish Med J 74:377-379, 1981

344. Ogawa K, Yoshida A: Throwing fracture of the humeral shaft. An analysis of 90 patients. Am J Sports Med 26:242-246, 1998

345. Oler M, Tomson W, Pepe H, et al: Morbidity and mortality in the martial arts: a warning. J Trauma 31:251-253, 1991

346. Olvey S: Auto racing, in Jordan B, Tsairis P, Warren R (eds): Sports Neurology. Philadelphia, Pa: Lippincott-Raven, 1998, pp 317-329

347. O'Neill DF, McGlone MR: Injury risk in first-time snowboarders versus first-time skiers. Am J Sports Med 27:94-97, 1999

348. Owens R, Ghadiali E: Judo as a possible cause of anoxic brain damage. J Sports Med Phys Fitness 31:627-628, 1991

349. Pappas A, Zawacki R, Sullivan T: Biomechanics of baseball pitching. A preliminary report. Am J Sports Med 13:33-35, 1985

350. Park KG, Dickson AP: BMX bicycle injuries in children. Injury 17: 34-36, 1986

351. Pasternack JS, Veenema KR, Callahan CM: Baseball injuries: a Little League survey. Pediatrics 98:445-448, 1996

352. Petracic B: Sportbedingte Kompressionssymptomatik des Nervus ulnaris. Sportschaden 3:133-134, 1989

353. Pettrone FA, Ricciardelli E: Gymnastic injuries: the Virginia experience 1982-1983. Am J Sports Med 15:59-62, 1987

354. Pieter W, Zemper ED: Injury rates in children participating in taekwondo competition. J Trauma 43:89-96, 1997

355. Pigozzi F, Santori N, Di Salvo V, et al: Snowboard traumatology: an epidemiological study. Orthopedics 20:505-509, 1997

356. Pino EC, Colville MR: Snowboard injuries. Am J Sports Med 17: 778-871, 1989

357. Povey LJ, Frith WJ, Graham PG: Cycle helmet effectiveness in New Zealand. Accid Anal Prev 31:763-770, 1999

358. Powell EC, Tanz RR: Tykes and bikes: injuries associated with bicycle-towed child trailers and bicycle-mounted child seats. Arch Pediatr Adolesc Med 154:351-353, 2000

359. Powell J, Barber-Foss K: Sex-related injury patterns among selected high school sports. Am J Sports Med 28:385-391, 2000

360. Powell JW, Barber-Foss KD: Traumatic brain injury in high school athletes. JAMA 282:958-963, 1999

361. Powell KE, Heath GW, Kresnow MJ, et al: Injury rates from walking, gardening, weightlifting, outdoor bicycling, and aerobics. Med Sci Sports Exerc 30:1246-1249, 1998

362. Prall JA, Winston KR, Brennan R: Severe snowboarding injuries. Injury 26:539-542, 1995

363. Prebble TB, Chyou PH, Wittman L, et al: Basketball injuries in a rural area. Womens Med J 98:22-24, 1999

364. Price C, Mallonee S: Hunting-related spinal cord injuries among Oklahoma residents. J Okla State Med Assoc 87:270-273, 1994

365. Puder DR, Visintainer P, Spitzer D, et al: A comparison of the effect of different bicycle helmet laws in three New York City suburbs. Am J Publ Health 89:1736-1738, 1999

366. Putukian M, Knowles WK, Swere S, et al: Injuries in indoor soccer. The Lake Placid Dawn to Dark Soccer Tournament. Am J Sports Med 24:317-322, 1996

367. Raisanen J, Ghougassian DF, Moskvitch M, et al: Diffuse axonal injury in a Rugby player. Am J Forensic Med Pathol 20:70-72, 1999

368. Ray J, McCoomb W, Sternes R: Basketball and volleyball, in Reider B (ed): The School Aged Athlete. Philadelphia, Pa: WB Saunders, 1991

369. Rayan G: Archery-related injuries of the hand, forearm, and elbow. South Med J 85:961-964, 1992

370. Renstrom P, Johnson RJ: Cross-country skiing injuries and biomechanics. Sports Med 8:346-370, 1989

371. Richards J, Liberi V: Presented at the U.S. Soccer Symposium on the Sports Medicine of Soccer, Orlando, Florida, 1994

372. Rimel R, Nelson W, Persing J: Epidural hematoma in lacrosse. Phys Sportsmed 11:140-144, 1983

373. Ringel S, Treihaft M, Carry M, et al: Suprascapular neuropathy in

pitchers. **Am J Sports Med** 18:80-86, 1990

374. Risk of injury from baseball and softball in children 5 to 14 years of age. **Pediatrics** 93:690-692, 1994

375. Rivara F: Traumatic deaths of children in the United States: currently available prevention strategies. **Pediatrics** 75:456-462, 1985

376. Rivara FP, Thompson DC, Thompson RS: Epidemiology of bicycle injuries and risk factors for serious injury. **Inj Prev** 3:110-114, 1997

377. Rivara FP, Thompson DC, Thompson RS, et al: Injuries involving off-road cycling. **J Fam Pract** 44:481-485, 1997

378. Roaf R: A study of the mechanics of spinal injuries. **J Bone Joint Surg (Br)** 42:810-823, 1960

379. Roberts J: Injuries, handicaps, mashies, and cleeks. **Phys Sportsmed** 6:121-123, 1978

380. Robertson J: Neck manipulation as a cause of stroke. **Stroke** 13:260-261, 1982 (Author's rebuttal in Letters to the Editor)

381. Rodd HD, Chesham DJ: Sports-related oral injury and mouthguard use among Sheffield school children. **Community Dent Health** 14:25-30, 1997

382. Rodriguez G, Francione S, Gardella M, et al: Judo and choking: EEG and regional cerebral blood flow findings. **J Sports Med Phys Fitness** 31:605-610, 1991

383. Rontoyannis GP, Pahtas G, Dinis D, et al: Sudden death of a young wrestler during competition. **Int J Sports Med** 9:353-355, 1988

384. Ross RJ, Casson IR, Siegel O, et al: Boxing injuries: neurologic, radiologic, and neuropsychologic evaluation. **Clin Sports Med** 6:41-51, 1987

385. Rossi F, Dragoni S: Lumbar spondylolysis: occurrence in competitive athletes. Updated achievements in a series of 390 cases. **J Sports Med Phys Fitness** 3:450-452, 1990

386. Rossi F, Triggs WJ, Gonzalez R, et al: Bilateral medial pectoral neuropathy in a weight lifter. **Muscle Nerve** 22:1597-1599, 1999

387. Roth E, Teichner W, Craig R: Compendium of human responses to the aerospace environment. **NASA Contractor Rep** 11:7-9, 1968

388. **Rule Book of the MIAA.** Milford: MIAA, 1996

389. Sacco DE, Sartorelli DH, Vane DW: Evaluation of alpine skiing and snowboarding injury in a northeastern state. **J Trauma** 44:654-659, 1998

390. Sacks JJ, Holmgreen P, Smith SM, et al: Bicycle-associated head injuries and deaths in the United States from 1984 through 1988. How many are preventable? **JAMA** 266:3016-3018, 1991

391. Sacks JJ, Kresnow M, Houston B, et al: Bicycle helmet use among American children, 1994. **Inj Prevent** 2:258-262, 1996

392. Salai M, Brosh T, Blankstein A, et al: Effect of changing the saddle angle on the incidence of low back pain in recreational bicyclists. **Br J Sports Med** 33:398-400, 1999

393. Sammarco G: The foot and ankle in classical ballet and modern dance, in Jahss M (eds): **Disorders of the Foot.** Philadelphia, Pa: WB Saunders, 1982, pp 1626-1659

394. Sammarco G: The hip in dancers. **Med Prob Perf Artists** 2:5-14, 1987

395. Sammarco G: The lower extremity and spine in sports medicine, in Nicholas J, Hershman E (eds): **Dance Injuries.** St Louis, Mo: CV Mosby, 1986, pp 1406-1439

396. Sammarco G, Miller E: Forefoot conditions in dancers: part II. **Foot Ankle** 3:93-98, 1982

397. Sammarco G, Stephens M: Neurapraxia of the femoral nerve in a modern dancer. **Am Orthop Soc Sports Med** 19:413-414, 1991

398. Sane J: Maxillofacial and dental injuries in contact team sports. **Proc Finn Dent Soc** 84:1-45, 1988

399. Sankhala SS, Gupta SP: Spoke-wheel injuries. **Ind J Pediatr** 54:251-256, 1987

400. Santavirta S, Tallroth K, Ylinen P, et al: Surgical treatment of Bertolotti's syndrome: a follow-up of sixteen patients. **Arch Orthop Trauma Surg** 112:82-87, 1993

401. Scher A: Cervical spinal cord injury without evidence of fracture or dislocation. **S Afr Med J** 50:962-965, 1976

402. Scher A: The "double" tackle—another cause of serious cervical spinal injury in Rugby players. **S Afr Med J** 64:595-596, 1983

403. Scher A: The high Rugby tackle—an avoidable cause of cervical spinal cord injury. **S Afr Med J** 53:1015-1018, 1978

404. Scher A: Premature onset of degenerative disease of the cervical spine in Rugby players. **S Afr Med J** 77:557-558, 1990

405. Scher A: Rugby injuries of the spine and spinal cord. **Clin Sports Med** 6:87-99, 1987

406. Scher A: Rugby injuries to the cervical spine and spinal cord: a ten year review. **Clin Sports Med** 17:197, 1998

407. Scher A: Spinal cord concussion in Rugby players. **Am J Sports Med** 19:485-488, 1991

408. Scher AT: Bodysurfing injuries of the spinal cord. **S Afr Med J** 85:1022-1024, 1995

409. Scher AT: Diving injuries to the cervical spinal cord. **S Afr Med J** 59:603-605, 1981

410. Schmidt-Olsen S, Jorgensen U, Kaalund S, et al: Injuries among young soccer players. **Am J Sports Med** 19:273-275, 1991

411. Schneider R: **Head and Neck Injuries in Football.** Baltimore, Md: Williams & Wilkins, 1973

412. Schneider R: The syndrome of acute anterior spinal cord injury. **J Neurol Neurosurg Psychiatry** 21:216-227, 1958

413. Schultz JS, Leonard JA Jr: Long thoracic neuropathy from athletic activity. **Arch Phys Med Rehabil** 73:87-90, 1992

414. Schwartz ML, Hudson AR, Fernie GR, et al: Biomechanical study of full-contact karate contrasted with boxing. **J Neurosurg** 64:248-252, 1986

415. See LC, Lo SK: Cycling injuries among junior high school children in Taiwan. **J Formos Med Assoc** 96:641-648, 1997

416. Seward H, Orchard J, Hazard H, et al: Football injuries in Australia at the elite level. **Med J Aust** 159:298-301, 1993

417. Shae K, Shumsky I, Shae O: De Quervain's disease and off-road mountain biking. **Phys Sportsmed** 19:59-64, 1991

418. Shapiro MJ, Marts B, Berni A, et al: The perils of bungee jumping. **J Emerg Med** 13:629-631, 1995

419. Shealy J: Death in downhill skiing, in Johnson R, Mote C (eds): **Skiing Trauma and Safety.** Philadelphia, Pa: American Society for Testing and Materials

420. Shimizu J, Nishiyama K, Takeda K, et al: A case of long thoracic nerve palsy, with winged scapula, as a result of prolonged exertion on practicing archery. **Rinsho Shinkeigaku** 30:873-876, 1990

421. Shorter NA, Mooney DP, Harmon BJ: Snowboarding injuries in children and adolescents. **Am J Emerg Med** 17:261-263, 1999

422. Silver JR, Gill S: Injuries of the spine sustained during Rugby. **Sports Med** 5:328-334, 1988

423. Silver JR, Silver DD, Godfrey JJ: Injuries of the spine sustained during gymnastic activities. **Br Med J (Clin Res Ed)** 293:861-863, 1986

424. Silver M, Gelberman R, Gellman H, et al: Carpal tunnel syndrome: associated abnormalities in ulnar nerve function and the effect of carpal tunnel release on these abnormalities. **J Hand Surg** 10A:710-713, 1985

425. Sim FH, Simonet WT, Melton LJ, et al: Ice hockey injuries. **Am J Sports Med** 15:30-40, 1987

426. Sinson G, Zager EL, Kline DG: Windmill pitcher's radial neuropathy. **Neurosurgery** 34:1087-1090, 1994

427. Sliding-associated injuries in college and professional baseball—1990-1991. **MMWR Morbid Mortal Wkly Rep** 42:223, 229-230, 1993

428. Smith C: Physical management of muscular low back pain in the athlete. **Can Med Assoc J** 177:632, 1977

429. Snook GA: Injuries in women's gymnastics. A 5-year study. **Am J Sports Med** 7:242-244, 1979

430. Soler T, Calderon C: The prevalence of spondylolysis in the Spanish elite athlete. **Am J Sports Med** 28:57-62, 2000

431. Sorenson B: Bow hunter's stroke. **Neurosurgery** 2:259-261, 1978

432. Sorenson H: Scheuermann's juvenile kyphosis. Junksgaard, Copenhagen, 1974

433. Sovio O, Van Petegham P, Schweigel J: Cervical spine injuries in Rugby players. **Can Med Assoc J** 130:735-736, 1984

434. Sparks J: Half million hours of Rugby football. The injuries. **Br J Sports Med** 15:30-32, 1981

435. Stahl S, Kaufman T: Ulnar nerve injury at the elbow after steroid injection for medial epicondylitis. **Br J Sports Med** 21:69-70, 1997

436. Stallard M: Backache in oarsmen. **Br J Sports Med** 14:105-108, 1980

437. Steiner M, Micheli L: The use of a modified Boston brace to treat symptomatic spondylolysis. **Orthop Trans** 7:20, 1983

438. Stephenson S, Gissane C, Jennings D: Injury in Rugby League: a four year prospective survey. **Br J Sports Med** 30:331-334, 1996

439. Stewart J (ed): **Focal Peripheral Neuropathies.** New York, NY: Elsevier, 1987

440. Stover C, Wiren G, Topaz G: The modern gold swing and stress syndrome. **Phys Sportsmed** 4:42-47, 1976

441. Stricevic MV, Patel MR, Okazaki T, et al: Karate: historical perspective and injuries sustained in national and international tournament competitions. **Am J Sports Med** 11:320-324, 1983

442. Sugawara M, Ogino T, Minami A, et al: Digital ischemia in baseball players. **Am J Sports Med** 14:329-334, 1986

443. Sullivan JA, Gross RH, Grana WA, et al: Evaluation of injuries in youth soccer. **Am J Sports Med** 8:325-327, 1980

444. Sullum J: Leaping to conclusions. **Reason** 24:46-49, 1992

445. Sumi Y, Morita T, Kumazawa I, et al: Trends in snowboard injury in these eight seasons. **Clin Sports Med** 14:207-212, 1997

446. Sutherland AG, Holmes JD, Myers S: Differing injury patterns in snowboarding and alpine skiing. **Injury** 27:423-425, 1996

447. Svensson B, Schutz A, Nilsson A, et al: Lead exposure in indoor firing ranges. **Int Arch Occup Environ Health** 64:219-221, 1992

448. Sward L: The thoracolumbar spine in young elite athletes. Current concepts on the effects of physical training. **Sports Med** 133:357-364, 1992

449. Sward L, Hellstrom M, Jacobsson B, et al: Back pain and radiological changes in the thoracic-lumbar spine of athletes. **Spine** 15:1079, 1990

450. Sward L, Ericksson B, Peterson L: Anthropometric characteristics, passive hip flexion and spinal mobility in relation to back pain in athletes. **Spine** 15:124-129, 1990

451. Swart R: Hard facts about bicycle helmets. **Cycling Sci** 1:14-16, 1989

452. Szewczyk J, Hoffmann M, Kabelis J: [Meralgia paraesthetica in a body-builder]. **Sportverletz Sportschaden** 8:43-45, 1994 (Ger)

453. Takakuwa T, Hakozaki S, Hurukawa K, et al: [Penetrating craniocerebral injuries during downhill skiing]. **No Shinkei Geka** 22:477-479, 1994 (Jpn)

454. Takami H, Takahashi S, Ando M: Traumatic rupture of iliacus muscle with femoral nerve paralysis. **J Trauma** 23:253-254, 1983

455. Tanabe S, Nakahira J, Bando E, et al: Fatigue fracture of the ulna occurring in pitchers of fast-pitch softball. **Am J Sports Med** 19:317-321, 1991

456. Tanaka N, Hayashi S, Amagasa T, et al: Maxillofacial fractures sustained during sports. **J Oral Maxillofac Surg** 54:715-720, 1996

457. Tarazi F, Dvorak MF, Wing PC: Spinal injuries in skiers and snowboarders. **Am J Sports Med** 27:177-180, 1999

458. Tatlow W, Bammer H: Syndrome of vertebral artery compression. **Neurology** 7:331-340, 1957

459. Tator CH, Edmonds VE: Acute spinal cord injury: analysis of epidemiologic factors. **Can J Surg** 22:575-578, 1979

460. Taylor T, Coolican M: Spinal cord injuries in Australian Footballers. **Med J Aust** 147:112-118, 1987

461. Teitz C, Kilcoyne R: Premature osteoarthrosis in professional dancers. **Clin J Sport Med** 8:255-259, 1998

462. Tenvergert EM, Ten Duis HJ, Klasen HJ: Trends in sports injuries, 1982-1988: an in-depth study on four types of sport. **J Sports Med Phys Fitness** 32:214-220, 1992

463. Tertti M, Paajanen H, Kujala UM, et al: Disc degeneration in young gymnasts. A magnetic resonance imaging study. **Am J Sports Med** 18:206-208, 1990

464. Thompson DC, Patterson MQ: Cycle helmets and the prevention of injuries. Recommendations for competitive sport. **Sports Med** 25:213-219, 1998

465. Tongue JR: Hang gliding injuries in California. **J Trauma** 17:898-902, 1977

466. Toole J, Tucker S: Influence of the head position upon cerebral circulation: studies on blood flow in cadavers. **Arch Neurol** 2:616-632, 1960

467. Torg J, Pavlov H, Genuario S, et al: Neurapraxia of the cervical spinal cord with transient quadriplegia. **J Bone Joint Surg (Br)** 68:1354-1370, 1986

468. Torg JS, Corcoran TA, Thibault LE, et al: Cervical cord neurapraxia: classification, pathomechanics, morbidity, and management guidelines. **J Neurosurg** 87:843-850, 1997

469. Torg JS, Truex RC Jr, Marshall J, et al: Spinal injury at the level of the third and fourth cervical vertebrae from football. **J Bone Joint Surg (Am)** 59:1015-1019, 1977

470. Toro-Gonzalez G, Navarro-Roman L, Roman G, et al: Acute ischemic stroke from fibrocartilaginous embolism to the middle cerebral artery. **Stroke** 24:738-740, 1993

471. Torre P, Williams C, Blackwell T: Bungee jumper's foot drop peroneal nerve palsy caused by bungee cord jumping. **Ann Emerg Med** 22:1993

472. Tough SC, Butt JC: A review of fatal injuries associated with downhill skiing. **Am J Forensic Med Pathol** 14:12-16, 1993

473. Toy safety. **MMWR Morbid Mortal Wkly Rep** 34:755-762, 1985

474. Trammell T: Motor sports, in Watkins R (ed): **The Spine in Sports.** St Louis, Mo: CV Mosby, 1995

475. Trammell T, Olvey S, Reed D: Championship car racing accidents and injuries. **Phys Sportsmed** 14:114-120, 1986

476. Tripathi R, Sherertz P, Llewellyn G, et al: Reducing exposures to airborne lead in a covered, outdoor firing range by using totally copper-jacketed bullets. **Am Ind Hyg Assoc J** 51:28-31, 1990

477. Tsur A, Shahin R: [Suprascapular nerve entrapment in a basketball player]. **Harefuah** 133:190-192, 247, 1997 (Hebr)

478. Tudor R: Acute subdural hematoma following a blow from a basketball. **Am J Sports Med** 7(2):136, 1979

479. Tuominen R: Injuries in national karate competitions in Finland. **Scand J Med Sci Sports** 5:44-48, 1995

480. Tysvaer AT, Storli OV, Bachen NI: Soccer injuries to the brain. A neurologic and electroencephalographic study of former players. **Acta Neurol Scand** 80:151-156, 1989

481. Ungerholm S, Gustavsson J: Skiing safety in children: a prospective study of downhill skiing injuries and their relation to the skier and his equipment. **Int J Sports Med** 6:353-358, 1985

482. Urquhart C, Hawkins M, Howdieshell T, et al: Deer stands: a significant cause of injury and mortality. **South Med J** 84:686-688, 1991

483. U.S. Consumer Product Safety Commission: Head injuries. NEISS Data Highlights: CPSC Directorate for Epidemiology. **Consumer Products Safety Commission** 14:1-10, 1990

484. Van Dijk C, Lim L, Poortman A, et al: Injury rates from walking, gardening, outdoor bicycling, and aerobics. **Med Sci Sports Exerc** 30:1246-1249, 1998

485. van Elegem P: [Bicycling and chronic pathology]. **Acta Orthop Belg** 49:88-100, 1983 (Belg)

486. van Linschoten R, Backx F, Mulder O, et al: Epilepsy and sports. **Sports Med** 10:9-19, 1990

487. van Mechelen W, Hlobil H, Kemper HC: Incidence, severity, aetiology and prevention of sports injuries. A review of concepts. **Sports Med** 14:82-99, 1992

488. Vanderford L, Meyers M: Injuries and bungee jumping. **Sports Med** 20:369-374, 1995

489. Viano D, Andrzejak D, Polley T, et al: Mechanism of fatal chest injury by baseball impact: development of an experimental model. **Clin J Sports Med** 2:161-165, 1992

490. Vinger PF: Prevention of sports injuries. **J Ophthalmic Nurs Technol** 9:210-214, 1990

491. Vinger PF: Sports eye injuries a preventable disease. **Ophthalmology** 88:108-113 1981

492. Vinger PF, Knuttgen H: Eye injuries and eye protection in sports: a position statement. **Br J Sports Med,** 1989, p 23

493. Volski R, Bourguignon G, Rodriguez H: Lower spine screening in the shooting sports. **Phys Sportsmed** 14:101-106, 1986

494. Wadley GH, Albright JP: Women's intercollegiate gymnastics. Injury patterns and "permanent" medical disability. **Am J Sports Med** 21:314-320, 1993

495. Walsh M: Preventing injury in competitive canoeists. **Phys Sportsmed** 13:120-128, 1985

496. Ward A: Improving bicycle safety for children. **Phys Sportsmed** 15:203-208, 1987

497. Warme WJ, Feagin JA Jr, King P, et al: Ski injury statistics, 1982 to 1993, Jackson Hole Ski Resort. **Am J Sports Med** 23:597-600, 1995

498. Warren LW, Bailes JE: On the field evaluation of athletic head injuries. **Clin Sports Med** 17:13-25, 1998

499. Warren M, Brooks-Gunn J, Hamilton L, et al: Scoliosis and fractures in young ballet dancers: relation to delayed menarche and secondary amenorrhea. **N Engl J Med** 314:1348-1353, 1986

500. Warren W: The effects of exercise on the pubertal progression and reproductive function in girls. **J Clin Endocrinol Metab** 51:1150-1157, 1980

501. Wasserman RC, Waller JA, Monty MJ, et al: Bicyclists, helmets and head injuries: a rider-based study of helmet use and effectiveness. **Am J Publ Health** 78:1220-1221, 1988

502. Watson AW: Sports injuries in the game of hurling. A one-year prospective study. **Am J Sports Med** 24:323-328, 1996

503. Watts C, Jones D, Crouch D, et al: Survey of bicycling accidents in Boulder, Colorado. **Phys Sportsmed** 14:99-104, 1986

504. Webster DA, Bayliss GV, Spadaro JA: Head and face injuries in scholastic women's lacrosse with and without eyewear. **Med Sci Sports Exerc** 31:938-941, 1999

505. Weiss BD: Bicycle-related head injuries. **Clin Sports Med** 13:99-112, 1994

506. Weiss BD: Nontraumatic injuries in amateur long distance bicyclists. **Am J Sports Med** 13:187-192, 1985

507. Weiss BD: Preventing bicycle-related head injuries. **NY State J Med** 87:319-320, 1987

508. Wesson D, Spence L, Hu X, et al: Trends in bicycling-related head injuries in children after the implementation of a community-based bike helmet campaign. **J Pediatr Surg** 35:688-689, 2000

509. Whitlock MR, Whitlock J, Johnston B: Equestrian injuries: a comparison of professional and amateur injuries in Berkshire. **Br J Sports Med** 21:25-26, 1987

510. Wiesel S, Bernini P, Rothman R (eds): **The Aging Lumbar Spine.** Philadelphia, Pa: WB Saunders, 1982

511. Wilber CA, Holland GJ, Madison RE, et al: An epidemiological analysis of overuse injuries among recreational cyclists. **Int J Sports Med** 16:201-206, 1995

512. Wilberger JE: Athletic spinal cord and spine injuries. **Clin Sports Med** 17:113, 1998

513. Wilberger JE: Minor head injuries in American football. Prevention of long term sequelae. **Sports Med** 15:338-343, 1993

514. Wilkerson LA: Martial arts injuries. **J Am Osteopath Assoc** 97: 221-226, 1997

515. Williams P, McKibbon B: Unstable cervical spine injuries in Rugby—a 20-year review. **Injury** 18:329-332, 1987

516. Wilmarth M, Nelsen S: Distal sensory latencies of the ulnar nerve in long distance bicyclists: pilot study. **J Orthop Sports Phys Ther** 9: 370-374, 1988

517. Wiltse L, Widell E Jr, Jackson D: Fatigue fracture: the basic lesion in isthmic spondylolisthesis. **J Bone Joint Surg (Am)** 57:17-22, 1975

518. Wismach J, Krause D: [Spinal changes in artistic gymnasts]. **Sportverletz Sportschaden** 2:95-99, 1988 (Ger)

519. Wolf T: Injuries and physical complaints caused by golf. **Sportverletzung Sportschaden** 3:124-127, 1989

520. Woodhead ABD: Paralysis of the serratus anterior in a world class marksman. A case study. **Am J Sports Med** 13:359-362, 1985

521. Worrell J: BMX bicycles: accident comparison with other models. **Arch Emerg Med** 2:209-213, 1985

522. Wright J: Ski jumping injuries, in Casey M, et al (eds): **Winter Sports Medicine.** Philadelphia, Pa: FA Davis, 1990, pp 324-330

523. Wu J, Morris J, Hogan G: Ulnar neuropathy at the wrist: case report and review of literature. **Arch Phys Med Rehabil** 66:785-788, 1985

524. Wu WQ, Lewis RC: Injuries of the cervical spine in high school wrestling. **Surg Neurol** 23:143-147, 1985

525. Zagelbaum BM, Starkey C, Hersh PS, et al: The National Basketball Association eye injury study. **Arch Ophthalmol** 113:749-752, 1995

526. Zelisko J, Noble H, Porter M: A comparison of men's and women's professional basketball injuries. **Am J Sports Med** 10:297-299, 1982

527. Zollinger H, Gorschewsky O, Cathrein P: [Injuries in snowboarding—a prospective study]. **Sportverletz Sportschaden** 8:31-37, 1994 (Ger)

528. Zuckerman JD, Polonsky L, Edelson G: Suprascapular nerve palsy in a young athlete. **Bull Hosp Joint Dis** 53:11-22, 1993

CHAPTER 14

Traumatic Brain Injury in Boxing

BARRY D. JORDAN, MD, MPH

Traumatic brain injury (TBI) represents an inevitable consequence of boxing. Accordingly, the diagnosis, management, and prevention of TBI become essential. The acute, subacute, and chronic neurological sequelae secondary to boxing have been well recognized in the clinical literature. This chapter highlights these neurological consequences associated with boxing.

Acute Traumatic Brain Injury

Epidemiology

Studies analyzing the frequency of acute TBI in amateur boxing indicate that permanent and irreversible neurological dysfunction is rare. Blonstein and Clarke[2] assessed boxing injuries in amateur boxers over a 7-month period and found that 29 boxers (0.58%) were severely concussed or knocked out more than once. Injury reports of the 1981 and 1982 United States National Amateur Boxing championships noted that 48 (8.7%) of 547 bouts were stopped because of knockouts or blows to the head.[12] This yielded a rate of 4.38 head injuries per 100 personal exposures. In amateur boxing in Ireland, Porter and O'Brien[42] observed 33 cerebral concussions in 281 bouts, or 562 personal exposures, yielding 5.87 concussions per 100 personal exposures. Jordan et al[23] reviewed all boxing injuries sustained by amateur boxers at the U.S. Olympic Training Center during a 10-year period. Among a total of 477 injuries, 29 (6.1%) were brain injuries. In a survey of amateur boxers in Denmark, 5.7% to 7.8% of competitions resulted in a knockout (KO) and 0.8% to 5.4% of the bouts, respectively, were terminated because the referee stopped the contest secondary to head blows.[48] Welch et al[56] conducted a survey of boxing injuries that occurred during an institutional boxing program over a 2-year period at the U.S. Military Academy in West Point, New York. Of approximately 2100 cadets who received boxing instruction, 22 cases of blunt head trauma were reported, none of which resulted in neurological deficits.

Investigations documenting the frequency of acute TBI among professional boxers have been conducted in New York State. Jordan and Campbell[16] reviewed all acute boxing injuries among professional boxers in New York from August 1982 through July

1984. During this 2-year period, there were 3110 rounds fought and 376 injuries, of which 262 were head injuries. This yielded a frequency of 0.8 head injuries per 10 rounds fought and 2.9 injuries per 10 boxers. In a survey of a representative sample of active professional boxers in New York (n=143), the prevalence of a self-reported technical knockout (TKO) or KO was 42%.[18] Also observed in this study was a tendency for TKOs or KOs to occur in the earlier rounds. In 1 year, 122 (64%) of 189 bouts resulted in a TKO or KO, and 80% of these occurred within the first three rounds.[15]

Clinical Presentation

The knockout is synonymous with a cerebral concussion and is the most common acute neurological injury in boxing. The majority of concussions in boxing are not associated with a loss of consciousness and are most commonly associated with transient cognitive impairment and/or loss of motor tone. Cognitive impairment usually anticipated after a boxing match may include problems with attention, planning, and memory.[32] Characteristic of many knockouts seems to be an amnestic period with confusion,[29] but amnesia can occur without a knockout and should be regarded as evidence of serious injury.[35] Blonstein and Clarke[2] described a boxer who won a decision but was amnesic for the entire fight despite not being knocked out. Both retrograde and anterograde amnesia have been described following boxing matches.[10]

In addition to cognitive impairment, a variety of acute neurophysiological symptoms may be encountered. Sercl and Jaros[49] analyzed the acute neurological findings in 427 boxers involved in 1165 matches. In 336 boxers (79%), there were clinical abnormalities that resolved within several minutes, and 91 (21%) had neurological symptoms lasting up to 24 hours. The most common clinical finding was derangement of muscular tone (380 cases), followed by cerebellar and vestibular signs (319 cases) and pyramidal symptoms (253 cases). Other findings included extrapyramidal signs (191 cases), general muscular weakness (142 cases), and unconsciousness (112 cases). Cranial nerve lesions were rare (seven cases).

The concussion in boxing is typically not associated with any gross pathological changes. Microscopically, animal studies suggest that chromatolysis can occur after concussion.[57] However, when extrapolating to humans, the severity of the head trauma experienced by the experimental animals in these investigations may be more significant than what is typically encountered in boxing. In human studies, Oppenheimer[40] observed microscopic changes such as axonal retraction balls and myelin destruction in the setting of microglial clusters after a concussion. However, the contribution of anoxia to these neuropathological changes was difficult to assess. Accordingly, whether the uncomplicated concussion in boxing (i.e., without anoxia or reduced cerebral perfusion) results in structural damage remains to be determined.

Although uncommon, acute catastrophic pathological lesions such as diffuse axonal injury, subdural hematoma, epidural hematoma, cerebral contusion, intracerebral hemorrhage, injury to the carotid artery, and subarachnoid hemorrhage may be encountered in boxers.[28,55]

Pathophysiology

The concussive properties of a boxer's punch are related to the manner in which the punch is delivered and how the mechanical forces are transferred and absorbed through the intracranial cavity. Blows thrown from the shoulder, such as the roundhouse or the hook, tend to deliver more force than the straightforward jab. The force transmitted by a punch is directly proportional to the mass of the glove and the velocity of the swing, and is inversely proportional to the total mass opposing the punch.[41]

The essential feature of a concussive force is that it is sufficient to accelerate the skull. Rotational (angular) acceleration, linear (translational) acceleration, and impact deceleration can all play a role in the development of acute cerebral injury.[28] Angular acceleration occurs when a punch causes a rotational movement of the skull that can potentially stretch and tear cerebral blood vessels. Subdural hematomas typically result from tearing of the bridging veins secondary to rotational acceleration. Rotational acceleration is also responsible for diffuse axonal injury. Linear acceleration occurs with blows directly to the face that propel the skull in an anterior-to-posterior direction. Linear acceleration may result in gliding contusions.

Management

The treatment of acute TBI is dependent upon the type and severity of the injury. Since the overwhelming majority of acute brain injuries are concussions, typical management requires observation because these injuries are usually self-limited. However it is imperative for the clinician to be aware of more potentially dangerous injuries to the central nervous system (CNS). Indicators of more ominous neurological injuries include prolonged loss of consciousness (longer than a few minutes), focal neurological signs, seizures, and/or persistent postconcussion symptoms (longer than 24 hours). Any boxer suspected of having experienced an acute focal TBI during a competitive bout should be immediately transported via ambulance to the nearest hospital equipped with proper neuroradiological and neurosurgical services. Any boxer who experiences persistent postconcussion symptoms should be properly evaluated and not allowed to return to competition until he is asymptomatic. Traditional guidelines utilized for the return to competition after concussion in sports have not been routinely utilized in boxing.[1,14] The recommendations for rest or inactivity after a concussion tend to be longer in boxing than that recommended in other contact sports and at minimum should be 30 days.

Prevention

It is impossible to eliminate the incidence of acute TBI in boxing. However, the mainstay of prevention should be to minimize the severity of it. This goal could be accomplished by conducting proper prefight examinations in anticipation of identifying those individuals who may be predisposed to acute catastrophic brain injury. Boxers included in this classification are those with abnormal neurological and/or neuroradiological examinations indicative of a pre-existing brain lesion. In addition to performing the proper prefight examination, qualified medical personnel (including an ambulance) should be at ringside to provide medical assistance to an injured boxer. After a competition, all boxers should be briefly examined by the ringside physician. The referee is also instrumental in increasing medical safety in the ring. A qualified referee should be able to identify a boxer who is experiencing a concussion and should terminate the bout before additional neurological injury can occur. Overall, the entire boxing community (e.g., the trainer and promoter) should work together to increase medical safety in boxing.[14]

Second-impact Syndrome in Boxing

The second-impact syndrome represents an exaggerated, commonly fatal response to a second concussion while an athlete is symptomatic from an earlier concussion.[4,5,47] This syndrome, initially described by Saunders and Harbaugh,[47] has been noted primarily in tackle football. However, it can be anticipated in any contact sport and recently has been described in boxing.[5]

Epidemiology

The precise frequency of second-impact syndrome in sports is unknown, but it is believed to be relatively uncommon. Risk factors have not been clearly established.[34] However, any boxer or athlete who participates in a contact/collision sport while being symptomatic from a concussion appears to be at increased risk. In boxing, the second-impact syndrome may occur in a tournament setting where a boxer competes more than once over a selected time period (typically a few days to a week) or, less frequently, within a given bout associated with multiple concussive blows.

Clinical Presentation

Clinically, the athlete experiences a mild TBI (most typically a concussion) followed by persistent postconcussion symptoms that may include headache, dizziness, memory impairment, and other motor-sensory symptoms. While symptomatic from the first brain injury, the athlete returns to participation and sustains a second brain injury. According to Cantu and Voy,[5] this second traumatic impact may be remarkably minor and may not even involve direct head trauma. After sustaining this second impact, the athlete may collapse into coma with rapid brainstem compromise, respiratory failure, and possible death.[5]

According to McCory and Berkovic,[34] the following clinical criteria need to be fulfilled for the definitive diagnosis of second-impact syndrome:

- a medical review after a witnessed first impact;
- documentation of ongoing symptoms following the first impact up to the time of the second impact;
- witnessed second head impact, with a subsequent rapid cerebral deterioration; and
- neuropathological or neuroimaging evidence of cerebral swelling without significant intracranial hematoma or other cause for edema.

Pathology/Pathophysiology

The postmortem hallmark of the second-impact syndrome is massive cerebral edema. Although subdural hematomas may be encountered, they tend to be small and of no clinical significance.[5] The pathophysiological mechanism of this syndrome appears to be loss of vasomotor autoregulation leading to excessive hyperemia or cerebrovascular engorgement, resulting in massive cerebral swelling and brain herniation. Animal studies suggest that repetitive brain injury results in a breakdown of the blood-brain barrier and that the brain remains vulnerable for a period of time and is more susceptible to the effects of a second concussive blow.[30]

Prevention

In view of the high mortality and morbidity associated with it, prevention of the second-impact syndrome becomes paramount. The mainstay of preventive measures relies on the proper evaluation of the athlete. Any athlete who sustains an acute TBI should undergo a detailed neurological evaluation to determine the severity of the injury. In cases of cerebral concussion, the player should not be allowed to return to competition unless they are asymptomatic for a period of time. In individuals with more severe acute TBI, permanent or indefinite restriction of participation in contact sports may be indicated. Restriction of the symptomatic boxer from participating in sparring or competition should minimize the occurrence of this syndrome.

Chronic Traumatic Brain Injury in Boxing

Chronic TBI, also known as dementia pugilistica, chronic traumatic encephalopathy, chronic neurological injury, or the "punch drunk" syndrome, represents the long-term cumulative neurological consequences of repetitive concussive and subconcussive blows to the head. This syndrome was first described in the medical literature in 1928 when Martland[31] described a 38-year-old retired boxer with advanced parkinsonism, ataxia, pyramidal tract dysfunction, and behavioral changes. Chronic TBI is typically delayed in onset and occurs following a long exposure to the sport, usually after a boxer retires or late in the career of a boxer. As a result of this delayed onset, it represents the most difficult safety challenge in modern-day boxing.

Epidemiology

Among former professional boxers licensed by the British Board of Control for at least 3 years from 1929 through 1955, a 17% incidence of chronic TBI has been estimated, with the prevalence increasing as exposure to boxing increases.[43] More recent documentation of the prevalence among more modern-day boxers is nonexistent. Putative and established risk factors for chronic TBI are presented in Table 1. Documented risk factors in boxing include later retirement (i.e., over 28 years of age), increased duration of career (i.e., more than 10 years), and a greater number of bouts (i.e., more than 150 bouts).[43] Clinical studies suggest that risk factors for the development of chronic TBI include poor performance (i.e., second- or third-rate boxers), boxing style (i.e., being a slugger rather than a scientific, intelligent boxer), boxers who are notorious for their ability to "take" a punch, and being a professional boxer as opposed to an amateur.[10] The boxer's age at examination also influences the prevalence of chronic TBI. Boxers examined after the age of 50 had a higher prevalence than those examined before the age of 50.[43] Increasing sparring exposure may increase the risk of neurocognitive decline among professional boxers.[21] A history of a TKO or KO has also been reported to be associated with abnormal computed tomography (CT) of the brain.[18] In addition, progressive changes on CT have been noted in boxers who lose more than 10 bouts.[18]

TABLE 1

PUTATIVE AND DOCUMENTED RISK FACTORS FOR CHRONIC TRAUMATIC BRAIN INJURY

- total number of fights
- number of knockouts experienced
- number of losses
- duration of boxing career
- fight frequency
- age of retirement from boxing
- sparring exposure
- poor performance or skills

Clinical Presentation

In a comprehensive review of the neuropsychiatric aspects of boxing, Mendez[36] classified the clinical manifestations of chronic TBI into motor, cognitive, and psychiatric symptoms. The first, or early, signs may include dysarthria, mild incoordination, tremor, and decreased complex attention. Psychiatric symptoms may include emotional lability and other mild behavioral disturbances such as euphoria or hypomania and increased irritability. Although it has been observed that the initial manifestations are predominantly psychiatric or behavioral in nature,[27] it is the experience of the author that behavioral and personality disturbances may be difficult to assess early in the disease. This is particularly the case when the examiner lacks knowledge of the boxer's premorbid personality.

The second, or moderate, stage of chronic TBI is characterized by progression of the motor, cognitive, and/or behavioral symptoms.[36] Indications of motor dysfunction include signs of parkinsonism and/or progressive difficulty in coordination and ambulation. Cognitive deficits include mild deficits in memory, attention, and executive function. Psychiatric manifestations may include inappropriate behavior, morbid jealousy, paranoia, and violent outbursts.

The third, or severe, stage of chronic TBI is often referred to as dementia pugilistica.[27] During this phase, the boxer exhibits significant motor dysfunction characterized by prominent pyramidal, extrapyramidal, and/or cerebellar symptoms. Cognitive dysfunction as evidenced by amnesia, executive-frontal lobe dysfunction, and psychomotor retardation may be observed. Behaviorally, boxers may exhibit disinhibition, violent outbursts, hypersexuality, and psychosis.[27]

Neurodiagnostic testing demonstrates nonspecific findings in chronic TBI. Magnetic resonance imaging (MRI) and CT may demonstrate brain atrophy with or without a cavum septum pellucidum.[6,7,18,19,24,45,50] Electroencephalography may be normal or may demonstrate focal or diffuse slowing.[3,44,52] Single photon emission CT (SPECT) may exhibit perfusion deficits in the boxer that localize primarily to the frontal and temporal regions.[17,26]

Pathology

Pathologically, boxers with end-stage chronic TBI, or full-blown dementia pugilistica, may exhibit septal and hypothalamic anomalies, cerebellar changes, degeneration of the substantia nigra, and regional occurrence of Alzheimer's neurofibrillary tangles.[8,9] Boxers may exhibit a fenestrated septal cavum, the floor of the hypothalamus may appear to be stretched, and the fornix and mammillary bodies may be atrophied. The cerebellum may demonstrate scarring of the folia in the region of the cerebellar tonsils, and there may be a reduction in the number of Purkinje cells on the inferior surface of the cerebellum. The substantia nigra may lack pigment, and nerve cells may become gliosed. Neurofibrillary tangles primarily involving parts of the hippocampus and the medial temporal gray matter may also be encountered. Although not typically accompanied by senile neuritic plaques, neurofibrillary tangles may be accompanied by diffuse amyloid plaques.[44,53] Neurofibrillary tangles observed in boxers with chronic TBI are also immunoreactive for tau[53] and ubiquitin,[11] similar to those seen in Alzheimer's disease. Another similarity between chronic TBI and Alzheimer's disease is a significant reduction of choline acetyltransferase activity in the nucleus basalis of Meynert and in several regions of the cerebral cortex.[54]

Pathophysiology

The pathophysiology of chronic TBI is unknown; however, it has been speculated that it may share a similar pathogenic mechanism to that of Alzheimer's disease.[43] Any account of the pathophysiology would need to consider the pathological role of the formation of neurofibrillary tangles, abnormal amyloid deposition, and central cholinergic system dysfunction. It has been speculated that blows to the head could conceivably produce local changes in the blood-brain barrier that may enable the deposition of beta amyloid in the injured areas.[37] Alternatively, cerebral concussion may damage the blood-brain barrier, thus allowing extravasation of serum proteins that may serve as antigenic initiators of a secondary immune response that attenuates normal CNS function.[38] The role of the cholinergic system in the pathogenesis of chronic TBI remains to be determined. Animal studies indicate that concussive head injury has a profound effect on central cholinergic neurons.[46] Furthermore, the cholinergic system has been implicated in the pathophysiology of Alzheimer's disease and is probably involved in the physiological basis of learning and memory.[51]

Accordingly, any theory of the pathogenesis of chronic TBI must delineate the interactions between head trauma, neurofibrillary tangle formation, amyloid deposition, central cholinergic function, and subsequent cognitive impairment.

In addition to the foregoing factors, the potential role of the apolipoprotein E (APOE) e4 allele in the development of chronic TBI needs to be explored. Evidence suggests that the presence of the APOE e4 allele may promote the deposition of cerebral amyloid in individuals experiencing TBI.[39] Mayeaux et al[33] noted a 10-fold synergistic increased risk of Alzheimer's disease in individuals with TBI and the presence of APOE e4, whereas an addictive increased risk of Alzheimer's disease in patients with head trauma and APOE e4 was observed by Katzman et al.[25] Based on the author's observation of extensive parenchymal cerebral amyloid deposition and cerebral amyloid angiopathy in a demented boxer who harbored an APOE e4 allele,[20] a study was conducted to determine whether APOE e4 is associated with chronic TBI.[22] In an analysis of 30 active and retired boxers, the author and colleagues found that APOE e4 was associated with an increased severity of chronic TBI in high-exposure boxers (i.e., boxers with more than 12 professional bouts). This finding suggests that there may be a genetic predisposition to the untoward effects of a long boxing career.[22]

Management

A definitive treatment for chronic TBI has not been clearly established. In view of the pathological similarities between chronic TBI and Alzheimer's disease, standard treatments for the management of the cognitive and behavioral symptoms in Alzheimer's disease may be employed in chronic TBI. However, the efficacy of these interventions has not been determined. Boxers with parkinsonian features may be treated with conventional dopaminergic agents utilized in the management of Parkinson's disease.

Prevention

The mainstay of preventing chronic TBI in boxing is to limit exposure and identify boxers who may be at increased risk. Those boxers should undergo more detailed neurodiagnostic testing such as MRI, SPECT, and neuropsychological testing (Table 2). Whether APOE genotyping will prove useful in the prevention of chronic TBI remains to be determined, but it is extremely controversial.[13] Theoretically, boxers who are APOE e4-positive can be informed of the potential risks and followed more closely from the neurological standpoint. Nonetheless, the prevention of chronic TBI will be a medical challenge in the new millennium.

TABLE 2
CRITERIA FOR HIGH-RISK BOXERS
• age: 40 years of age or older
• duration of career: 350 rounds or more
• inactivity: 30 months or more
• consistent poor performances (15 or more losses, 6 consecutive losses, or 3 consecutive losses by knock out or technical knock out)
• severe concussion/knock out or technical knock out

Conclusion

Acute, subacute, and chronic TBI are major medical concerns in modern-day boxing. Despite the frequency of concussions in boxing, catastrophic acute TBI is relatively infrequent and is minimized by proper pre- and postbout medical evaluations. The proper management of boxers with postconcussion symptoms will limit the frequency of the second-impact syndrome. Chronic TBI, which shares many similarities with Alzheimer's disease, represents the most significant public health concern in boxing. The identification of high-risk boxers who would be subjected to more detailed neurological testing may help to lower the prevalence of chronic TBI. The role of genetic testing in preventing brain injury in boxing remains to be determined.

References

1. American Academy of Neurology: Practice parameter. The management of concussion in sports (summary statement). **Neurology 48:** 581-585, 1997
2. Blonstein JL, Clarke E: Further observations on the medical aspects of amateur boxing. **Br Med J 1:**362-364, 1957
3. Brooker KH, Iti T, Jordan BD: Electrophysiologic testing in boxers, in Jordan BD (ed): **Medical Aspects of Boxing.** Boca Raton, Fla: CRC Press, 1993, pp 207-214
4. Cantu RC: Guidelines for return to contact sports after a cerebral concussion. **Phys Sportsmed 14(10):**75-83, 1986
5. Cantu RC, Voy R: Second impact syndrome: a risk in any contact sport. **Phys Sportsmed 23(6):**172-177, 1995
6. Casson IR, Sham R, Campbell EA, et al: Neurological and CT evaluation of knocked-out boxers. **J Neurol Neurosurg Psychiatry 45:** 170-174, 1982
7. Casson IR, Siegel O, Sham R, et al: Brain damage in modern boxers. **JAMA 251:**2663-2667, 1984
8. Corsellis JAN: Posttraumatic dementia in Alzheimer's disease, in Jatzman R, Terry RD, Bick K (eds): **Senile Dementia and Related Disorders.** New York, NY: Raven Press, 1978, pp 125-133
9. Corsellis JAN, Bruton CJ, Freeman-Browne C: The aftermath of boxing. **Psychol Med 3:**270-303, 1973
10. Critchley M: Medical aspects of boxing, particularly from a neurological standpoint. **Br Med J 1:**357-362, 1957
11. Dale GE, Leigh PN, Luthert P, et al: Neurofibrillary tangles in dementia pugilistica are ubiquinated. **J Neurol Neurosurg Psychiatry 54:** 116-118, 1991
12. Estwanik JJ, Boitano M, Ari N: Amateur boxing injuries at the 1981 and 1982 USA/ABF national championships. **Phys Sportsmed 12:** 123-128, 1984
13. Jordan BD: Genetic susceptibility to brain injury in sports. A role for genetic testing in athletes. **Phys Sportsmed 28(2):**25-26, 1998
14. Jordan BD: Increasing medical safety in boxing, in Jordan BD (ed): **Medical Aspects of Boxing.** Boca Raton, Fla: CRC Press, 1993, pp 17-21
15. Jordan BD: Professional boxing: experience of the New York State Athletic Commission, in Cantu RC (ed): **Boxing and Medicine.** Champaign, Ill: Human Kinetics, 1995, pp 177-185
16. Jordan BD, Campbell E: Acute boxing injuries among professional boxers in New York State: a two-year survey. **Phys Sportsmed 16:** 87-91, 1988
17. Jordan BD, Dane SD, Rowen AJ, et al: SPECT scanning in professional boxers. **J Neuroimaging 9:**59-60, 1999
18. Jordan BD, Jahre C, Hauser WA: Serial computed tomography in professional boxers. **J Neuroimaging 2:**181-185, 1992
19. Jordan BD, Jahre C, Hauser WA, et al: CT of 338 active professional boxers. **Radiology 185:**509-512, 1992
20. Jordan BD, Kanick AB, Horwich MS, et al: Apolipoprotein e4 and fatal cerebral amyloid angiopathy associated with dementia pugilistica. **Ann Neurol 38:**698-699, 1995
21. Jordan BD, Matser E, Zimmerman RD, et al: Sparring and cognitive function in professional boxers. **Phys Sportsmed 24(5):**87-98, 1996
22. Jordan BD, Relkin NR, Ravdin LD, et al: Apolipoprotein E e4 associated with chronic traumatic brain injury in boxing. **JAMA 278:** 136-140, 1997
23. Jordan BD, Voy RO, Stone J: Amateur boxing injuries at the United States Olympic Training Center. **Phys Sportsmed 18(2):**80-90, 1990
24. Jordan BD, Zimmerman RD: Computed tomography, magnetic resonance imaging comparisons in boxers. **JAMA 263:**1670-1674, 1990
25. Katzman R, Galosko DR, Saitoh T, et al: Apolipoprotein e4 and head trauma: synergistic or additive risks? **Neurology 46:**889-892, 1996
26. Kemp PM, Houston AS, Macleod MA, et al: Cerebral perfusion and psychometric testing in military amateur boxers and controls. **J Neurol Neurosurg Psychiatry 59:**368-374, 1995
27. LaCava G: Boxer's encephalopathy. **J Sports Med Phys Fitness 3:**87-92, 1963
28. Lampert PW, Hardman JM: Morphological changes in brains of boxers. **JAMA 251:**2676-2679, 1984
29. Larson LW, Melin KA, Nordstrom-Ohrberg G, et al: Acute head injuries in boxing. **Acta Psychiatr Neurol Scand 95 (Suppl):**1-42, 1954
30. Laurer HL, Scherbel U, Raghupathi R, et al: Second impact syndrome: myth of pathologic sequelae? **J Neurotrauma 16:**956, 1999
31. Martland HAS: Punch drunk. **JAMA 91:**1103-1107, 1928
32. Matser EJT, Kessels AGH, Lezak MD, et al: Acute traumatic brain injury in amateur boxing. **Phys Sportsmed 28(1):**87-92, 2000
33. Mayeaux R, Ottoman R, Maestre G, et al: Synergistic effects of traumatic head injury and apolipoprotein e4 in patients with Alzheimer's disease. **Neurology 45:**555-557, 1995
34. McCory PR, Berkovic SF: Second impact syndrome. **Neurology 50:** 677-683, 1998
35. McCunney RJ, Russo PK: Brain injuries in boxers. **Phys Sportsmed 12:**53-67, 1984
36. Mendez MF: The neuropsychiatric aspects of boxing. **Int J Psychiatry 25:**249-262, 1995
37. Merz Brown: Is boxing a risk factor for Alzheimer's? **JAMA 261:** 2597-2598, 1989
38. Mortimer JA, French LR, Hutton JT, et al: Head injury as a risk factor for Alzheimer's disease. **Neurology 35:**264-267, 1985
39. Nicoll JAR, Roberts GW, Graham DI: Apolipoprotein e4 allele is associated with deposition of amyloid beta protein following head injury. **Nat Med 1:**135-137, 1995
40. Oppenheimer DR: Microscopic lesions in the brain following injury. **J Neurol Neurosurg Psychiatry 31:**299-306, 1968
41. Parkinson D: The biomechanics of concussion. **Clin Neurosurg 29:** 131-145, 1982
42. Porter M, O'Brien M: Incidence and severity of injuries resulting from amateur boxing in Ireland. **Clin J Sport Med 6:**97-101, 1996
43. Roberts AH: **Brain Damage in Boxers.** London: Pitman, 1969
44. Roberts GW, Allsop D, Bruton C: The occult aftermath of boxing. **J Neurol Neurosurg Psychiatry 53:**373-378, 1990
45. Ross RJ, Cole M, Thompson JS, et al: Boxers—computed tomography, EEG and neurosurgical evaluation. **JAMA 249:**211-213, 1983
46. Saija A, Hayes RL, Lyeth BG, et al: The effects of concussive head injury on central cholinergic neurons. **Brain Res 452:**303-311, 1988
47. Saunders RL, Harbaugh RE: The second impact in catastrophic contact-sports head trauma. **JAMA 252:**538-539, 1984
48. Schmidt-Olsen S, Jensen SK, et al: Amateur boxing in Denmark: the effect of some preventive measures. **Am J Sports Med 18:**98-100, 1990
49. Sercl M, Jaros O: The mechanisms of cerebral concussion in boxing and their consequences. **World Neurol 3:**351-357, 1962
50. Sironi VA, Scotti G, Ravagnati L, et al: CT scan and EEG findings in professional pugilists: early detection of cerebral atrophy in young boxers. **J Neurosurg Sci 26:**165-168, 1982
51. Smith CM, Swash M: Possible biochemical basis of memory disorder in Alzheimer's disease. **Neurology 3:**471-473, 1978
52. Thomassen A, Juul-Jensen P, Olivarius B, et al: Neurological electroencephalographic and neuropsychological examination of 53 former amateur boxers. **Acta Neurol Scand 60:**352-362, 1979
53. Tokuda T, Ikeda S, Yanugesa N, et al: Re-examination of ex-boxer's brain using immunohistochemistry with antibodies to amyloid beta protein and tau protein. **Acta Neuropathol 82:**280-285, 1991
54. Uhl GR, McKinney M, Hedreen JC, et al: Dementia pugilistic: loss of basal forebrain cholinergic neurons and cortical cholinergic markers. **Ann Neurol 12:**99, 1982
55. Unterhamsheidt F: About boxing: review of historical and medical aspects. **Tex Rep Biol Med 28:**421-495, 1970
56. Welch MJ, Sider M, Kroeten H: Boxing injuries from an instructional program. **Phys Sportsmed 14:**81-89, 1986
57. Windle WF, Groat RA: Disappearance of nerve cells after concussion. **Anat Rec 93:**201-209, 1945

CHAPTER 15

Spinal Cord and Brain Injuries in Ice Hockey

CHARLES H. TATOR, CM, MD, PHD, FRCSC

Ice hockey is one of the most injury-prone sports[10,18,32] because of frequent collisions, high speed by players and the puck, sharp skate blades, and the presence of the hockey stick and unyielding surfaces such as the ice, goal posts, and boards.[19] Although several different types of injuries can be incurred in organized ice hockey and recreational hockey ("shinny"), they occur much more commonly in organized leagues and pose a considerable public health problem, both in financial and in human terms.[11,24] For example, ice hockey injuries accounted for 1.77% of all visits to a Canadian emergency hospital from October 1985 until March 1986.[11] In a study of 287 adult male recreational ice hockey players, 32% of reported injuries were to the head, neck, and facial area, and 42% of these occurred as a result of penalizable behavior.[62] Many of these injuries, especially spinal injuries, can be extremely costly.[38,50]

Although peripheral nerve injuries occur in ice hockey (e.g., skate blade injuries to the sciatic nerve), they are not very common and, thus, this chapter concentrates on brain and spinal cord injuries, which unfortunately are common in ice hockey. Comparing ice hockey to football, the incidence of head injuries is equal, but that of major spinal cord injuries (SCIs) is higher. There is evidence that during the 1980s, ice hockey produced three times more quadriplegia injuries in Canada than occurred in football in the United States on a per capita basis.[52] Violence may be an important factor in the etiology of both head and spinal injuries in hockey,[50,53] and there is now widespread public concern about the level of violence in ice hockey.[22]

In spite of the increased use of protective equipment such as helmets in ice hockey, surprisingly, in most countries, both brain and spinal injuries have increased during the past 30 years.[5] There are several mechanisms that are common to both brain and spinal cord injuries, although there are also some important differences. For example, striking the boards headfirst is one of the most common mechanisms of both head and spinal injuries, and increased violence and aggressive play are important factors for both types of injury. In contrast, fighting and elbowing are frequent causes of head injuries, but seldom lead to spinal injury.

The recording of data concerning spinal injuries in hockey in Canada has been undertaken by SportSmart Canada since 1981; recently, this organization has collected data on spinal injuries in the U.S. and Europe. However, there is no national or international counterpart for the recording of brain injury data in ice hockey. In contrast to football, there is no comprehensive system for reporting head injuries and deaths in hockey and, thus, it is not possible to state the annual incidence of fatalities. However, it has been estimated that the risk of fatality and injury among hockey participants is much greater than in football.[19]

Methods of Data Collection: Spinal Cord Injury

The SportSmart data have been collected retrospectively by questionnaires sent at 2- to 3-year intervals to all neurosurgeons, orthopedic surgeons, sports medicine specialists, and physical medicine and rehabilitation specialists in Canada requesting information about major spinal injuries to hockey players. The definition of a major spinal injury in hockey includes neurological deficits due to spinal injury and any fracture or dislocation of the spine with or without a permanent neurological deficit. Beginning in 1987, cases of transient paralysis and/or transient sensory loss have also been collected. Minor spinal injuries such as strains or whiplash were excluded. The demographic details were augmented in some cases by information obtained from players, coaches, and league officials.

Spinal Cord Injuries in Ice Hockey

In most countries, sports and recreation account for up to 20% of SCIs, with diving being one of the most frequent sports and recreational activities leading to injury.[55] Prior to 1979, hockey was a rare cause of SCI in Canada; however, since then there have been approximately 14 major spinal injuries annually, despite prevention programs to educate the hockey public about the mechanisms of injury.

Demographics of Spinal Injuries

For the years 1966-1996, the SportSmart registry contained information on approximately 300 ice hockey players worldwide who had sustained spinal injuries, approximately 250 of which occurred in Canada, 35 in the U.S., and 15 in Europe.[50] Major spinal injuries in ice hockey were rare in the 1960s and 1970s, but beginning in 1980, the annual incidence has increased markedly, and from 1981 to 1996, has averaged 14 cases per year with a maximum of 18 injuries during both 1990 and 1992. Six players are known to have died as a result of their injuries. Complete motor injuries were suffered in approximately 25% of the players. Approximately 75% of the injuries occurred during organized games, with the reminder during practice or shinny games.

The age range was 11-47 years, with a median age of 17 years and a mean age of 20.4 years. Approximately 2% of the injured players were females. Burst fractures and fracture-dislocations were the most frequent types of vertebral injuries recorded (Figure 1). Burst fractures were usually due to axial compression which caused comminution of the vertebra, displacement of bony fragments posteriorly into the spinal canal, and neurological deficit.[26] Acute disc ruptures were found in several players (Figure 2), many with evidence of pre-existing cervical spondylosis.

The most frequent precipitating mechanism was a push or check from behind (40%). In most instances, the injured player was unsuspecting and was hurled horizontally into the boards, with the cervical spine crushed by an axial-loading force applied to the head.[58] In addition to a push or check from behind, other mechanisms of injury include a push or check but not from behind (25%), a trip on the ice (20%), sliding on the ice (9%), and being tripped by another player (5%). Impact with the boards accounted for 77% of the injuries, impact between players for 16%, and impact with the ice or goal post was less frequent. Approximately 85% of the injuries involved the cervical spine, and the remainder were equally distributed over the thoracic, thoracolumbar, and lumbosacral regions.

Etiology of Spinal Injuries

Several etiological factors contribute to spinal injuries in hockey.[49,53,54] Social and psychological factors include increased aggressiveness and willingness to take risks, a feeling

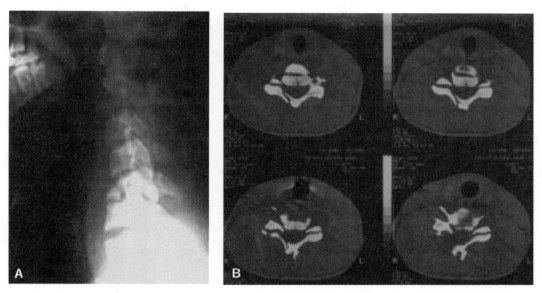

Figure 1: A) Lateral cervical spine x-ray of an ice hockey player who struck the boards head first and sustained a burst fracture of C5 and an incomplete SCI. **B)** CT myelography of the same player showing a burst fracture of the body of C5, with some posterior displacement and mild spinal cord compression. There is also a fracture of the lamina of C5.

of invincibility often related to equipment, and a lack of awareness of the possibility of SCI. In many cases, the victims were injured during illegal play, especially illegal checking or pushing from behind. Indeed, SportSmart Canada was the first to identify checking or pushing from behind as a major cause of SCI in hockey and to advocate specific rules against this illegal play. The increased body weight and speed of contemporary players magnify the forces generated during collisions and are important contributing factors. Poor neck muscle development, especially in younger players, has also been identified as a contributing factor. Another factor in the etiology of injury is the insufficient instruction by hockey coaches regarding the risks of spinal injury and the defensive methods of protecting the spine against injury. It is possible that head protection may have increased the incidence of spinal trauma by contributing to more aggressive

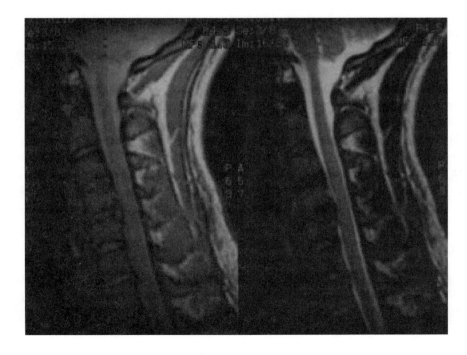

Figure 2: MRI of a player who collided head-first with another player and sustained a radiculopathy without SCI due to an acute disc rupture at C4-5. Plain x-rays demonstrated evidence of moderate cervical spondylosis. The radiculopathy resolved, and the player resumed playing several months later.

behavior,[40] but it should be noted that there is no evidence that the helmet contributes to spinal injury on the basis of biomechanics.[6]

Although there appears to be an association between larger ice surface size and decreased overall rates of injury, there is no relationship between ice surface size and neurotrauma.[63]

Prevention

Unfortunately, screening of participants is of limited value in terms of injury prevention in sports and recreation. Routine radiological examination of the spine in all athletes is not cost-effective, although there are specific exceptions. For example, atlantoaxial dislocation is a recognized complication in Down's syndrome[12,42] and in some cases of Klippel-Feil syndrome and other congenital anomalies; therefore, all such patients should have flexion-extension views prior to participation. Fortunately, the incidence of SCI in the Special Olympics is very low.[37]

The issue of routine radiological screening in high-risk sports such as football and hockey has not been settled. There is no definite evidence that certain presumed radiological risk factors such as the ratio of the diameter of the cervical spinal canal to the cervical body, other measures of spinal stenosis, or the features of the so-called "spear tackler's spine" are proven contraindications to play.[59-61] Lumbar spondylolisthesis has been shown to be present in a high proportion of gymnasts,[7,48] but it has not been shown that this is a proven contraindication to participating. Progressive degenerative spondyloarthropathies are common in sports such as hockey and football. In these conditions, the pain and neurological deficits associated with disc protrusion and osteophyte that produce radiculopathy and/or myelopathy may prevent a return to play.

The education of players, coaches, trainers, referees, and the administrators of hockey leagues and associations is an important aspect of injury prevention. The teaching should emphasize respect for the health and safety of all players, including the opponents. Awareness of specific risk factors in hockey is essential, and repeated safety messages can be given via coaching sessions, videos, and posters. Players should be warned about highly dangerous maneuvers such as checking from behind. There is mounting evidence that prevention measures can reduce the incidence of SCI in sports such as football and hockey.[33,49] Proper conditioning also has value, especially neck muscle conditioning in young players. Adherence to appropriate return-to-play guidelines as outlined below will also help reduce the incidence of catastrophic spinal injury.

Prevention can also be promoted by attention to the structural and physical aspects of the sports venue and the availability of special equipment, such as breakaway goalposts, that has been developed to enhance hockey safety, although absolute proof of their effectiveness is lacking. There is also a need for improved helmet design. More research is required to determine the best shape and padding for energy deflection and energy absorption, respectively. As noted above, there is no definitive evidence that helmets have led to an increase in SCI in hockey or that improved helmets can actually reduce the incidence of SCI. Although it may be true that "helmets can neither cause nor prevent serious neck injuries,"[13] it is the view of this author that proper helmet fit, design, and use can reduce the incidence and severity of SCI in sports such as hockey.

Return-To-Play Guidelines

In general, the neurosurgeon or orthopedic surgeon should treat athletes the same as the general population of patients. However, the practitioner should anticipate that athletes will treat themselves differently from the general population and should be pre-

TABLE 1

SPINAL INJURIES TO HOCKEY PLAYERS: CRITERIA AND GUIDELINES FOR RETURN/NON-RETURN TO PLAY

	Allow Return to Play	Advise Never Return to Play
Neurological injury	No neurological symptoms or deficit Single transient SCI or spinal cord concussion Neurological deficit that recovers to normal Neurological deficit related to root injury only	Residual neurological deficit related to SCI Repeated transient SCI or spinal cord concussion
Spinal column injury	Stable spinal column Minor fracture (e.g., spinous process or single-body compression fracture) Spinal column stability restored by conservative or operative treatment	Unstable spinal column Major fracture (e.g., burst fracture with canal compromise)
Congenital lesions	Minor spinal stenosis Congenital or operative fusion of one motion segment	Major spinal stenosis Atlantoaxial dislocation congenital or operative fusion of two or more motion segments
Acquired lesions	Mild cervical spondylosis or other arthropathy	Severe cervical spondylosis or other arthropathy
MRI findings	Normal MRI	T2-weighted signal changes in cord; syrinx

pared to resist intimidation by relatives, coaches, trainers, league officials, and players' agents. Many factors need to be considered when advising athletes about return to play after sports and recreational injuries of the spine. Although there have been attempts to develop reliable guidelines,[2,39,59] there is still a great deal of uncertainty. The decision about return to play depends primarily on the nature and severity of the neurological and spinal column injuries (Table 1).

Players with neurological injuries pose special problems compared with those with spinal column injuries alone. After a permanent SCI, it is best to advise no return to contact sports. However, if the cord injury is transient or if the neurological injury involves only a root and there is no significant spinal column injury, the player may return to play. If the spinal column injury is stable, such as a spinous or transverse process fracture or a mild compression fracture, return to play most likely can be allowed, with or without surgical treatment. In the case of an unstable injury, the player should not be permitted to return to play until stability can be restored by either conservative or operative means. Players who have had operative fusions involving one spinal motion segment or who have required a single corpectomy for burst fracture may be eligible for return to play in 6-12 months. Most players with a radiculopathy due to a herniated disc can be allowed to return to play after conservative or operative treatment.

Players who require surgery such as a cervical or lumbar fusion are permitted a gradual return to activity, with progression from walking only in the first month, then floor exercises and bicycling. In the second month, postoperative weight training can begin and swimming is encouraged. In the third month, treadmill workouts can be allowed, with return to aerobic exercises in the fourth month. Usually, players should wait until next season to return to play following a cervical or lumbar fusion or a disc removal.

In summary, players should not return to play if there is a persisting neurological deficit and/or spinal column instability. In those with a neurological deficit, return to play may be permitted if there is full recovery of the neurological deficit and if the spinal column is stable. In those without a neurological deficit, return to play may be permitted if the spinal column is stable.

Brain Injuries in Ice Hockey

Although fatal[15,16] and other major[21] brain injuries have occurred in ice hockey players, the incidence has been very small. Helmets are very effective in reducing this incidence in hockey players, and facemasks have resulted in a remarkable reduction of eye and dental injuries.[36] Although there is some evidence that the incidence of concussions can be reduced in some younger age groups by helmet usage,[23] there is rising concern that concussions are increasing in other age groups and in professional players.[5] Some investigators found no evidence that facemasks are related to an increase in head and neck injuries,[30] although others have some concerns.[47]

Demographics of Brain Injuries

In the author's series, there were 22 males and 3 females, ranging from 16 to 37 years of age (average 22 years). Of 11 players known to be wearing a helmet at the time of their most recent head injury, three reported losing it upon impact or during a fight. Nineteen players (76%) were enrolled in advanced-level hockey leagues (professional n=6; Ontario Hockey League n=5; college or university hockey n=5; and junior A hockey n=3). As reported by others,[19,25] head injuries were much more frequent in games than in practices. Based on the classification of concussion established by the American Academy of Neurology,[1] 15 players had a Grade 2 concussion and 10 had a Grade 3 concussion with respect to their most recent injury (see Table 3 in Chapter 2 for a description of the grading system). Twenty-two players (88%) had sustained more than one concussion in their hockey careers: four had one previous concussion; seven had two to five previous concussions; and 11 had six to 10 previous concussions. The overall average for the players in the study was 4.5 previous concussions per player. These 25 players sustained 137 head injuries, with the most recent mechanisms of head injury being stick contact to the head or face in 24%, fighting in 20%, elbowing in 16%, collisions including body checks or boarding in 16%, checking from behind in 8%, goalies kicked in the head 8%, and puck contact to the head or face in 4%; in 4%, the mechanism of injury was unknown. The most common posttraumatic symptoms were amnesia (72%), headaches (72%), dizziness (48%), and nausea (40%). Four players had brain injuries (mostly contusion and intracerebral hematoma) detectable on magnetic resonance imaging (MRI) or computed tomography (CT). In terms of recovery, only eight of the 25 players had fully recovered from the most recent head injury at the time of the consultation, six required less than 4 weeks to recover, and two required more than 8 weeks. The remaining 17 players had not fully recovered at the time of consultation, and in 11 of these, the injuries had occurred more than 8 weeks prior to the consultation. The average time from injury to consultation in this group was 20 weeks.

Seventeen players were advised to permanently stop playing hockey. The average time between the last head injury and the recommendation to permanently stop playing hockey was 4.7 months, and 16 these players had sustained multiple concussions in their careers, at an average of 5.8 previous concussions per player. Most, but not all, of the players complied with this recommendation. In contrast, the eight players who were allowed to resume playing hockey had an average of 1.8 previous concussions per player.

Etiology of Brain Injuries

It was alarming to find that 20% of the most recent concussions were due to fighting and 16% due to elbowing. Indeed, 28% of this sample reported fighting and/or elbowing as mechanisms of injury for at least one concussion in their career. In contrast, checking from behind, which accounted for 8% of the most recent concussions in the author's

---

Methods of Data Collection: Brain Injury

There is no organized registry that tracks the incidence of brain injuries in hockey, although some epidemiological studies of this issue have been performed. Gerberich and colleagues[20] documented the incidence of head injuries in 12 high-school hockey teams in Minnesota in a 2-year period (1982-1984) and found that 9% of the players sustained a concussion, accounting for approximately 10% of the total types of injuries sustained. Head and neck injuries were the most frequent injuries, comprising 22%-25% of all injuries.[20] In college sports in the U.S., one injury registry listed ice hockey as the sport with the second highest incidence of concussions, with an annual incidence of 3.7 concussions per 100 athletes, while football had the highest incidence at 6.1 concussions per 100 athletes per year.[13] The rates for a Danish study of head injuries in hockey were also high.[25]

The author recently summarized his experience from 1995-1999 in managing 25 consecutive Canadian ice hockey players with concussion or other brain injuries.[56] Many of these players underwent formal neuropsychological evaluations, CT, and MRI. The data were gathered by a retrospective review of the medical records. Much of the information about head injuries in this chapter is from this study.

sample, was not as significant a cause of head injury as it was for spinal injury.[51] Other reports, such as a study by Tegner and Lorentzon[57] of Swedish elite ice hockey players, found that collisions (checking or boarding) and stick contacts were the most common causes of concussions. Similarly, Muller and Biener,[34] in their study of ice hockey injuries in Switzerland, found stick contact, puck contact, and collision as the leading causes of injury, 42% of which involved the head or face and included concussions. Although the author's study also found stick contact and collision to be frequent mechanisms of injury, accounting for 24% and 16%, respectively, of the most recent head injuries, these findings differ from those in other countries by also identifying fighting and elbowing as significant causes of concussion. Clearly, both fighting and elbowing have the potential for causing serious brain injury that can occur directly from a punch or an elbow to the face or head, or subsequently, when the falling player's head strikes the ice or boards.

As with spinal injuries, head injuries in ice hockey are more frequent in organized games than in "shinny" or practice. In addition, all types of hockey injuries, including concussions, are more frequent in tournaments than in regular season games.[41]

Prevention

Helmets have been shown to reduce the incidence of concussion.[23,29] However, players must be cautioned repeatedly by coaches and league officials that helmets do not eliminate the risk of concussion and other brain injuries, since most of the players in the author's study sustained their head injuries while wearing a helmet.

Measures must be taken to ensure that helmets remain in place, especially after collisions with other players or the boards, upon impact with the ice, or during fights. Straps should be tightly fastened at all times during play. In three players, the helmets came off after the first impact and thus there was no head protection during the second impact, and the outcomes were serious. The CT and MRI of one of these players are seen in Figure 3. This individual sustained a Grade 3 concussion and other serious brain injuries due to a fight during which he sustained a punch to the head leading to a fall to the ice and a second impact to his unprotected head.

Specific measures are required to reduce the incidence of both fighting and elbowing in ice hockey. It is highly probable that improved coaching and player attitudes, combined with stricter enforcement of current rules regarding these two infractions, would reduce the incidence of head injuries due to these mechanisms.

Although there is no evidence that wearing facial protection such as a full-face shield decreases the risk of a head injury such as a concussion,[30] there is strong evidence that such facial protection markedly reduces the incidence of eye, dental, and other facial injuries such as lacerations.[4] There is much less scientific certainty about the role of the mouthguard in preventing concussions,[3] although it seems likely that mouthguards will dissipate some of the energy from blows to the face in the absence of a full-face shield. It is not certain that a mouthguard would reduce the incidence of injury to the brain from a blow to the head.

The author's experience appears to be in accordance with the observation by Honey[23] that there is a correlation between the level of hockey and the incidence of concussion: the higher the level of play, the faster and rougher the sport becomes, and the greater the frequency of concussion. In the author's case series the more serious concussions and brain injuries occurred at higher levels of hockey. For example, all but one of the players with a Grade 3 concussion were playing in either a professional hockey league, the Ontario Hockey League, a university/college hockey program, or a junior A hockey league.

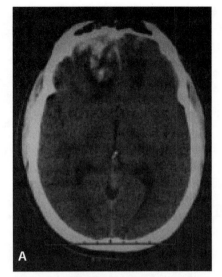

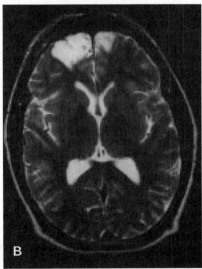

Figure 3: A) CT scan of a player who sustained a head injury after he was struck in the jaw by a punch that knocked off his helmet. He fell to the ice and struck the back of his head and sustained bilateral frontal contrecoup contusions and intracerebral hematomas. The scan was performed shortly after the injury. **B)** MRI obtained several months after the injury.

Definitions and Classifications of Concussion

There have been several systems of classification of head injuries in athletes, each with its own guidelines for allowing return to play (see Chapter 2 for additional information).[8,9,45,46] In 1997, the American Academy of Neurology published a report on the management of concussion in which concussion was defined as "a trauma-induced alteration in mental status that may or may not involve loss of consciousness."[1] This definition differs with the long-standing view that loss of consciousness is the hallmark feature of concussion. According to this new classification, a concussion with loss of consciousness is considered a Grade 3 concussion. Less severe concussions (no loss of consciousness) are classified as Grade 1 or 2, depending upon whether the transient symptoms of altered mental status resolve in less or more than 15 minutes, respectively.[1] This classification should be endorsed, and athletic trainers, sports medicine specialists, and family physicians should be encouraged to adopt it. A universally accepted protocol for the classification of concussion would be an important step toward improved management of concussion. Indeed, it would be advantageous for sports if a single classification system was used and evaluated over time. Most important is the recognition that concussion can occur without loss of consciousness.

Prevention of Cumulative Damage

A major feature and concern about concussion is that the neurological damage is cumulative and renders the player increasingly vulnerable to future incidents and to permanent neurological deficits. Studies have shown that repeated concussions can cause cumulative neuropsychological and neuroanatomical damage.[28] Indeed, a recent study in college football players demonstrated that a history of two or more concussions was associated with reduced cognitive performance on neuropsychological testing.[14] This is a crucial point in the management of patients with concussions; in the author's series described above, several patients with a history of multiple concussions and permanent neurological deficits had not been previously advised to quit playing hockey. If a player is allowed to return to play too soon after a concussion, there is a risk of the second-impact syndrome[44] in the event of a subsequent concussion. This syndrome is characterized by cerebrovascular congestion and loss of autoregulation, which may lead to brain swelling, raised intracranial pressure, and death.[28] In fact, there is one case in the literature describing a high-school football player who died of diffuse brain swelling after repeated concussions without loss of consciousness.[27] It is essential to allow enough time for the postconcussion symptoms to subside, which can only be achieved by preventing return to play until well after the symptoms resolve. The duration of abstinence from play and the time required for complete disappearance of symptoms and return to normal function depend on the severity and number of concussions sustained.[1,28]

Return-To-Play and Permanent Withdrawal Guidelines

It is often difficult to determine whether an athlete should be advised to permanently stop playing hockey after one or more head injuries. For example, there is much controversy and little scientific evidence to guide the practitioner about the number and severity of concussions that a player can tolerate before suffering a permanent neurological deficit.[43] Furthermore, some players are unreliable about conveying the extent of their current symptoms and providing an accurate concussion history given the various factors involved, such as the dependence of some players on hockey for a livelihood. Table 2 lists the criteria and guidelines for deciding whether a player should be advised to permanently stop playing hockey following a brain injury. Persistent neurological deficits of any nature (including persistent postconcussion symptoms) preclude a return to play.[9] A his-

TABLE 2

BRAIN INJURIES TO HOCKEY PLAYERS: CRITERIA AND GUIDELINES FOR RETURN/NON-RETURN TO PLAY

	Allow Return To Play	Advise Never Return To Play
Neurological examination	No neurological deficits	Presence of any neurological deficits or significant symptoms
Number, pattern, and severity of previous concussions	Small number, dispersed in time, low severity (Grades 1-2) with complete recovery	Multiple, over a short period of time, high severity (Grades 2-3)
Length of time to achieve recovery	Short duration (days)	Long duration (months)
Neuropsychological evaluation	No cognitive deficits	Presence of cognitive deficits
MRI/CT findings	No abnormalities	Presence of lesions

tory of multiple, recent, and severe concussions (Grades 2-3) occurring over a short period of time should be considered incompatible with continuing play. The length of time required for full recovery from the most recent and each previous concussion is an important criterion: the longer the recovery period, the more vulnerable the player will be if allowed to return. Neuropsychological evaluations can be of great assistance, especially when the patient exhibits persistent memory deficits with respect to average normative values, or more importantly, relative to the individual player's own baseline values. Significant neuropsychological deficits preclude a return to play. It is of interest that the National Hockey League, alarmed by the increased incidence of concussions in hockey, has recently required several hundred of its players to undergo a preseason baseline neuropsychological evaluation to facilitate the future management of concussion. The National Football League has a similar study underway. The presence of traumatic brain lesions detected on CT or MRI is usually sufficient reason to advise against playing hockey. Significant deficits or findings in any one of the five criteria presented in Table 2 or less severe deficits or findings in more than one criteria dictates permanent withdrawal from hockey.

Management of Spinal Cord and Brain Injuries

It is important for physicians associated with sports teams or athletic or recreational events to have the necessary equipment and training to provide first aid safely and effectively. Such personnel should engage in practice sessions because preparation for the management of a catastrophic spinal or head injury is important for quality performance.[31] Rapid management of any compromise of airway, breathing, or circulation is essential. Endotracheal intubation at the playing venue has occasionally been required for major brain or cord injury, and there have also been instances of on-ice emergency requirement for tracheostomy or cricothyrotomy. The attending physician or athletic trainer should quickly obtain a thorough history of the injury, inquiring specifically for cognitive ability, spinal pain, muscle weakness, and sensory loss, followed by a specific examination of the nervous system including motor power and sensation. With a spinal injury, the athletic trainer or physician should perform gentle manual palpation of the entire spine, examining for tenderness and deformity. Effective first aid includes prevention of a secondary injury, such as occurs with anoxia. These measures will prevent the worsening of neurological deficits or the initiation of a neurological deficit such as may occur in a player with an unstable spinal injury.

It is essential to ensure absolute immobilization of the entire spine during any required transfers and transport. Special attention must be given to the careful documentation of all previous injuries, as this information is required for deliberations regarding return to play. With respect to brain injury, coaches, trainers, and medical personnel should be skilled in administering rinkside assessments of mental status which should be performed serially, and medical personnel should also record the patient's Glasgow Coma Scale score.[45,46]

With few exceptions, the first aid and subsequent hospital management of the athlete with an acute cord or brain injury are identical to the management of other patients with these injuries.[31] In hockey, as in football, one of the specific differences relates to helmet removal in injured players wearing shoulder pads, in which case the helmet should not be removed first. If there is a problem with airway management, only the facemask should be removed, and this can be accomplished with heavy wire cutters. Removal of the helmet first in a player wearing shoulder pads may cause extension of the neck because of the thickness of the shoulder pads, resulting in a cervical cord injury in a player with an unstable cervical spine. Thus, it is recommended that the shoulder pads and helmet be removed simultaneously while maintaining the neck in axial alignment with the trunk.[17,35]

The subsequent in-hospital management of players with spinal cord or brain injury is no different from other individuals with these injuries. However, the issue of return to play presents a specific management challenge in players, as outlined above. As with other injuries to the brain or spine, athletic injuries of a significant degree should be thoroughly investigated by imaging to detect evidence of previous injury to the brain or spine and spinal cord. In players with spine injuries, efforts should be made to detect previous ligamentous injury and to detect spinal instability and intracanalicular space-occupying lesions such as herniated discs. Liberal use of MRI is recommended to detect ligamentous injury and subtle evidence of previous or current cord injury, sometimes evident only on high-resolution T2-weighted images. With brain injury, gradient echo MRI techniques have been helpful in detecting iron deposits in the brain from previous cerebral contusions or intracerebral hemorrhages.

References

1. American Academy of Neurology: Practice parameter. The management of concussion in sports (summary statement). **Neurology 48:** 581-585, 1997
2. Bailes JE, Hadley MN, Quigley MR, et al: Management of athletic injuries of the cervical spine and spinal cord. **Neurosurgery 29:**491-497, 1991
3. Barth JT, Freeman JR, Winters JE: Management of sports-related concussions. **Dent Clin North Am 44:**7-83, 2000
4. Benson BW, Mohtadi NGH, Rose MS, et al: Head and neck injuries among ice hockey players wearing full face shields vs. half face shields. **JAMA 282:**2328-2332, 1999
5. Biasca N, Simmen HP, Bartolozzi AR, et al: Review of typical ice hockey injuries. Survey of the North American NHL and Hockey Canada versus European leagues. **Unfallchirurgie 98:**283-288, 1995
6. Bishop PJ, Norman RW, Wells RP, et al: Changes in the centre of mass and moment of inertia of a headform induced by a hockey helmet and face shield. **Can J Appl Sport Sci 8:**19-25, 1983
7. Caine DJ, Lindner KJ, Mandelbaum BR, et al: Gymnastics, in Caine DJ, Caine CG, Linder KJ (eds): **Epidemiology of Sports Injuries.** Champaign, Ill: Human Kinetics, 1996, pp 213-246
8. Cantu RC: Guidelines for return to contact sports after a cerebral concussion. **Phys Sportsmed 14:**75-83, 1986
9. Cantu RC: Return to play guidelines after a head injury. **Clin Sports Med 17:**45-60, 1998
10. Cantu RC, Mueller F: Catastrophic spine injury in football 1977-1989. **J Spinal Disord 3:**227-231, 1990
11. Carson JD, Reesor D: A survey of hockey injuries in an emergency department. **Mod Med Can 43:**145-150, 1988
12. Chang FM: The disabled athlete, in Stanitski CL, DeLee JC, Drez D (eds): **Pediatric and Adolescent Sports Medicine.** Philadelphia, Pa: WB Saunders, 1994, Vol 3, pp 48-76
13. Clarke KS, Jordan BD: Sports neuroepidemiology, in Jordon BD, Tsairis P, Warren RF (eds): **Sports Neurology, 2nd ed.** Philadelphia, Pa: Lippincott-Raven Press, 1998, pp 3-13
14. Collins MN, Grindel SH, Lovell MR, et al: Relationship between concussion and neurophysiological performance in college football players. **JAMA 282:**964-970, 1999
15. Fekete JF: Severe brain injury and death following minor hockey accidents: the effectiveness of the "safety helmets" of amateur hockey players. **Can Med Assoc J 99:**1234-1239, 1968
16. Feriencik K: Case report: depressed skull fracture in an ice hockey player wearing a helmet. **Phys Sportsmed 7:**107, 1979
17. Ford M: Neck, spinal cord and back injuries, in Bull RC (ed): **Handbook of Sports Injuries.** New York, NY: McGraw-Hill, 1999, pp 55-71
18. Gerberich SG, Brust JD, Burns SR, et al: Ice hockey, in Jordan BD, Tsairis P, Warren RF (eds): **Sports Neurology, 2nd ed.** Philadelphia, Pa: Lippincott-Raven, 1998, pp 407-421
19. Gerberich SG, Finke R, Madden M, et al: An epidemiological study of high school ice hockey injuries. **Childs Nerv Syst 3:**59-64, 1987
20. Gerberich SG, Priest JD, Grafft J, et al: Injuries to the brain and spinal cord—assessment, emergency care and prevention. **Minn Med 65:**

691-696, 1982

21. Gibbs RW: Unsafe headgear faulted in critical hockey injuries. **Phys Sportsmed** 2:39-42, 1974

22. Grossman S, Hines T: National Hockey League players from North America are more violent than those from Europe. **Percept Motor Skills** 83:589-590, 1996

23. Honey CR: Brain injury in ice hockey. **Clin J Sport Med** 8:43-46, 1998

24. Janda DH: Prevention has everything to do with sports medicine. **Clin J Sport Med** 2:159-160, 1992

25. Jorgensen U, Schmidt-Olsen S: The epidemiology of ice hockey injuries. **Br J Sports Med** 20:7-9, 1986

26. Kaye JJ, Nance EP Jr: Thoracic and lumbar spine trauma, in Dalinka MK (ed): **Radiol Clin North Am** 28:361-377, 1990

27. Kelly JP, Nichols JS, Filley CM, et al: Concussion in sports. Guidelines for the prevention of catastrophic outcome. **JAMA** 266:2867-2869, 1991

28. Kelly JP, Rosenberg JH: Diagnosis and management of concussion in sports. **Neurology** 48:575-580, 1997

29. Kraus JF, Anderson BD, Mueller CE: The effectiveness of a special ice hockey helmet to reduce head injuries in college intramural hockey. **Med Sci Sports** 2:162-164, 1970

30. LaPrade RF, Burnett QM, Zarzour R, et al: The effect of the mandatory use of face masks on facial lacerations and head and neck injuries in ice hockey. A prospective study. **Am J Sports Med** 23:773-775, 1995

31. Leidholt JD: Spinal injuries in athletes: be prepared. **Orthop Clin North Am** 4:691-707, 1973

32. Montelpare WJ, Pelletier RL, Stark RM: Ice hockey, in Caine DJ, Caine CG, Linder KJ (eds): **Epidemiology of Sports Injuries.** Champaign, Ill: Human Kinetics, 1996, pp 247-267

33. Mueller F, Zemper ED, Peters A: American football, in Caine DJ, Caine, CG, Lindner KJ (eds): **Epidemiology of Sports Injuries.** Champaign, Ill: Human Kinetics, 1996, pp 41-62

34. Muller P, Biener K: [Ice hockey accidents.] **Minerva Med** 66:1325, 1975 (Ital)

35. Palumbo M, Hulstyn MJ, Fadale PD, et al: The effect of protective football equipment on alignment of the injured cervical spine: radiographic analysis in a cadaveric model. **Am J Sports Med** 24:446-453, 1996

36. Pashby TJ, Pashby RC, Chisholm LDJ, et al: Eye injuries in Canadian hockey. **Can Med Assoc J** 113:663-666, 1975

37. Pizzutillo PD: Klippel-Feil syndrome, in The Cervical Spine Research Society Editorial Committee: **The Cervical Spine, 2nd ed.** Philadelphia, Pa: JB Lippincott, 1987, pp 258-271

38. Rampton J, Leach T, Therrien SA, et al: Head, neck, and facial injuries in ice hockey: the effect of protective equipment. **Clin J Sport Med** 7:162-167, 1997

39. Rappoport LH, Cammisa FP Jr, O'Leary PF: Fractures and dislocations of the cervical spine, in Jordan BD, Tsairis P, Warren RF (eds): **Sports Neurology, 2nd ed.** Philadelphia, Pa: Lippincott-Raven Press, 1998, pp 157-179

40. Reynen PD, Clancy WG Jr: Cervical spine injury, hockey helmets, and face masks. **Am J Sports Med** 22:167-170, 1994

41. Roberts WO, Burst JD, Leonard B: Youth ice hockey tournament injuries: rates and patterns compared to season play. **Med Sci Sports Exer** 31:46-51, 1999

42. Robson HE: The Special Olympic games for the mentally handicapped—United Kingdom 1989. **Br J Sports Med** 24:225-230, 1990

43. Ross R: Guidelines for managing concussion in sports. **Phys Sportsmed** 24:67-74, 1996

44. Saunders RL, Harbaugh RE: The second impact in catastrophic contact-sports head trauma. **JAMA** 252:538-539, 1984

45. Schwartz ML, Tator CH: Head injuries and concussions, in Bull RC (ed): **Handbook of Sports Injuries.** New York, NY: McGraw-Hill, 1999, pp 3-12

46. Schwartz ML, Tator CH: Head injuries in athletics, in Harries M, Williams C, Stanish ED, et al (eds): **Spinal Problems in Sports. Oxford Textbook of Sports Medicine.** New York, NY: Oxford University Press, 1994, pp 57-67

47. Sim FH, Simonet WT, Melton LJ III, et al: Ice hockey injuries. **Am J Sports Med** 15:30-40, 1987

48. Sward L: The thoracolumbar spine in young elite athletes. Current concepts on the affects of physical training. **Sports Med** 13:357-362, 1992

49. Tator CH, Carson JD, Cushman R: Spinal injuries in Canadian ice hockey players, 1966-1996, in Cantu RC (ed): **Neurologic Athletic Head and Spine Injuries.** Orlando, Fla: WB Saunders, 2000 (In press)

50. Tator CH, Carson JD, Edmonds VE: New spinal injuries in hockey. **Clin J Sport Med** 7:17-21, 1997

51. Tator CH, Carson JD, Edmonds VE: Spinal injuries in ice hockey. **Clin Sports Med** 17:183-194, 1998

52. Tator CH, Edmonds VE: National survey of spinal injuries in hockey players. **Can Med Assoc J** 130:875-880, 1984

53. Tator CH, Edmonds VE, Lapczak L: Spinal injuries in ice hockey: review of 182 North American cases and analysis of etiologic factors, in Castaldi CR, Bishop PJ, Hoerner EF (eds): **Safety in Ice Hockey.** Philadelphia, Pa: American Society for Testing and Materials, 1993, pp 11-20

54. Tator CH, Edmonds VE, Lapczak L, et al: Spinal injuries in ice hockey players, 1966-1987. **Can J Surg** 34:63-69, 1991

55. Tator CH, Edmonds VE, New ML: Diving: a frequent and potentially preventable cause of spinal cord injury. **Can Med Assoc J** 124:1323-1324, 1981

56. Tator CH, Tawadros PS: The etiology and management of concussion and other brain injuries in 25 professional and amateur Canadian ice hockey players with emphasis on return/non-return to play guidelines. **Clin J Sport Med** (In press)

57. Tegner Y, Lorentzon R: Concussion among Swedish elite ice hockey players. **Br J Sports Med** 30:251-255, 1996

58. Torg JS: **Athletic Injuries to the Head, Neck and Face.** Philadelphia, Pa: Lea & Febiger, 1982

59. Torg JS, Glasgow SG: Criteria for return to contact activities following cervical spine injury. **Clin J Sport Med** 1:12-26, 1991

60. Torg JS, Pavlov H: Cervical spine stenosis with neuropraxia and transient quadriplegia. **Clin Sports Med** 6:115-133, 1987

61. Torg JS, Sennett B, Pavlov H, et al: Spear tackler's spine: an entity precluding participation in tackle football and collision activities that expose the cervical spine to axial energy inputs. **Am J Sports Med** 21:640-649, 1993

62. Voaklander DC, Saunders LD, Quinney HA, et al: Epidemiology of recreational and old-timer ice hockey injuries. **Clin J Sport Med** 6:15-21, 1996

63. Watson RC, Nystrom MA, Buckolz E: Safety in Canadian junior ice hockey: the association between ice surface size and injuries and aggressive penalties in the Ontario Hockey League. **Clin J Sport Med** 7:192-195, 1997

CHAPTER 16

Helmet Design for Brain Protection

T. BLAINE HOSHIZAKI, PhD

Protecting the head has been a concern of humans for thousands of years. In the book *Impact Head Injury,* Gurdjian[5] referred to the first recorded helmet as being a gift offered to a pharaoh during the 15th century BC. Head protection fashioned from animal hides, wood, and metals have appeared continually in drawings during subsequent centuries. The persistent use of head protection over such a long period of time attests to the need and efficacy of such accouterments. The most common application of head protection involved protective devices used in warfare. Helmets have become an integral part of a soldier's dress, originating when combatants first discovered that a sharp blow to the head rendered an opponent incapacitated and easy to dispose. As a result, head protection has become the one piece of protective equipment that was developed early in the art of war and remains in use today.

As methods of transportation became more sophisticated, the demand for better head protection followed. The first helmets were a reflection of the manufacturer's experience and best guess as to what provided protection of the head. Inconsistent performance between helmets and the often tragic results led consumers to demand a method of standardizing minimal protection levels. As a result, helmet standards have been developed for head protection while partaking in such activities as motor sports, bicycling, United States football, construction, and ice hockey, as well as a variety of recreational activities, such as alpine skiing and skateboarding. Standards for each type of helmet have been adapted to the hazards encountered in the particular environment. The standards were applied to certification programs enforced by a variety of levels of government, leagues, and consumer groups.

Human Tolerance to Head Impacts

Gennarelli[4] described the two most common mechanisms of head injuries in sport to be the result of rapidly applied mechanical input to the head from an impact. The first mechanism was described as the result of local factors beneath the site of the impact causing deformation to the skull and resulting in shockwave propagation through the

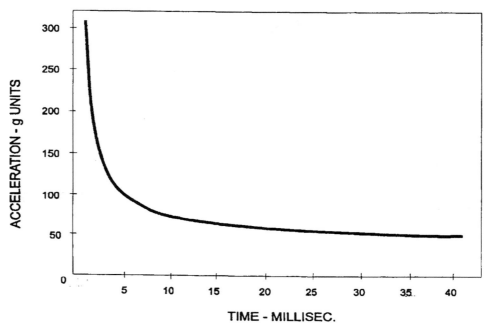

Figure 1: Acceleration vs. time. The Wayne State Tolerance Curve.

skull and brain. The magnitude and the direction of the impact, and the size of the impacting device are factors that affect the damage. Resulting skull deformation can cause fracture and underlying cerebral contusion. Diffusing the impacting forces over the surface of the head can minimize damage from contact phenomena of impact. The second mechanism involves the acceleration or deceleration of the head, resulting in shear, tensile, and compression strains created in the brain.

Research investigating the effects of impacts on injuries to the brain has provided data useful in setting acceptable levels of insult to the brain. The Wayne State Tolerance Curve[6] in Figure 1 is arguably the most influential data used for setting human tolerances. Data were collected using human cadaver heads impacted with a drop test and a rotary hammer. The presence of a linear skull fracture is the criterion used to define what was described as a moderate to severe concussion.

It can be seen in Figure 1 that impacts resulting in accelerations of very short duration (<0.002 sec) required skull accelerations of 200 to 300 g to result in fractures. In accelerations lasting longer than 0.002 sec, the required peak acceleration resulting in a skull fracture dropped from 200 to 50 g very quickly. It is obvious from the data that, if a helmet is able to keep the peak acceleration at a lower level, the possibility of a person withstanding injury without serious effect becomes multiplied several fold. The importance given to the data in setting tolerance levels relating to brain concussion deserves the following observations. The Wayne State Tolerance Curve was developed based on the relationship between intracranial pressure and skull acceleration, and the nature of the impact (the angle and location of impact and the shape of the impact surface) influences the characteristics of the curve.

Newman[12] observed that one might expect to be able to correlate head injury to acceleration when:

- the stress-inducing (hence, injury-inducing) mechanism is dominant of an inertial characteristic;
- the skull deformation is small; and
- head motion-limiting features are controlled.

Newman[12] goes on to provide an excellent summary of the criteria for head injury based upon measures of acceleration:

1. The maximum acceleration during impact must not exceed some limiting value: $a_{max} < c_1$.

    This form of the criteria is employed, for example, in some motorcycle helmet standards.[16]

2. Given a certain total duration of the pulse, the average acceleration during the impact may not exceed some value: $a_{avg} < c_2$.

    The Wayne State Tolerance Curve was the initial basis for the inclusion of both maximum acceleration and time; this was also confirmed in work by Ono et al.[13] The formulae defined by Ono and coworkers are depicted as JARI Head Injury Tolerance Curve (JHTC) in Figure 2.[12] It should be noted that this type of dependent variable does not take into account the acceleration waveform shape. The use of the average acceleration versus time duration as the factor resulting in head injury has not been fully resolved.

3. Given a certain a(t), the time during which "a" exceeds a limiting value may not be exceeded. Examples of this are CMVSS Part 111[1] and FMVSS No. 218.[2] Examples of these criteria include the following:

    • MVSS 201: The deceleration of the test headform shall not exceed 80 g continuously for more than 3 msec.

    • MVSS 218: i) peak acceleration shall not exceed 400 g; ii) acceleration in excess of 200 g shall not exceed a cumulative duration of 2.0 msec; and iii) acceleration in excess of 150 g shall not exceed a cumulative duration of 4.0 msec.

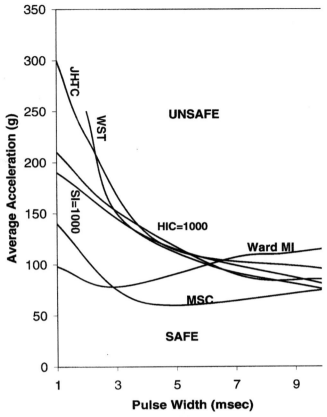

Figure 2: Tolerance boundary predictions using various head injury models: JHTC = JARI Head Injury Tolerance Curve; MSC = maximum strain criteria; Ward MI = finite model based on the 24 PSI unit; HIC = head injury criteria; SI = severity index; WST = Wayne State Tolerance Curve.

The intention of the first example is to limit the bulk of the deceleration to below 80 g, with only brief excursions above it. The rationale is that decelerations of greater than 80 g but shorter than 3 msec are not deemed dangerous. The rationale for limiting short bursts to less than 3 msec as part of a longer pulse is questionable.

In the second example, Newman[12] remarks that the purpose of the specifications is not absolutely clear. Limiting peak headform acceleration to 400 g is in effect limiting the peak force that can be applied through a helmet to 4400 lb (the test headform usually weighs 11 lb). The imposition of the 200- and 150-g acceleration level has the effect of shaping the waveform to some presumably desirable shape. It should be noted that it is possible to tailor the headform response to meet the standard without necessarily producing a better helmet.

A third form of a(t) and t correlation to head injury severity is that the value of some functional relationship between the two may not be exceeded. Examples of this are the Gadd severity index[3] ($\int a(t)^{2.5} dt \leq 1000$) and the head injury criteria[18] ($((1/t_2-t_1 \int_{t_1}^{t_2} a(t)dt)^{2.5} (t_2-t_1) \leq 1000$), where t_1 and t_2 are chosen to maximize the head injury criteria.

Naham et al[11] developed a brain model using a finite element modeling technique to simulate the response of the brain to dynamic loading. The model uses peak intracranial pressure as the factor directly related to brain injury. Moderate brain injury was correlated with 24 psi and severe brain injury with 35 psi. Figure 2 compares the predicted $a_{avg.}$ vs. T of the finite element model to those other models. The Ward MI[19] wave represents the finite model based on the 24-psi limit. Also included in Figure 2 is the lumped parameter model of Stalnaker et al[17] called the "maximum strain criteria," the Gadd severity index, the head injury criteria, and the Wayne State Tolerance Curve.

The Wayne State Tolerance Curve[6] has had an immense influence in setting the benchmark for linear acceleration tolerance values for the brain. However, a number of very persuasive arguments have been presented for lowering acceptable acceleration levels. The problem with the data supporting these proposals is that they originate from experiments using dogs, pigs, and primates as subjects. Unless humans are used as subjects, concussions are not easily recognizable in the absence of a skull fracture or bleed in the brain. However, using behavioral data collected on human subjects, it has been well documented that brain injuries (concussions) occur before the advent of a skull fracture or bleed in the brain.[9] The interpretation of the human tolerance response to impact data is confused by the complexity of the problem. The skull has an irregular geometry with inconsistent wall structures. The brain, as well, is inconsistent in its geometry and matter. Therefore, the skull/brain system has a very unpredictable response to impacts of varying characteristics. The application of an impact to the front of the skull at 30° does not describe the resulting effect of an impact of the same energy applied at a different location of the skull or even at a different angle. While the above observation is well established by the unpredictability of the brain to various forms of impact, the solution is not simple. Research involving injuries to the brain is outside the realm of acceptable protocols when involving humans. The use of data collected from head-impact injuries in humans and research conducted on animals has established the principles used to understand the mechanism of brain injuries resulting from head impacts.

An important summary observation by Newman follows, "In spite of the dramatic differences in the predictions of these various models, one feature is common: For any given time duration, head injury severity or likelihood increases with average (or peak) acceleration."[12]

Rotational Injuries

The studies described above investigated translational accelerations as the mechanism of injury using the relationship between skull acceleration and fracture; however, they did not consider brain trauma related to rotational injuries. Sano et al[14] demonstrated the limited protection afforded by the design of today's ice hockey helmets in mitigating rotational accelerations to the brain (Figures 3 and 4). The results of their study confirmed concerns of previous researchers regarding the lack of methods for evaluating the performance of head protection in mitigating rotational accelerations. Without validated procedures for evaluating, rotational accelerations have been limited to the development of a knowledge base in this particular area. As a result, design innovation to manage angular accelerations to the brain during impact has been largely ignored.

Helmet Mass

Research involving the influence of helmet mass on potential injury has been undertaken by a number of research groups, with differing results. A Swedish study concluded that helmet weight had a negative effect, causing fatigue in children and resulting in undue neck flexion and increased vulnerability to neck injuries. Similar studies undertaken by Smith et al[15] concluded that the mass in existing ice hockey helmets was not high

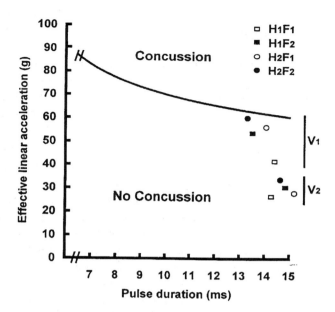

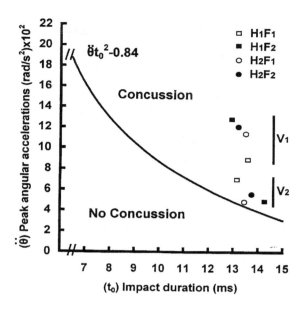

Figure 3: Plot of translational accelerations using the Wayne State Tolerance Curve.

Figure 4: Plot of rotational accelerations using the Wayne State Tolerance Curve.

enough to be a factor in neck fatigue. A search of the literature did not provide any studies implicating mass of existing helmets as an important factor in head and neck injuries. Helmets weighing under a mass of 1200 gm were considered safe. It must be mentioned that nearly all authors recognized that, at some point, the mass of the helmet would become a factor in the wearer's safety. However, helmets manufactured today generally weigh between 400 and 1500 gm, well below the levels sited as possibly causing neck fatigue. The investigators pointed out that, when possible, designers should consider minimum helmet mass as a design objective.

In order to protect the brain from impact, helmet designs have had to incorporate the following principles: decrease peak skull acceleration, decrease the duration of the acceleration pulse to the brain, minimize rotational accelerations, and maintain the helmet mass as low as possible. It should also be noted that the helmet design must address the unique hazards of the activity for which it is to be used. To design a helmet based solely on human tolerance data as described above would be negligent. For example, ice hockey helmet designers must consider hazards such as pucks impacting at over 160 km per hour, incidental stick impacts, as well as the inertial head impacts described above. Each activity presents a unique set of criteria that must be prioritized and balanced in a helmet design. Repeated accelerations and constant head movement to monitor the flow of the game require helmets that do not have high mass or moment of inertia. In addition, the larger the helmet, the greater the opportunity of contact with other players or the playing area and increased moment arms to generate high rotational forces.

Helmets are not designed to protect the wearer from all possible head injuries; in fact, helmets are designed primarily to mitigate head injuries. Crashing a bicycle into a building, being hit by a car, sliding into the sideboards in ice hockey, and collisions in football all have the potential to generate impact energies many fold the level that the helmet is designed to manage. However, helmets do protect the head from impact, and standards are intended to provide parameters to ensure that helmets are designed to provide optimal protection for particular activities. It is essential to design helmets to meet the particular requirements of the intended use.

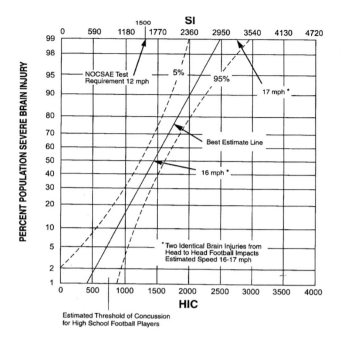

Figure 5: The percent of population expected to experience a brain injury of AIS level 4 or greater due to frontal head impacts as a function of head injury criteria.

The challenge facing helmet designers is to optimize the protective qualities of the helmet design by balancing often-competing protective elements. In order to manage high-energy impacts, liner thickness must be increased. Unfortunately, a large helmet increases the moment arm around the neck, resulting in higher forces acting on the neck during impact.[6] Larger helmets are also larger targets and harder to protect from being hit, especially in contact sports. As a result, designers are faced with the challenge of balancing a helmet's energy attenuation qualities with increased helmet size and mass.

It is also important to understand that the energy levels used to set standards for protective helmets range from 35 to 55 J. Even crash helmets, which are designed primarily for high-energy impacts, are tested at joules. Designing helmets to withstand all impacts that may be encountered during an activity is not realistic. Figure 5 provides an indication of the risk involved when an individual receives an impact with a head injury criteria of 1500 concussion threshold.[10] If a head injury criteria of 1500 is considered the level at which a concussion occurs,[3] then an estimated 55% of the population is at risk of a level 4 brain injury as classified by the American Spinal Injury Association Impairment Scale (AIS) (Figure 5).[10]

Helmet Type

Helmets can be divided into two fundamental classifications. In the first classification, the crash helmet is designed to protect the wearer during a single high-energy impact. Activities where head impacts are not considered an integral part of the sport, but the risk of an accidental head impact necessitates the use of crash helmets. Crash helmets are used for head protection in cycling, motorcycling, and, in North America, alpine skiing. This type of helmet generally employs expanded polystyrene as the impact attenuation material. Once the expanded polystyrene has received a high-energy impact, the absorbent quality of the helmet is severely diminished and the helmet is no longer safe to use. A crash helmet must be replaced after receiving an impact. During impact, the structured cells are crushed, destroying the material absorbing energy.

The second type of helmet is referred to as a multiple-impact helmet and is designed to attenuate many impacts at the same site. Classic examples of multiple-use helmets are those used in ice hockey and U.S. football. Materials used to absorb impact energies are elastic in nature and regain their shape after the impact, allowing the liner to protect against multiple impacts. Typically, multiple-impact helmets are tested using a minimum of three consecutive impacts at the same site.

Hodgson[7] tested four types of helmets as a means of comparing nonpenetrating impact characteristics. Figure 6 depicts the top-loading characteristics of a skateboard helmet, a crash helmet, an ice hockey helmet, and a U.S. football helmet. Also shown are two horizontal lines, the lower line at 8.9 kN and the upper at 10 kN, representing the dynamic load that would produce 200- and 225-gm acceleration, respectively. This is the range of peak accelerations, depending on pulse shape, at which the severity index exceeds the 1500 concussion limit recommended by Gadd.[3] The skateboard helmet wave reflects the following characteristics: it accomplishes very little work (area under the curve) and has a precipitous load increase reflecting a bottoming out at 0.75-cm displacement. The ability of the helmet to manage only small energies (5.8 J) and a sudden transition to high loads reflects poor protection afforded the wearer. The loading curve of the hockey helmet reflects a greater capacity to do work (26 J) and a less precipitous transition to compression saturation compared to the skateboard helmet. Hodgson observed that the geometry of the hockey helmet shell was designed to absorb energy. The football helmet, which relies primarily on a 3-cm thick resilient liner, is reflected in the resulting curve. The work done to compress the liner was 88 J, with 34 J absorbed under the concussion level. The transition to compression saturation was even more gradual than the hockey helmet curve.

The loading curve of the crash helmet (motorcycle) is indicative of a stiffer system and a more efficient energy absorber than the other three. The total work up to 16 kN was 193 J. However, only 44 J of work was completed below the concussion line and, consequently, much of the protective capabilities against impact would be expected to be above the level at which serious head injury could occur. The steep slope on the load-deflection curve also indicates that abrupt loading (jerk) is likely to occur while wearing this helmet during impact. In a paper investigating the efficacy of motorcycle helmets, Hurt et al[8] concluded that, in general, the helmets studied were effective in mitigating head injuries such as abrasion, contusion, fracture, laceration, and pain. However, in the case of concussion, helmet protection was not significant. These findings are reflective of the tendency to engineer helmets that address high-energy impact injuries without consideration for low-energy impacts.

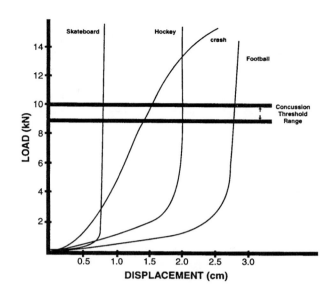

Figure 6: A comparison of static load-deflection curves of four types of helmets: a skateboard helmet, an ice hockey helmet, a crash (motorcycle) helmet, and a U.S. football helmet.

These papers provided an interesting comparison of helmet designs, reflecting fundamental differences in energy-absorbing properties. They make clear that the setting of criteria for the design of particular helmets must coincide with the nature of the impact energies that the helmet will be required to manage.

Summary

Helmet designers must consider the limitations of the science of protecting the head. To consider that certification standards would be the benchmark in helmet protection is folly and will surely lead to abuse. In addition, optimizing one safety parameter (e.g., peak linear acceleration during high-energy impacts) at the expense of other safety criteria is dangerous. Helmet design/engineering teams are responsible for the safety performance of the helmet and should not use safety standards as a shield for ignorance. Understanding human tolerances to brain injury, environmental hazards, injury mechanisms, material and part physical characteristics, and consumer product performance expectations are essential in helmet design.

Safe helmets are the result of incorporating the above criteria into helmet designs. Consumers must be educated as to the performance limits of helmets in protecting against head injuries. Few athletes make a distinction between skull fracture injuries and concussion when choosing head protection. It is troubling that the public does not understand that crash helmets as a whole provide poor protection from concussion injuries, although they perform very well in attenuating linear acceleration of a high-energy impact. To suggest that helmets do not protect the head from injury is incorrect; however, to give the impression that the helmets presently available are designed to prevent concussive injuries is also deceptive. Understanding the limitations of head protection and making design/engineering decisions in the interest of the consumer are the bases for safe product development.

In the absence of understanding the science defining the principles of head injuries, helmet designers risk developing and promoting inferior products. To employ one or two safety criteria as the sole objective in designing a helmet is irresponsible and could prove dangerous. Educating consumers regarding the limits of helmets in protecting against head injuries is an important element in decreasing injuries that is often overlooked by helmet manufacturers.

References

1. CMVSS: Part III. Occupant Protection/Head Impact Area. 1979, pp 200-201
2. FMVSS No. #18: Motorcycle helmets. **Federal Register, Vol 38, No 160,** 1973
3. Gadd CW: Use of a weighted impulse criterion for estimating injury hazard. Proceedings of the 10th Conference of the Society of Automotive Engineers, New York, NY, 1966, pp 164-174, Paper No. 660793
4. Gennarelli TA: Head injury mechanisms, in Torg JS (ed): **Athletic Injuries to the Head, Neck and Face, 2nd ed.** St Louis, Mo: Mosby-Year Book, 1991, pp 232-240
5. Gurdjian ES: **Impact Head Injury.** Springfield, Ill: Charles C Thomas, 1975, pp 303-359
6. Gurdjian ES, Roberts VL, Thomas LM: Tolerance curves of accelerations and intracranial pressure and protective index in experimental head injury. **J Trauma** 6:600-604, 1966
7. Hodgson VR: Approaches and evaluative techniques for helmets. A Symposium on Biomechanical Assessments of Sports Protective Equipment. The 9th Congress of the International Society of Biomechanics, Waterloo, Canada, 1988, pp 23-28
8. Hurt HH Jr, Oullet JV, Thom DR: **Motorcycle Accident Cause Factors and Identification of Counter Measures, Volumes 1 and 2. Final Report.** Washington, DC, Department of Transportation, 1981, HS-805, p 862
9. Kelly JP, Rosenberg JH: Diagnosis and management of concussion in sports. **Neurology** 48:575-580, 1997
10. Mertz HJ, Weber DA: Interpretations of the impact responses of a three-year-old dummy relative to child injury potential. Proceedings of the 9th International Technical Conference of Experimental Safety Vehicles, Kyoto, Japan, 1961
11. Naham AM, Ward C, Smith R, et al: Intracranial pressure relationships in the protected and the unprotected head. Proceedings of the 23rd STAPP Car Crash Conference, 1979, SAE Paper No. 791024
12. Newman JA: Tissue stress tolerances and injury indices. A Symposium on Biomechanical Assessments of Sports Protective Equipment. The 9th Congress of the International Society of Biomechanics, Waterloo, Canada, 1988, pp 11-20
13. Ono K, Kikuchi A, Nakamura M, et al: Human head tolerance to sagittal impact reliable estimation deduced from experimental head injury using subhuman primates and human cadaver skulls. Proceedings of the 24th STAPP Car Crash Conference, 1980, SAE Paper No. 801303
14. Sano K, Nakamura N, Hirakawa K, et al: Correlative studies of dynamics and pathology in whiplash and head injuries. **Scand J Rehabil Med** 4:47-54, 1972
15. Smith AW, Bishop PJ, Wells RP: Alterations in head dynamics with the addition of a hockey helmet and face shield under inertial loading. **Can J Applied Sports Sci** 10:1985
16. Snell Memorial Foundation: **Standard for Protective Headgear,** 1980
17. Stalnaker RL, McElhaney JH, Roberts VL: MSC Tolerance curves for human head impacts, 1971, ASME Paper 71-WA/BHF-10
18. Versace J: A review of the severity index. Proceedings of the 15th STAPP Car Crash Conference, 1971, SAE Paper No 710881
19. Ward C, Chan M, Naham A: Intracranial pressure—a brain injury criterion. Proceedings of the 24th STAPP Car Crash Conference, 1980, pp 161-185, SAE Paper No 801304

CHAPTER 17

Research and Trends in Sports Medicine

MONIQUE H. OLESNIEWICZ, MS, and
J. CHRISTOPHER DANIELS, MD

In 1904, 19 American football players were killed or paralyzed during competition, leading President Theodore Roosevelt to threaten to ban the playing of football in the United States. This prompted the establishment of the National Collegiate Athletic Association (NCAA) to serve as a governing body creating rules for safer athletic competition.[7] Then as well as now, injuries and deaths incurred while playing football received more media attention than in any other sport. From the time when the American Football Coaches Association began an annual survey of football fatalities in 1931 until 1998, there have been 966 deaths directly attributed to football in the U.S.,[40] with more than two thirds of these due to head injury.[11] In the past 40 years, various researchers have attempted to discern the mechanism and incidence of head injuries, develop sturdier equipment and tackling techniques to reduce the rate, and more effectively identify, assess, and manage head injuries that occur while playing football and other sports.

Because of the intentional contact inherent in tackling and blocking while playing football, the sport can be regarded as an ideal environment for clinical trauma research. Head injuries, or more specifically traumatic brain injuries, are quite common in football. The Centers for Disease Control have estimated that of the 300,000 sports-related traumatic brain injuries occurring each year, 100,000 are in football.[49] These numbers are conservative. With underreporting being common due to the desire to keep playing, as well as the amnestic effects of the injury itself, the actual number of brain injuries sustained while playing football may be closer to 250,000 per year.[19] Reasonable estimates report that between 4% and 20% of college and high school football players will sustain a brain injury during the course of a season. In comparison, 1%-5% of soccer players sustain a brain injury each season; other sports with lower participation among the population but with significant incidences of brain injury include ice hockey, wrestling, diving, and gymnastics. Brain injuries are also commonly identified among children and adolescents in recreational activities such as skiing, sledding, skating, and bicycling. In professional boxers, the rates of reported brain injuries are reported to be as high as 79%, with the rates of injuries in amateur boxing even higher.[23]

The overwhelming majority of traumatic brain injuries sustained in football are concussions, although in greater than 90%, there is no loss of consciousness (LOC). This does not mean that persons who do not sustain an intracranial bleed or, at a minimum, lose consciousness are not significantly affected.[7] In fact, the absence of LOC does not appear to reduce the risk of the second-impact syndrome, the postconcussion syndrome, or other significant sequelae. The signs, symptoms, and potential sequelae of a concussion include one or more of the following: amnesia, confusion, headache, easy distractibility, poor vigilance, incoordination, a vacant stare, delayed motor or verbal responses, slurred or incoherent speech, and/or emotional lability.

In a study of 2992 mild closed-head injury patients for whom the Glasgow Coma Scale score was 15 points and computed tomography (CT) was normal, 2.3% had early seizures within 1 week of injury.[25]

Days, weeks, and months after a concussion, symptoms and signs that persist may include: decreased information processing speed, short-term memory impairment, irritability, depression, fatigue, vertigo, tinnitus, diminished hearing, taste and/or smell, visual difficulties, insomnia, and a general feeling of "fogginess." In the absence of further injury, most patients who have sustained concussions appear to recover within a few months, but may suffer postconcussion syndrome. Postconcussion syndrome is characterized by the persistence of symptoms that may last days, weeks, or months following a concussion. In as many as 24% of concussed subjects, some symptoms may persist for 4 or more years.[17] Although the player may certainly be functional, he/she may suffer a "subclinical" postconcussion syndrome. Subtle cognitive deficits can be detected on computerized neuropsychological testing (the Automated Neuropsychological Assessment Metrics) years after an injury, even in those who have "recovered."[3]

In 1973, Schneider[47] first reported a case of what was later termed second-impact syndrome by Saunders and Harbaugh.[46] This syndrome, with a mortality rate of greater than 50% and a morbidity rate of 100%, results from a secondary blow to the head following an initial head injury in which the symptoms have not abated and is believed to be due to disruption of cerebrovascular autoregulation by the first injury. Typically, within 2-5 minutes of the second (frequently very mild) concussion, there is a rapid increase in intracranial pressure, uncal herniation (or herniation of the cerebellar tonsils through the foramen magnum), and brainstem failure.[8] Some authors, including Cantu, believe that a "malignant brain edema syndrome" is a separate process in children, although this may be a variant of the same syndrome.[38] Cantu has noted the increased reporting of cases in the 1990s, with at least 17 between 1992 and 1997 and only seven prior to 1992.[8] It is unlikely that this increase is due to an increase in incidence; it is more probable that it is due to an increased awareness of the condition. With continued efforts toward educating coaches, athletic trainers, and sports medicine professionals, it is hoped that this phenomenon could be completely eliminated in the next decade.

Researchers are studying the roles of genetic make-up, multiple concussions, and preexisting learning disabilities in predisposing athletes to increased risk of severe or long-term sequelae from concussion.[13] Educational and diagnostic efforts are underway to increase the early identification of concussion. Finally, neuropsychological and neuroradiological assessment tools are being developed and refined to improve immediate management and to track recovery. All of these initiatives share the common goal of reducing the significant acute and long-term sequelae of concussions and other traumatic brain injuries.

This chapter reviews research conducted during the past decade, discusses the current status, and speculates on future research and management of concussion in sports as we enter the next millennium.

Guidelines for Return to Play

Although medical professionals agree that no athlete should enter an environment that exposes oneself to potential head injury while symptomatic from a concussion, "return-to-play" guidelines have not been universally accepted by coaches, athletic trainers, and sports medicine professionals. At the Sports Related Concussion and Nervous System Injuries Conference held in Orlando, Florida in 1999, many sports medicine professionals and athletic trainers expressed a preference to maintain a team-specific standard method of assessment for concussions, rather than adopting one universally accepted guideline. This may prove to be problematic because without universal acceptance of a standard method of assessment and care for head injuries, confusion in taxology between caregivers may continue to occur and patients may not receive optimal care.

During the 1997-1999 football seasons, a consortium of researchers representing healthcare professionals and research institutions throughout San Diego worked together to disseminate information to players, parents, coaches, athletic trainers, team physicians, and administrators regarding the identification and assessment of concussion in sports, called the High School Head Injury Project. This infrastructure for dissemination has proved to be ineffective in maintaining a complete triage of knowledge and procedure. Key personnel involved in the care of athletes were not using the most updated guidelines and definitions of concussion to identify and assess athletes who sustained head injury, specifically Emergency Medical Technicians (EMTs) and urgent-care physicians. The following are specific, nonfictional examples not meant to be generalized or to stereotype medical professionals. They are included to illustrate the need for overall educational dissemination and universal acceptance of guidelines among all persons in contact with sports-related concussion.

Within one football season, two incidences of confusion were experienced when diagnosing concussion in two adolescent football players from a high school participating in the High School Head Injury Project. In one athlete, EMTs were the first point of contact following a head injury during the initial event. The athlete was dazed, confused, experiencing headaches and nausea, and did not come to his feet immediately after injury. The EMTs performed a brief neurological examination and concluded that there was neither injury nor concussion and the player was allowed to return to play. Five to 10 minutes following the initial evaluation, the school athletic trainer noticed the player sitting on the bench holding his head. After learning more about the injury, following a period of questioning of the athlete regarding his symptoms, the athletic trainer administered the Sideline Assessment of Concussion and recorded symptom history to determine the extent of the head injury. The player experienced symptoms until the end of the game and into the next morning. Using the Colorado, the American Academy of Neurology (AAN), and Cantu's guidelines, this concussion was classified as a Grade 2 concussion. The appropriate management includes removal from competition and a week's rest once symptoms of concussion have abated.

Another incident involved an urgent-care physician and an athletic trainer. The school athletic trainer diagnosed a Grade 1 concussion in a player because the player's score on the Standardized Assessment of Concussion improved and the symptoms cleared within 15 minutes of injury. Following the football game, the parents took their son to urgent care. The urgent-care physician told the parents that the player had experienced a mild traumatic brain injury, not a concussion. The physician explained that a concussion included strictly LOC and since the player did not suffer from concussion, he was cleared to return to play. In the past, students in medical school institutions were trained to identify concussion by the presence of LOC; since that time, researchers have discovered that any alteration in mental status constitutes a concussion. The following morning, the player was still experiencing headaches from his injury. At practice that

TABLE 1

A COMPARISON OF CONCUSSION GRADING SYSTEMS

Grading System	Grade 1 (Mild)	Grade 2 (Moderate)	Grade 3 (Severe)
Cantu (ACSM)	PTA <30 minutes; no LOC	LOC <5 or PTA >30 minutes	LOC >5 minutes or PTA >24 hours
Wilberger and Maroon	PTA <20 minutes; minimal or no LOC	LOC <5 or PTA >20 minutes	LOC >5 minutes or PTA >12 hours
Kelly (Colorado)	confusion without amnesia/LOC	confusion plus amnesia	LOC (any duration)
AAN (Kelly and Rosenberg)	all symptoms and mental status abnormalities resolve within 15 minutes; no LOC	any symptoms and/or mental status abnormalities persist after 15 minutes; no LOC	any LOC (two subsets: brief (seconds) and prolonged (minutes))

*PTA = posttraumatic amnesia.

day, the athletic trainer re-examined the athlete and recommended that the player be managed as having a Grade 2 concussion and not be allowed to return to play until 1 week later.

In both instances, the players, coaches, and athletic trainers appropriately managed the injury; however, other medical professionals not educated in or updated with the same guidelines had not identified or assessed the injury correctly and had put the athlete at risk of second-impact syndrome. A universally accepted guideline for the management of concussion in sports needs to be adopted and disseminated to ensure that these instances do not occur in the future.

Ideally, the adoption of a standard methodology of assessment and management by the sports medicine community would mean that athletic trainers, school nurses, emergency room personnel, and physicians could discuss early management of patients with traumatic brain injuries without ambiguity and facilitate the transfer and recovery of such patients. Upon identification of an injury, the first point of contact (i.e., the athletic trainer, coach, or nurse) would immediately evaluate the patient using this standardized method of assessment. Using the immediate assessment report, EMT personnel would be able to make faster and better triage decisions. This will allow the physician to receive a report of the immediate and delayed assessment of the injury and to make a recommendation based on the current information about concussion.

In Chapter 2 of this book, Cantu has described several grading guidelines for concussion evaluation and return-to-play criteria being used across the nation, including those of Cantu (American College of Sports Medicine, ACSM), Kelly (Colorado Medical Society), Wilberger and Maroon, and the AAN.[37] Most use the presence or duration of LOC and posttraumatic amnesia to grade concussion, and all are based on opinions of experts or groups of experts, rather than on evidence-based data. Guidelines were established to assist nonmedical personnel with the means to appropriately identify the severity of concussion and then to determine the appropriate duration of observation and recovery. The objective is to allow athletes to fully recover before returning to play. Most guidelines distinguish between three grades of concussion: Grade 1 (mild), Grade 2 (moderate), and Grade 3 (severe), and a few use a 4th grade. The guidelines differ mostly in *how* they distinguish between these grades. Table 1 demonstrates some of the differences between the guidelines.

The most commonly used guidelines for evaluation and management of concussion in sports are those of Cantu and the AAN. The main differences among these guidelines are the time interval of posttraumatic amnesia between Grade 1 and Grade 2 concussions, and the length of LOC between Grade 2 and Grade 3 concussions. Cantu uses a 30-minute posttraumatic amnesia time interval to distinguish between a Grade 1 and Grade 2

TABLE 2

A COMPARISON OF MINIMAL CRITERIA FOR RETURN TO PLAY

Guidelines	Grade 1 (Mild)	Grade 2 (Moderate)	Grade 3 (Severe)
Cantu (ACSM)	in selected cases, same day if asymptomatic	within 2 weeks if asymptomatic for 1 week	after a minimum of 1 month if asymptomatic for 1 week
Wilberger and Maroon	after asymptomatic for 1 week	after asymptomatic for 2 weeks	after asymptomatic for 1 month; normal CT
Kelly (Colorado)	after asymptomatic for for 20 minutes	after asymptomatic for 1 week	after 1 month if asymptomatic for 2 weeks
AAN (Kelly and Rosenberg)	after 15 minutes, if asymptomatic	after asymptomatic for 1 week	after asymptomatic for 1 week (brief LOC) or 2 weeks (sustained LOC)

2 concussion, while the AAN uses a 15-minute parameter. The sole parameter used by the AAN classification to distinguish between a Grade 3 and a Grade 1 or 2 concussion is LOC. If a player were knocked unconscious, regardless of the duration of LOC, the AAN guidelines would classify the player as having a Grade 3 concussion. One acknowledged drawback of the AAN guidelines is that concussion in a patient who does not lose consciousness, but has prolonged amnesia or other symptoms, is considered to be Grade 2, while another patient with a brief LOC whose symptoms resolve quickly is considered to have a Grade 3 concussion. However, the recommendations on return to play take this into account; the latter patient would return sooner than the former.

Regardless of the guidelines used, periodic reassessment and maintaining a high index of suspicion is warranted. Minimum criteria for return-to-play recommendations following a first concussion based on the above guidelines are listed in Table 2 (disposition becomes more cautious with multiple concussions). The common thread on all confirmed cases of second-impact syndrome is the persistence of symptoms at the time of the second injury, so all authorities agree that *any* symptoms (at rest or with exertion) should preclude a return to collision sports.

It is important to keep in mind the reason that these guidelines were established, which is to give nonmedical personnel a method by which to initially identify, evaluate, and triage head-injured athletes in the absence of trained medical personnel. Additionally, it is crucial that all persons, medical or nonmedical, who care for athletes playing "at risk" sports be knowledgeable of the definition and management of concussion in sports. There is no "gold standard," as research has not validated any of these guidelines, although this is an aim of the future. For the present, caregivers (e.g., athletic trainers or team physicians) should choose a guideline that they are comfortable and proficient using, that can easily educate persons potentially involved in the care of the athletes, and that can be used consistently.

Immediate and Early Assessment of Concussion Severity

A patient with a single concussion has as much as a fourfold risk of incurring a second one.[19] Recurrent concussions are more likely to result in postconcussion syndrome[10,17] and greater cognitive deficits.[13,20] Repeat concussions occurring soon after the first can result in the frequently fatal second-impact syndrome. Is it possible that some cases of death, or for that matter, of intracranial hemorrhage and severe postconcussion syndrome following concussion were actually the result of recurrent head injuries following unreported prior concussions? Although all current management guidelines agree in not allowing an athlete with persistent symptoms to resume play, is the mere absence of symptoms an adequate predictor of decreased risk, especially since subtle cognitive deficits may persist much longer than symptoms?

In October 1999, a junior varsity football player died following a concussion; it was reported that the player was diagnosed with a blood clot in his brain. The only indication of a prior concussion had taken place 4 weeks prior to his death. The player was cleared to return to play by a doctor several weeks after suffering an initial concussion. It is not yet known whether or not this injury is attributed to second-impact syndrome (F. Mueller, personal communication, 1999).[33] Are there **any** concussed patients who can be reassured? These questions point to the need for optimal detection and assessment of concussion.

On the Field: Advanced Trauma Life Support Evaluation, Mini-Mental Status Examination, and Balance Testing

All sports medicine physicians should be familiar with basic Advanced Trauma Life Support (ATLS) principles and be prepared to identify and stabilize a severe injury, which may not always be apparent on initial examination. The primary survey of any injured patient involves the "ABCDs." This includes airway (with cervical spine control), breathing, circulation, and disability. The latter refers to a brief neurological evaluation and includes the level of consciousness (AVPU-Alert, responsive to Vocal stimuli, responsive to Pain, or Unresponsive), pupil size, and reaction. This is immediately followed, in the case of an isolated head injury, by a "mini-neurological" examination as part of the secondary survey. The top priority is to determine whether a patient needs immediate transport to a trauma facility for an emergency or urgent neurosurgical procedure. This is more likely if the patient is comatose, has a lateralized motor deficit, and/or pupil asymmetry. Frequent re-evaluation of the player is paramount.[1] Emergency stabilization and management are critical and are discussed elsewhere in this book.

In addition to the primary and secondary surveys, specific screening for amnesia, orientation, concentration, and gait is warranted. Such evaluation and serial re-evaluation helps rule out more-severe injuries and allows for an assessment of severity, facilitating return-to-play decisions. Commonly, a player who suffers a concussion will not associate his/her symptoms with concussion or will deliberately not report them due to societal pressures of playing competitive sports (e.g., self-motivation to continue playing, coaching pressure, or peer pressure). Due to the potential for mortality and significant morbidity of athletes who resume play while symptomatic from concussion, research in this area has focused on efforts to standardize and improve sideline assessment. In recent years, standardized instruments have been developed for immediate confirmation and assessment of concussion severity.[21,35,36,51] Although the various management guidelines agree that a player needs to be asymptomatic before returning to play, researchers continue to collect data to determine which objective tests or collection of tests are the most effective for identifying immediate and long-term effects of concussion.

For years, sports medicine professionals have performed individualized versions of sideline assessment, focusing on event-specific orientation (e.g., the score of the game or the last play call), concentration, and short-term memory. One of the first specific tools to be developed for immediate sideline triage and assessment of sports concussion, and probably the most widely utilized, is the Standardized Assessment of Concussion (SAC).[36] This 5-minute mini-mental status examination contains four scored components: orientation, immediate memory, concentration, and delayed memory, as well as sections on brief neurological screening and exertional maneuvers. The SAC is fully described in Chapter 8. Statistically sound and easy for nonmedical personnel to administer, it has demonstrated 89% sensitivity and 95% specificity to concussion for up to 48 hours after an injury.[35] It can be clinically useful in identifying immediate cognitive impairment, screening for those who need full neuropsychological evaluation, and assisting in return-to-play decisions. Many sports teams at the high school, college, and professional levels are now obtaining baseline (preseason) SAC scores on their players, so that there is objective data for comparison when a concussion occurs. More recently, another sideline tool, the Field Mental Status Examination, has been developed by Lovell and colleagues with five scored components: orientation, anterograde amnesia, retrograde amnesia, concentration, and word list memory. This test is described more fully in Chapter 12.

Although the Romberg test can detect only gross equilibrium deficits, it has been frequently used in postconcussion assessment. Guskiewicz and colleagues have studied alternatives to the Romberg test to measure postural stability following concussion,[21] including the Balance Error Scoring System (see Chapter 9 for additional information). This postural stability test consists of the following stances performed once on a firm surface and once on a foam surface: double leg (narrow), single leg (nondominant), and tandem (heel to toe). If during this test, the athlete lifts their hands off their iliac crests; opens their eyes; steps, stumbles, or falls; moves their hips into more than 30° of flexion or abduction; lifts forefoot or heel; or remains out of testing positions for more than 5 seconds, an error is recorded. The Balance Error Scoring System is calculated by adding one point for each error during the nine 20-second tests. Their preliminary data show that single-leg (nondominant) and tandem (heel to toe) stances on a firm surface and double-leg (narrow) and tandem stances on foam of medium density are sensitive to subtle deficits of concussion. This measure of postural stability can be useful when used in conjunction with an immediate sideline evaluation of concussion.[21]

Neuroradiological Assessment

The National Federation of State High School Associations requires a written release from a physician before any football player with LOC can resume practice or competition.[51] However, in the absence of persistent symptoms or focal neurological deficits, there are no clear data to support an early assessment of the risk of sequelae following a first concussion, with or without LOC. Thus, some authors recommend that neuroradiological studies be performed following any concussion before allowing return to play.[46] Magnetic resonance imaging (MRI) in particular has been found to be quite sensitive for detecting small subdural hematomas and diffuse axonal injury patterns in mild head injuries. A subset of 134 hospitalized patients with mild head injuries (Glasgow Coma Scale score 13-15), in a larger study comparing MRI with CT in acute head injuries, revealed MRI abnormalities in 62% vs. 45% with CT abnormalities.[53] A blinded comparison of MRI and CT in 107 closed head injuries of mixed severity referred from an emergency department showed 96.4% sensitivity by MRI vs. 63.4% by CT in detecting contusion, shearing injury, subdural and epidural hematoma, and sinus involvement.[41] In a study of 20 patients with mild head injury (score 13-15) and normal findings on CT, six had white matter abnormalities on MRI.[39] Finally, six of 58 patients discharged from an emergency department after mild head injuries had abnormalities on MRI when read blindly by two radiologists. In two patients, the results of CT were normal but subdural hematomas were present on MRI; the four other players did not undergo CT, but three had cortical contusions while one had a small subdural hematoma. There were no significant differences in symptoms between those with and without abnormal scans. Of note, this study was done in 1990, when some of our more sensitive MRI techniques were not yet available.[16]

Although CT is not as sensitive as MRI for subtle injuries such as small brain contusions and hematomas, it is fast, accurate, generally less expensive, and almost universally available in the U.S. Furthermore, it is less likely to miss a skull fracture than MRI and is more sensitive at detecting subarachnoid hemorrhage. CT can be used to expeditiously define or rule out most life-threatening large focal lesions. The most widely and readily available imaging medium in the U.S. following acute traumatic brain injuries is the CT scan. MRI is typically used for patients with persistent altered mental status or significant amnesia. Skull x-rays are recommended only in penetrating head injury or when CT or MRI is unavailable.

A new method for structural imaging for sports head injury research is magneto-encephalography (MEG). This method for assessing spontaneous brain activity will be used during the 1999 football season at the University of Utah on 83 college athletes in conjunction with the MRI and neuropsychological testing.[12]

Other scanning methods used to identify structural impairments in traumatic brain injury patients are electroencephalography (EEG), single photon emission CT (SPECT), and positron emission tomography (PET). None of these methods is commonly used for clinical purposes. The EEG is not generally used to assess the effect of head injury because the reading would usually be abnormal immediately following head injury and then quickly return to normal. SPECT perfusion imaging and PET are very sensitive tests of a patient's physiological activity; however, they are currently limited to research work.

Traditional and Computerized Neuropsychological Assessment

Cognitive function following traumatic brain injury has been studied for many years, with postinjury neuropsychological testing in the general population dating back to the 1980s.[22,32,44] Findings from this population served as a starting point to identify neuropsychological instruments sensitive for detecting subtle cognitive deficits following concussion in athletes. While desiring this sensitivity, other challenges facing neuropsychologists and researchers include time, cost, practicality, and standardization of assessment tools. The consequences of ignoring these factors include high rates of attrition among players and teams, the potential for an increase in the number of unreported head injuries, and methodological inconsistencies. While a traditional neuropsychological evaluation utilizes an extensive battery of tests that can take up to 6 hours to complete, the development and refinement of a much shorter assessment process have been considered a prerequisite for deployment with sports teams. The apparent inconsistency of achieving brevity, yet maintaining both sensitivity and specificity, can be resolved by collecting baseline data on an entire sports team. This allows a player to be compared to his/her own baseline score, as opposed to a normative databank.

Several research studies have assessed the utility of neuropsychological tools in determining the effects of concussion in sports. Some of the more commonly used traditional neuropsychological measures to assess postconcussion cognitive functioning are the Trail Making Test Parts A and B, the Paced Auditory Serial Addition Task, the Symbol Digit Modalities Test, and the Hopkins Verbal Learning Test. These tests have been used for assessment following concussion among professional, college, and high school athletes and are described more fully in Chapters 11 and 12. Other researchers have deviated from the use of these traditional neuropsychological tests in order to minimize the cost and time needed to assess athletes.

Generally, traditional neuropsychological assessment batteries are sensitive for measuring impairments in information processing, memory, speech fluency, decision-making, attention, concentration, and word retrieval at 1 to 5 days after concussion.[22,29,30,32] In most reported studies of adult athletes, performance improves by 5 to 10 days and recovery is mostly complete by 1 to 3 months, while impairment in reaction time impairment resolves by 6 months.[9,17,31] A potential limitation of some of the traditional neuropsychological tests is that they may have limited reliability when used repeatedly, due to practice effects; this can be offset somewhat by using control subjects. For example, Macciocchi et al[30] reported that cognitive performance significantly improved in some subtests among concussed college athletes from their preseason testing, but these athletes exhibited significantly less improvement than did their nonconcussed peers. Of note, these authors also reported that some athletes did not return to their premorbid level of performance. This, along with more recent studies using computerized neuropsychological testing, suggests that there is a subpopulation of athletes with subtle but persistent cognitive deficits following concussion.

There is currently no clear consensus in the literature as to the most appropriate postconcussion assessment protocol, and studies using similar protocols have concluded different findings. For example, three research studies were reviewed.[28,29] Each protocol utilized an abbreviated traditional neuropsychological test battery developed to monitor memory, speech fluency, decision-making, word retrieval, attention, and concentration in football players at least 18 years of age before and after head injury. Additionally, each player was given the test battery before the season and at 24-48 hours, 5 days, and 10 days following injury.

Each of these studies found that postconcussion symptoms as measured by traditional neuropsychological test batteries began to return to baseline at 5 days postinjury. However, the similarities ended here. In a study by Lovell[28] of professional athletes who sustained concussions ranging in severity from Colorado Grade 1 to 3, decreased performance was noted from baseline to 24-48 hours postinjury on all subtests of the neuropsychological test battery. This same protocol was replicated among three NCAA Division 1A football players treated by Olesniewicz and colleagues.[29] In the study by Olesniewicz, athletes who suffered Colorado Grade 2 concussions showed cognitive deficits on five of the six subtests used by Lovell at 24-48 hours postinjury. Those players who had sustained a Grade 1 concussion did not show any cognitive impairments postinjury, except for one player whose scores reflected cognitive impairment on one subtest at 24 hours postinjury. In the study by Lovell and Collins,[29] decreased performance was observed among some but not all subtests at 24 to 48 hours following concussion. Unfortunately, the grades of concussion were not reported in the latter article.

As mentioned previously, computerized neuropsychological test batteries are becoming more commonly used in posttraumatic cognitive assessment and research. Among other potential advantages, computerized assessment is time- and cost-efficient, is reliable for repeated testing, and is practical for use in large group settings. Furthermore, it maintains better standardization, since instructions can be presented on a computer monitor rather than by psychometricians. Perhaps the most powerful argument for computerized testing is the potential for increased sensitivity to subtle and/or persistent cognitive impairment. By allowing for reaction time to be measured accurately in units of milliseconds, subtle deficits have been observed retrospectively in concussed patients, even years after injury.[3,14,24]

Two computerized neuropsychological test batteries that have been utilized in sports concussion assessment research are a sports-concussion version of the Automated Neuropsychological Assessment Metrics (ANAM) and the Computerized Neuropsychological Testing for Athletic Concussion (CONTAC).[12] The CONTAC test battery was utilized in conjunction with MRI, MEG, and traditional neuropsychological assessments among college athletes at Michigan State University during the 1999 season. The ANAM test battery has been validated against traditional neuropsychological tests.[4] The ANAM, along with the previously discussed SAC, was administered prior to the beginning of the season to 270 high school football players. Athletes who sustained a concussion and noninjured matched controls (matched by age, grade point average, reaction time, and baseline SAC scores) completed these tests at 0-3 days (usually SAC on the field immediately after injury and ANAM the following day), 2 weeks, and 7 weeks. The mean SAC scores of injured athletes significantly decreased from 27.8 (of a high of 30) to 24.3 (P= .02) at 0-3 days postinjury, while no change in mental status was detected at 2 and 7 weeks postinjury using the same tool. ANAM detected cognitive impairment among concussed players at each of these evaluations. The impairment scores at 7 weeks were greater among those who had performed the worst (alpha ~ .05) in four ANAM subtests administered at 0-3 days postinjury. Thus, at least in this sample, the SAC was found to be useful for detecting immediate cognitive impairment, the ANAM was useful in discerning more subtle but persistent impairment (at 7 weeks), and an early ANAM was able to predict the severity of this persistent impairment.[50]

Traumatic Brain Injury in the Adolescent

Professional, college, and sandlot athletes make up only 17% of the estimated 1.8 million football participants in the U.S. each year.[40] The overwhelming majority of football players are high school students. However, relatively little has been published regarding high school football players and concussion.

Much of the work that has been published concerning traumatic brain injury among high school football athletes is epidemiological. In a classic study by Gerberich and colleagues,[19] comprehensive questionnaires about injuries and illnesses during the 1979 football season were mailed to individual football players in 103 Minnesota secondary schools. Retrospectively, 19% were identified as having sustained concussion. Many of these injuries had not been identified or evaluated previously and some of these players were still experiencing symptoms 6 to 9 months following the season. Concussion represented 24% of all identified injuries, which contrasts with a 1970 study in which only 4% of all injuries reported among 9- to 15-year-old football players were concussions[45] and a 1982 study that noted only 25 concussions among 1000 football injuries evaluated in emergency rooms.[43] More recently, using National Athletic Trainers' Association data from the 1995 through 1997 seasons, Powell and Barber-Foss[42] reported a 3.9% minor traumatic brain injury incidence rate among high school football players (see Chapter 1 for additional data). These authors[42] cite improvements in helmet design (due to the implementation of National Operating Committee for Safety in Athletic Equipment standards in 1980) as one possible factor in the difference between their 3.9% rate and the 19% rate of Gerberich and colleagues. This explanation is consistent with the fact that both subdural hematoma rates and mortality due to brain injuries sustained in football have dropped significantly from the 1970s to the 1990s.[40] Another factor that cannot be dismissed, however, is that there are still a significant (although difficult to quantify) number of players who suffer traumatic brain injury but do not seek medical attention. Gerberich et al[19] reported that players did not, in many cases, associate symptoms of loss of awareness, transient amnesia, or LOC with the word "concussion." In 1998, Boswell distributed a postseason concussion questionnaire to seven high schools in San Diego County to determine the percentage of players who experienced symptoms of concussion, including confusion, difficulty concentrating, blurred vision, ringing in ears, dizziness, headache, or nausea during the football season. It was concluded that 81% of the athletes from the participating seven high schools reported having experienced symptoms of concussion.[48] Despite increased awareness among sports medicine professionals, athletes continue to not report their injuries, highlighting the need for education among players, administrators, physicians, emergency medical technicians, athletic trainers, coaches, and parents about the seriousness of concussion in sports.

Research conducted on the adult population should not be presumed to generalize to the adolescent population, since the adolescent brain may respond to brain injury differently than the adult brain. Some authors hypothesize that undeveloped aspects of cognition in the adolescent brain are spared from immediate impairment, while cognitive impairments can emerge years later, when the injured area matures.[27] The Glasgow Coma Scale, which is used as an index for severity of head injury in adults, may not be a valid measure in children and adolescents, even when it is modified for such use.[26,34,52] Additionally, duration of LOC, which has been regarded by some researchers to be an indication of injury severity in adults, is not considered reliable in children.[6,18] In fact, children can experience very severe injury and not lose consciousness.[2] It has also been suggested that the effects of traumatic brain injury in adolescents may be due not only to the neuropathological characteristics of the damage, but also to the developmental tasks disrupted at the time of injury.[2] For example, in a study of language function in mildly brain-injured children and adolescents, younger children showed a differential pattern of impairment in written language when compared to an adolescent group.[18] This age-related differential pattern of cognitive performance has been identified not only among brain-injured subjects, but also in noninjured adolescent athletes. In a study by Daniel and colleagues,[15] high school football players underwent testing both before and after the football season. Improvements were noted in cognitive efficiency on three ANAM subtests among those who were not concussed ($P < 0.001$). Additionally, during both pre- and postseason testing, older adolescents generally demonstrated greater cognitive efficiency on these same subtests than younger adolescents.[15] All of these findings suggest that developmental factors should be considered when concussed adolescents are evaluated.

The Future of Research and Assessment of Sports Concussions

As mentioned previously, none of the current return-to-play guidelines is empirically based. Which combination of the following measures are significant predictors of brain injury severity: 1) the presence and/or duration of LOC and of posttraumatic amnesia; 2) SAC scores; 3) postural stability assessment; 4) neuropsychological testing (preferably in a streamlined, concise, yet reliable form, administered on a laptop computer on the sideline); or 5) duration of symptoms without or with exertion? Should variability in cognitive performance be a determining factor for return to play?[3] What will be the appropriate role of MEG or MRI? Are some athletes at greater risk of serious or persistent sequelae of concussion based on learning disability, prior concussions, or APOE polymorphism?[12,13] Large-scale prospective trials, with the potential to follow the course of hundreds of traumatic brain injuries, would be an optimal way to gather the necessary data to answer these questions satisfactorily. It is quite possible that an entirely different grading scale, based on composite data from multiple measures, will replace the current "mild/moderate/severe" or Grade 1, 2, or 3 scenarios.

Finally, with continued emphasis on education and awareness by organizations such as the Brain Injury Association, the Defense and Veterans Head Injury Program, the American Academy of Neurology, and the National Football League Players Association, we may hope for all concussions in sports to be reported, identified, and assessed in the near future. The authors are optimistic that great strides will be made to eliminate second-impact syndrome, minimize the severity of postconcussion syndrome, and change the cultural thinking regarding the seriousness of concussion in the third millennium.

References

1. **Advanced Trauma Life Support Instructor Course Manual.** Chicago, Ill: American College of Surgeons, 1997
2. Beers SR: Cognitive effects of mild head injury in children and adolescents. **Neuropsychol Rev** 3:281-320, 1992
3. Bleiberg J, Halpern EL, Reeves D, et al: Future directions for the neuropsychological assessment of sports concussion. **J Head Trauma Rehabil** 13:36-44, 1998
4. Bleiberg J, Kane RL, Reeves DL, et al: Factor analysis of computerized and traditional tests used in concussion research. (In press)
5. Bohnen NI, Jolles J, Twijnstra A, et al: Late neurobehavioral symptoms after mild head injury. **Brain Inj** 9:27-33, 1995
6. Boll TJ, Barth JT: Neuropsychology of brain damage in children, in Filskov SB, Boll TJ (eds): **Handbook of Clinical Neuropsychology.** New York, NY: John Wiley & Sons, 1981, pp 418-452
7. Cantu RC: Head injuries in sport. **Br J Sports Med** 30:289-296, 1996
8. Cantu RC: Second-impact syndrome. **Clin Sports Med** 17:37-44, 1998
9. Capruso DK, Levin HS: Cognitive impairment following closed head injury. **Neurol Trauma** 10:879-893, 1992
10. Carlson GS, Svardsudd K, Welin L: Long-term effects of head injuries sustained during life in three male populations. **J Neurosurg** 67: 197-205, 1987
11. Clarke KS: Epidemiology of athletic head injury. **Clin Sports Med** 17: 1-12, 1998
12. Collins MW: A multi-site college football project. Presented at the Sports Related Concussion and Nervous System Injuries Conference, Orlando, Florida, May 29, 1999
13. Collins MW, Grindel SH, Lovell MR, et al: Relationship between concussion and neuropsychological performance in college football. **JAMA** 282:964-970, 1999
14. Cremona-Meteyard SL, Geffen GM: Persistent visuospatial attention deficits following mild head injury in Australian Rules football players. **Neuropsychologia** 32:649-662, 1994
15. Daniels JC, Olesniewicz M, Reeves DL, et al: Repeated measures of cognitive processing efficiency in adolescent athletes: implications for monitoring recovery from concussion. **Neuropsychiatry Neuropsychol Behav Neurol** 12:167-169, 1999
16. Doezema D, Espinosa MC, King JN, et al: Magnetic resonance imaging in minor head injury. **Ann Emerg Med** 20:449, 1991
17. Evans RW: The postconcussion syndrome and the sequelae of mild head injury. **Neurol Clin** 10:815-847, 1992
18. Ewing-Cobbs L, Miner ME, Fletcher JM, et al: Neuropsychological sequelae following pediatric head injury, in Ylvisaker M (ed): **Head Injury Rehabilitation: Children and Adolescents.** San Diego, Calif: College Hill, 1985, pp 71-90
19. Gerberich SG, Priest JD, Boen JR, et al: Concussion incidences and severity in secondary school varsity football players. **Am J Publ Health** 73:1370-1375, 1983
20. Gronwall D, Wrightson P: Cumulative effect of concussion. **Lancet** 2: 995-997, 1975
21. Guskiewicz KM: Alternative methods of concussion assessment. Presented at the Sports Related Concussion and Nervous System Injuries Conference, Orlando, Florida, May 28, 1999
22. Hugenholtz H, Stuss DT, Stethem LL, et al: How long does it take to recover from concussion? **Neurosurgery** 22:853-857, 1988
23. Jordan BD: Boxing, in Jordan BD (ed): **Sports Neurology, 2nd ed.** Philadelphia, Pa: Lippincott-Raven, 1998, pp 351-366
24. Kane R, Reeves D: Computerized test batteries, in Horton A, Wedding D, Webster J (eds): **The Neuropsychology Handbook.** New York, NY: Springer-Verlag, 1997
25. Lee ST, Lui TN: Early seizures after mild closed head injury. **J Neurosurg** 76:435-439, 1992
26. Levin H, Benton A, Grossman R: **Neurobehavioral Consequences of Closed Head Injury.** New York, NY: Oxford University Press, 1982
27. Levin H, Eisenberg H, Benton A: **Mild Head Injury.** New York, NY: Oxford University Press, 1989
28. Lovell MR: Neuropsychological assessment in the National Football League—an update. Presented at the Sports Related Concussion and Nervous System Injuries Conference, Orlando, Florida, February 9, 1997
29. Lovell MR, Collins MW: Neuropsychological assessment of the college football player. **J Head Trauma Rehabil** 13:9-26, 1998
30. Macciocchi SN, Barth JT, Alves W, et al: Neuropsychological functioning and recovery after mild head injury in collegiate athletes. **Neurosurgery** 39:510-514, 1996
31. MacFlynn G, Montgomery EA, Fenton GW, et al: Measurement of reaction time following minor head injury. **J Neurol Neurosurg Psychiatry** 47:1326-1331, 1984
32. Maddocks D, Saling M: Neuropsychological deficits following concussion. **Brain Inj** 10:99-103, 1996
33. Martinez M: Teenager's death from head injury rocked young. **San Jose Mercury News,** 1999 (Internet, October 28, 1999)
34. Martini DR, Beers SR, Ryan CM: Long-term neuropsychologic sequelae of mild head injury in young children: effects of locus of injury and biomedical complications. Presented at the North Coast Society of Pediatric Psychology Annual Meeting, Detroit, Michigan, North Coast Society of Pediatric Psychology, 1990
35. McCrea MA: Sideline assessment of the high school athlete. Presented at the Sports Related Concussion and Nervous System Injuries Conference, Orlando, Florida, May 29, 1999
36. McCrea MA, Kelly JP, Randolph C, et al: Standardized Assessment of Concussion: on-site mental status evaluation of the athlete. **J Head Trauma Rehabil** 13:27-35, 1998
37. McCrory PR: Were you knocked out? A team physician's approach to initial concussion management. **Med Sci Sports Exerc (Suppl 7)** 29: S207-S212, 1997
38. McQuillen JB, McQuillen EN, Morrow P: Trauma, sport and malignant cerebral edema. **Am J Forensic Med Pathol** 9:12-15, 1988
39. Mittl RL, Grossman RI, Hiehle JF, et al: Prevalence of MR evidence of diffuse axonal injury in patients with mild head injury and normal head CT findings. **AJNR** 15:1583-1589, 1994
40. Mueller FO, Diehl JL: **Annual Survey of Football Injury Research 1931-1998.** Waco, Tx: American Football Coaches Association, NCAA, and National Federation of State High School Associations, 1999
41. Orrison WW, Gentry LR, Stimac GK, et al: Blinded comparison of cranial CT and MR in closed head injury evaluation. **AJNR** 15: 351-356, 1994
42. Powell JW, Barber-Foss KD: Traumatic brain injury in high school athletes. **JAMA** 282:958-963, 1999
43. Pritchett JW: A statistical study of physician care patterns in high school football injuries. **Am J Sports Med** 10:96-99, 1982
44. Rimel RW, Giordani B, Barth JT, et al: Disability caused by minor head injury. **Neurosurgery** 9:221-228, 1981
45. Roser LA, Clawson DK: Football injuries in the very young athlete. **Clin Orthop** 22:219-222, 1970
46. Saunders RL, Harbaugh RE: The second impact in catastrophic contact-only sports head trauma. **JAMA** 252:538-539, 1984
47. Schneider RC: **Head and Neck Injuries in Football: Mechanisms, Treatment, and Prevention.** Baltimore, Md: Williams & Wilkins, 1973
48. Schrock B, Tam D, Daniel JC, et al: Concussion rates high among teen athletes. **Sharp, One Step Ahead, Future Directions in Rehabilitation.** Vol 3(1), September 1999, pp 1-7
49. Sports-related recurrent brain injuries—United States. **MMWR** 46: 224-227, 1997
50. Tam DA, Olesniewicz MH, Daniel JC, et al: Neuropsychologic assessment in sports-related concussion. Academic Research Competition, Naval Medical Center, San Diego, California, April 8, 1999
51. Wilberger JE: Minor head injuries in American football: prevention of long term sequelae. **Sports Med** 15:338-343, 1993
52. Winogron HW, Knights RM: Neuropsychological deficits following head injury in children. **J Clin Neuropsychol** 6:268-279, 1984
53. Yokota H, Kurokawa A, Otsuka T, et al: Significance of magnetic resonance imaging in acute head injury. **J Trauma** 31:351-357, 1991

Index

Page numbers for figures and tables are followed by *f* and *t* respectively.

Julian E. Bailes, Jr., MD, graduated from Louisiana State University in 1978 with a Bachelor of Science degree and earned his medical degree from Louisiana State University School of Medicine in New Orleans in 1982. He completed a General Surgery Internship at Northwestern Memorial Hospital in 1983 and a Neurological Surgery residency at Northwestern University in Chicago in 1987. He also completed a fellowship in Cerebrovascular Surgery at the Barrow Neurological Institute in Phoenix.

In 1988, Dr. Bailes accepted the position of Chief of Cerebrovascular Surgery at Allegheny General Hospital, Pittsburgh, Pennsylvania. He was Associate Professor of Neurosurgery at the Medical College of Pennsylvania and Hahnemann University, and also served as Clinical Assistant Professor with the Department of Neurosurgery at West Virginia University.

Beginning in 1997, Dr. Bailes served as Director of Neurosurgery at the DisneyWorld Celebration Health Hospital, Senior Vice President and Medical Director for the Orlando Regional Healthcare System, Medical Director of Emergency Medical Services in Osceola County, Florida, and Assistant Professor for the College of Health and Public Affairs for the University of Central Florida.

Dr. Bailes is currently Professor and Chairman for the Department of Neurosurgery at West Virginia University. In 1999, he co-edited *Sports-Related Concussion* published by Quality Medical Publishing, Inc. His primary areas of interest include cerebrovascular surgery, neurological sports injury, spinal injury, and neurosurgical research.

Arthur L. Day, MD, is Professor, Co-Chairman, and Residency Program Director of the Department of Neurological Surgery at the University of Florida. Dr. Day graduated from Louisiana State University Medical School in 1972 and completed his neurological surgery residency training at the University of Florida in 1977. After a fellowship in brain tumor immunology at the University of Florida, he joined the neurosurgery faculty in 1978, and now holds the James and Newton Eblen Eminent Scholar Chair in Cerebrovascular Surgery.

Dr. Day has served as president of the Florida Neurosurgical Society, and his membership in professional organizations includes the Congress of the Neurological Surgeons, the Joint Section of Cerebrovascular Surgery of the American Association of Neurological Surgeons/CNS, the Sports Medicine Section of the AANS/CNS, and the Alachua County Medical Society. He has served as a member of the board of directors of the American Association of Neurological Surgery and as Chairman of the AANS/CNS Washington Committee. He is a director on the American Board of Neurological Surgery.

For the past 20 years, Dr. Day has served as a consulting physician for the University of Florida Athletic Department and for several Southeastern Conference and National Football League teams.